Experimental Therapeutics

Contents

Contributors

Sarah K Branch
Senior Pharmaceutical Assessor, Medicines and
Healthcare products Regulatory Agency,
Market Towers, 1 Nine Elms Lane, London
SW8 5NQ, UK

John Connelly
Metabometrix Ltd, RSM, Prince Consort Road,
London SW7 2BP, UK

Sir Colin Dollery
Senior Consultant R&D, GlaxoSmithKline
Pharmaceuticals, R&D, New Frontiers Science
Park, Third Avenue, Harlow, Essex
CM19 5AW, UK

Paul M Grasby
MRC Clinical Sciences Centre, Imperial College
School of Medicine, Hammersmith Campus,
Du Cane Road, London W12 0NN, UK

Andrew J Hutt
Department of Pharmacy, King's College
London, Franklin-Wilkins Building, Stamford
Street, London SE1 9NN, UK

Rebecca Kristeleit
Research Fellow, Cancer Research UK,
Hammersmith Hospital, Du Cane Road,
London W12 0NN, UK

Anthony Lynch
Safety Assessment, GlaxoSmithKline R&D,
Park Road, Ware SG12 0DP, UK

Christian Meisel
Institute of Clinical Pharmacology, University
Hospital Charité, Humboldt-University of
Berlin, Schumannstr. 20-21, D-10098 Berlin,
Germany

James J Oliver
Clinical Pharmacology Unit and Research
Centre, University of Edinburgh, Western
General Hospital, Crewe Road South,
Edinburgh EH4 2XU, UK

Colin NA Palmer
Biomedical Research Centre, Ninewells
Hospital and Medical School,
Dundee DD1 9SY, UK

Eugenii A (Ilan) Rabiner
GlaxoSmithKline, Division of Translational
Medicine and Technologies, Addenbrooke's
Centre for Clinical Investigation,
Addenbrooke's Hospital, Hills Road,
Cambridge CB2 2GG, UK

Punit Ramrakha
Section of Clinical Pharmacology, Imperial
College School of Medicine, Hammersmith
Hospital, Du Cane Road, London W12 0NN,
UK

Andrew G Renwick
Professor of Biochemical Pharmacology,
Clinical Pharmacology Group, University of
Southampton, Biomedical Sciences Building,
Bassett Crescent East, Southampton SO16 7PX,
UK

Matthias Schwab
Dr Margarete Fischer-Bosch-Institute of Clinical
Pharmacology, Auerbachstr. 112, D-70367
Stuttgart, Germany

Rashmi R Shah
Senior Medical Assessor, Medicines and
Healthcare products Regulatory Agency,
Market Towers, 1 Nine Elms Lane, London
SW8 5NQ, UK

Christopher Steele
Senior Preclinical Assessor, Medicines and
Healthcare products Regulatory Agency,
Market Towers, 1 Nine Elms Lane, London
SW8 5NQ, UK

David J Webb
Clinical Pharmacology Unit and Research
Centre, University of Edinburgh, Western
General Hospital, Crewe Road South,
Edinburgh EH4 2XU, UK

Martin R Wilkins
Professor of Clinical Pharmacology, Imperial
College, Hammersmith Hospital, Du Cane
Road, London W12 0NN, UK

Foreword

The discovery and successful development of biopharmaceutical products have, during the past century, progressed in leaps and bounds, revolutionising the practice and goal of medicine in a remarkable way. Yet, many common illnesses remain inadequately treated and others could certainly benefit from improved therapies. Even in situations where highly effective medicines do exist, their use may not have been fully evaluated in the whole range of patient populations or potential indications. Such observations underpin the importance of continued efforts to understand the basis of disease and produce ever more specific and effective therapeutic agents.

It is obvious to anyone who seeks to understand the discovery and development of a new medicine that it is a multifaceted and multidisciplinary process which requires advanced scientific skills and highly professional standards. The process starts with the identification of a defined medical need. Even this can be a complex analysis, requiring the expertise of clinicians, epidemiologists, biologists, health economists and marketing specialists. Definition of biological targets and possible therapeutic approaches involves biologists from a variety of sub-disciplines working together with medicinal chemists and biotechnologists. The development of a new drug candidate calls on a very wide range of expertise – pharma-cists, chemists, toxicologists, kineticists, clinicians, statisticians, regulatory affairs and pharmacovigilance professionals together with a variety of other scientific, legal and commercial roles. Bringing a newly-developed drug to the point of widespread clinical use involves yet further teams of professionals – those involved in manufacture, marketing, health education, healthcare delivery and regulatory approval. And, of course, the patients themselves have an ever-increasing role in defining what is safe, effective and generally acceptable.

The above lists are not exhaustive but they do illustrate certain key aspects of drug discovery and development – the need for high-level professional education, the role for continuing research into therapeutics and the symbiotic relationships between various sectors of society: academia, the biopharmaceutical industry, government departments or agencies and multiple healthcare systems. The complexity of such interactions is impressive, and it is not at all surprising that many individuals do not have a clear understanding of the roles or objectives of colleagues working at other steps of the process. Add to this the fact that each stakeholder constituency has its own knowledge base which is constantly developing and it becomes evident that the overall process must change constantly and often in a step-wise manner as new needs or technological possibilities arise.

For example, the recent decoding of the human genome will undoubtedly aid, over time, the discovery of medicines targeted more specifically at the root causes of disease. In some situations, it may even be possible to individualise treatment. Such opportunities will require major changes in the philosophies underlying many aspects of drug development, particularly the clinical evaluation, statistical analysis and regulatory approval criteria employed. The opportunity to use drugs to improve quality of life poses yet further challenges for the traditionalists and raises important questions about patient choice, clinical judgment and third-party payment.

The above observations also point to the very significant costs associated with drug discovery and development. Sadly, while costs in the bio-pharmaceutical sector are rising, there is little evidence that productivity is increasing at a proportionate rate. Hence, there is an urgent need for the development of tools which aid in the early screening out of poor candidate mol-

ecules and provide cost-effective indication of clinical utility. To such ends, a variety of in vitro, transgenic, non-invasive imaging and surrogate marker technologies are being developed. I have no doubt that, given time, new paradigms for drug discovery, development and regulatory approval will emerge. However, rigorous validation has to be carried out in each case and, hence, there is ample room for fundamental research into the utility of each such tool.

While no book can hope to cover all the issues I have described, the pages that follow do bring clarity to the state of the art in this essential pursuit. Demystification of the processes involved in improving therapeutics is essential if coherent visions of future medical possibilities are to be developed and realised.

Sir Richard B Sykes DSc FRS
Rector
Imperial College London

Preface

Primum non nocere – Hippocrates, 460–355 BC

All things are poisons and there is nothing that is harmless, the dose alone decides that something is no poison – Paracelsus, 1493–1541

The development and use of new medicines remain a formidable challenge. In 2001 the industry spent $44 billion on research and development (R&D).[1] How well that money was spent will not be apparent for another decade or more. Analysis from the Tufts Centre for the Study of Drug Development suggests it now costs an average of £550m (around $800m) to bring a drug to market, more than twice as much as in 1987. Much of this money (perhaps up to 70%) is spent on drugs that fail on the path to licensing. As a rule of thumb, for every 10 000 molecules screened in a given programme in the laboratory, only one will survive to launch.

Paradoxically, the rapid advances made in molecular biology, genetics and technology serve to enhance this problem. Novel drug targets have been identified and those involved in early drug development are facing a tidal wave of new chemical entities for consideration as medicines. Unfortunately, this intensifies the major dilemma, which is how to spot a potentially successful drug, as only a few can progress into human studies and fewer still into clinical trials in patients. To minimize costs, companies need to catch potential failures – due to either lack of clinical effect or toxicity – in early discovery phase, long before they reach patients.

In addition to the financial pressures, pharmaceutical companies need to satisfy the stringent criteria laid down by regulatory authorities on safety and efficacy. These authorities are there to protect the public, whose demands are high. In a recent MORI poll (March 2002), over 60% of the public questioned expected scientists to provide a 100% guarantee over the safety of medicines. Clearly, this is unrealistic and the authorities can only be expected to require data to show a reasonable risk–benefit. This will vary with the condition, with greater leeway given to the treatment of life-threatening disorders for which there are no or few treatment options.

The regulatory authorities and the pharmaceutical industry have to remain in dialogue. The regulatory authorities need to keep abreast of the implications of new concepts and practices in therapeutics so that the right questions can be posed. For example, which pre-clinical tests are appropriate for drugs designed specifically for human targets (i.e. drugs with poor affinity for tissues from mammalian species)? Does the targeting of drugs to patients with specific genotypes really reduce the risk of

toxicity? What are the risks of innovative therapeutic approaches, such as antisense and gene
therapies? These advances require the continuous evaluation and adjustment of guidelines, of
which pharmaceutical companies need to be
kept informed.

This book is written primarily for clinicians
and scientists with an active interest in experimental medicine as an introduction to this
dynamic and competitive discipline. It is divided
into three sections. The first section is an
overview of drug development from three perspectives – the clinical pharmacologist, the toxicologist and the regulatory body. Colin Dollery
has extensive experience of both academic medicine and the pharmaceutical industry and is well
placed to discuss the evolution of a therapeutic
agent from the birth of an idea to its rigorous
examination in human studies. Anthony Lynch
and John Connelly are actively engaged in safety
assessment and provide an up-to-date account of
the current battery of tests designed to identify
and evaluate the risk of adverse drug responses.
Rashmi Shah, Sarah Branch and Christopher
Steele work for the Medicines and Healthcare
products Regulatory Agency and describe the
package of data that needs to be assembled for
the application of a product licence. While there
is inevitable overlap in their content, these chapters give individual insights into how the various phases of the drug discovery and
development process are viewed by those
involved in bringing a drug to market.

The second section brings together and
expands on concepts and practices in clinical
pharmacology that are mentioned but not often
discussed in any detail in traditional pharmacology textbooks. Andy Renwick opens the section
with a well-illustrated and refreshing introduction to pharmacokinetics. Christian Meisel and
Matthias Schwab then discuss the exciting
potential for tailoring drug therapy according to
a patient's genotype and Andrew Hutt explores
the role of chirality in drug action, recently the
subject of the Nobel prize for chemistry. The last
two chapters in this section tackle two
approaches to the problem of demonstrating the
desired pharmacological activity in humans at
an early stage in development. This is an area

now fashionably known as translational medicine and it is an extremely important phase of
drug development, as it can enable rational
decisions to be made about which one of a family of compounds to progress as a drug and
which dose(s) to investigate in larger studies.
James Oliver and David Webb define and examine the role of surrogate clinical endpoints in
clinical studies, while Ilan Rabiner and Paul
Grasby summarize the advantages of positron-
emission tomography in the investigation of
receptor occupancy in neuroscience.

The third section introduces three novel therapeutic developments. This is not exhaustive
but provides a flavour of the new opportunities
that are emerging in disease management and
the new challenges facing those involved in
assessing efficacy and safety in therapeutics.
Drugs that act on nuclear receptors have been
around for many years, but the discovery and
synthesis of agents that act on peroxisome
proliferator-activated receptors (PPARs) has
expanded this category. Colin Palmer and
Martin Wilkins consider how these potent
chemicals are providing new insight into
human physiology and disease and are seeking
a place in the management of diabetes, atherosclerosis and cancer. Finally, as basic science
enters the clinical laboratory, it is appropriate
that we consider treatment strategies for
the future. Punit Ramrakha summarizes the
progress that has been made with bringing antisense oligonucleotide technology to the bedside
and Rebecca Kristeleit and Martin Wilkins look
at vectors for gene therapy and the issues surrounding their use in clinical studies.

Web-sites are referenced in each chapter to
enable readers to pursue topics of interest in
more detail and in some cases view animated
explanations of concepts and their application.
Collectively, it is hoped that this book will act
as a useful primer for anyone with a novel idea
for advancing the pharmacological management of disease.

Martin R Wilkins
January 2003

1. *The Economist.* 11 July 2002.

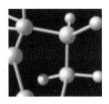

Section 1
Drug Discovery and Development

1

The clinical pharmacologist's view: drug discovery and early development

Sir Colin Dollery

SUMMARY

Drug discovery and development is one of the most complex processes undertaken by man. It involves close teamwork by scientists from many different disciplines and, despite their best efforts, the majority of projects fail to achieve their goal of creating a new therapeutic agent. Only 1–2% of early exploratory studies at the bench ever make it to a marketed product. Even when a compound progresses to the point of first administration to man between 70% and 95% fail depending upon the degree of novelty of the project. The account that follows is necessarily an over-simplification but is intended to give an introduction to the processes involved from the birth of an idea to proof of concept in man. The exact terminologies used to describe these steps vary in different pharmaceutical companies but the underlying processes have strong similarities. This is not a complete account of every step but attempts to cover the main points.

1. INTRODUCTION

Major research-based pharmaceutical companies adopt a matrix organization and create a multidisciplinary team to advance a concept or a compound to bring together the information from a great variety of disciplines in a timely fashion. These disciplines range from molecular pharmacology to experimental medicine, from laborious multi-step syntheses of microgram quantities in discovery chemistry to multi-kilogram batches in chemical development, from early studies of distribution and metabolism in animals to complex techniques such as positron emission tomography to gain comparable information in man, from early use of drug in solution to complex formulations in Phase II trials, from careful search of patent literature to complex negotiations with regulatory authorities, from basic epidemiology about disease prevalence and severity to hard-headed commercial assessment of market opportunity and potential competition years later when the product is marketed. And that is not a complete list!

Because the process is so complex and the different pieces interlock, it is often not possible to proceed in a sequential manner. The whole process would take far too long. In all except a few instances, where the risk of failure is exceptionally high, the watchword is 'Planning for Success'. In practical terms this means that a great deal of work (writing protocols, ordering supplies, booking slots with internal providers or external contractors) is undertaken on the assumption that the compound will pass all the preceding stages successfully. There is also great pressure to carry out all these steps as quickly as possible, avoiding unnecessary delay in the writing-up of reports, etc. A saying in the pharmaceutical industry is that if a compound will enjoy peak year sales of US $400 million, every day of delay in getting to market before the patent expires costs over a million dollars. Of course this fails to take into account the high failure rate of projects and only applies to those that actually achieve such sales, but time pressure in drug development is intense and unrelenting.

2. THE BIRTH OF AN IDEA

The ideas that trigger a new exploratory research project can come from many different directions. Many come from the scientists within the company but not a few originate with external advisers, the scientific literature or commercial recognition of an opportunity. These ideas can be divided broadly into 'pioneer' or 'unprecedented' projects where there is no existing marketed agent with that particular type of action and 'fast followers' or 'precedented' where there is an existing agent on the market but someone has an idea for a worthwhile improvement upon it. Such is the competition within the global pharmaceutical industry that the same 'pioneer' idea may occur to several different companies more or less simultaneously. There is great pressure to 'differentiate' the product during development so that it has a demonstrable clinical and/or commercial advantage, e.g. greater efficacy, less frequent dosing, fewer side-effects, etc.

2.1 Pioneer projects

Scientists in industry and academic researchers with an eye to starting their own company are very alert to new patentable discoveries that might form the starting point for a new therapeutic project. These days many of the new ideas come from genomics. Sequencing the human genome has disclosed a large number of potential targets in the shape of many hundreds of hitherto unknown G-protein-coupled receptors (GPCRs), kinases and proteases. Many of these discoveries are now made 'in silico' by bio-informatics specialists scanning newly published sequences. These pose both an opportunity and a challenge for industry (see Box 1.1). The opportunity to launch a research project against a target that may be unknown to competitors until patents are published is very attractive. The problem is that the amount of biological knowledge that exists about the target, at this early stage, may be very small and the hypothesis connecting it to modification of a disease mechanism may be highly speculative. Put simply, a target that has been in the public domain for a number of years may have attracted the attention of hundreds of academic researchers and thereby generated a large body of literature and personal expertise into which industry can tap. A new target discovered by a company in house may have been investigated by only a handful of biologists with a correspondingly slender file of data. Validation of novel targets before committing large resources in drug discovery is one of the major challenges facing industry today (see section 2.4 'Target validation').

2.2 Fast followers

The history of therapeutics has been that pioneer compounds are followed by many other compounds that have a similar basic action but have improved properties. For example, amoxycillin over benzyl penicillin, amlodipine over nifedipine, atorvastatin over pravastatin, etc. This process is often criticized under the derogatory label of 'me too' products but it ignores the fact that most scientific progress is incremental rather than quantal. A pharmaceutical company that deliberately sets out to imitate an existing product with no improvements would be unlikely to recover its investment unless the market for that therapeutic area was enormous or some means of differentiating it from the market leader could be found.

A fast follower strategy requires speed, as other companies are likely to be following the same strategy, but even more than that it requires a very clear set of objectives in the target product profile. Those objectives will define even stricter 'Go' and 'No go' criteria than are applied to the generality of drug discovery projects.

2.3 Target product profile (TPP)

The time period from the inception of a new idea to marketing a product derived from it is very long, a minimum of 10 years, and often considerably longer. Most projects will fail but it is much cheaper to fail them early than in late phase trials when tens or even hundreds of millions of US dollars may have been expended. One of the most important ways of deciding whether or not a compound should progress lies in whether it has achieved minimum requirements set out in the target product profile (TPP).

The TPP is essentially a list of commercial, medical and scientific requirements. These include the therapeutic indication (what disease(s) and where in the severity spectrum of the target disease is the compound positioned), frequency of dosing (once a day is almost essential for many drugs intended for long-term use), speed of onset of action (a hypnotic that was slowly absorbed and the peak concentration only reached after 4 hours would be of little use), duration and durability (e.g. no tachyphylaxis) of effect, relative efficacy required against a marketed drug, acceptable safety and side-effect profile, acceptable and unacceptable contra-indications in the label, lack of interactions with food and other drugs, stability and shelf-life, and so on. All these properties have to be judged against existing and anticipated competing molecules. From the

TPP a series of essential characteristics will be formulated into 'Go' and 'No go' criteria for different stages that will be used to judge whether the project should progress or terminate.

There are some obvious problems with the TPP. It can easily become an unrealistic wish list. At a time long before a compound has gone into man it may be impossible to foresee all the side-effects. Furthermore, the requirements written into a TPP at the inception of a project may become much less relevant as a result of the introduction of other competing compounds, new scientific knowledge, etc. TPPs are bound to have to be revised over the course of a project and there is a temptation to mould the TPP to the unfolding properties of the compound. This is a temptation to be resisted as it can lead to an unpromising molecule being progressed further than its properties warrant.

> **Box 1.1   Identifying a useful drug target**
>
> ***Is there an unmet medical need?***
> Consider:
> - The prevalence of the disease
> - The role of any existing treatments
> - The economic costs of managing the disease
>
> ***Is the target appropriate?***
>
> Consider:
> - Is it already a target for other drugs?
> - The effect of pre-existing ligands – natural and pharmacological
> - Does expression of the target change in diseased tissues?
> - The effect of knocking it out in animal models
> - Evidence from 'experiments of nature' – polymorphisms, mutations, etc.

2.4 Target validation

Target validation for a 'fast follower' is usually easy because the target and much of the development strategy have been defined by the lead compound. Target validation for a pioneer compound is much more difficult. For the purpose of this discussion let us suppose that a new orphan G-protein-coupled receptor has been identified and it is predominantly expressed in an area of the brain thought to be related to long-term memory. The initial working hypothesis is that stimulating or antagonizing the receptor might have therapeutic utility in age-related cognitive impairment or Alzheimer's disease. How can this hypothesis be validated to the extent that it is worth investing substantial sums of money in a drug discovery programme? There are a number of possible strategies.

One possibility is to find the natural ligand and investigate its physiological role. This can sometimes be achieved by a technique known as ligand fishing, where the high affinity of the receptor for its ligand is used to concentrate the ligand from a crude tissue extract. This was the method used to discover orexin.[1] Once the ligand is identified, it can be used in standard physiological, pharmacological and behavioural studies.

Another possibility is to 'knock out' the receptor in a mouse embryo and see how this affects the phenotype of the animal. Although scientifically attractive such data can be difficult to interpret. On the one hand the knockout may be lethal and on the other adaptations during development may mask the effect of the lost receptor system. An alternative is to produce a 'conditional knockout' – for example, using the Cre-Lox method[2] to inactivate a gene in a particular tissue at a defined moment in an adult animal.

Yet another approach is to study changes in the expression of the gene in animal models of the candidate disease. Unfortunately, animal models, although very valuable, do not necessarily reproduce the aetiological mechanism operating in man, even for an apparently straightforward condition such as hypertension. A few diseases such as schizophrenia have no animal model and this is an impediment to the development of new drugs.

The reality is that none of these methods is very robust in predicting the relevance of the target to human disease. A more direct method is to look for human polymorphisms of the ligand/receptor/effector system concerned and seek to identify associations with the target disease. These may strengthen the case that malfunction of the target system is involved in the aetiology of the disease. As more polymorphisms and haplotypes are identified, this method will gain in utility but at present it is only rarely helpful. The most direct method is to carry out experimental medicine studies in patients with the disease concerned using the most sensitive markers available. However, such data cannot be obtained until the project has been in use for a number of years and this approach is therefore of little help in making decisions in the early stages of a truly pioneer project.

Serendipity based on clinical observation has had, and still has, an important role in revealing unexpected actions of drugs. For example, the antihypertensive agent diazoxide that caused diabetes when administered orally over a few weeks found a new use in the treatment of patients with insulin-secreting tumours. The discovery of antipyschotic and antidepressant agents owed much to alert clinical observation.

2.5 Commercial assessment

Pharmaceutical companies are in business to make money. Apart from identified charitable projects a pharmaceutical company will only undertake a project if the commercial assessment suggests that it will be profitable if it succeeds. One consequence is that there is little incentive to discover drugs for very rare diseases. However, these may benefit as the indications for an established drug are progressively expanded and there is always the chance of finding new and unexpected applications of potent pharmacological agents. Furthermore, if there is a serious disease with no effective treatment, a new drug can command a very high price and that will go some way to offsetting the fact that the number of patients suffering from that particular disease is not very large.

Because of its importance, product development now always involves close interaction with strategy groups capable of making a full commercial assessment of the opportunity. The commercial evaluation function is usually fully integrated with the R&D operation and it will specify the target product profile and have a major influence on the choice of therapeutic areas for research.

A complete commercial assessment involves use of epidemiological data about the disease, current patterns of treatment and their cost. Various aspects of the proposed TPP will be discussed with focus groups of physicians, patients and providers such as health maintenance organizations. How will the value of the product be affected if it has to be taken twice a day rather than once or if it has to be given by injection rather than by mouth? How many patients are there with the disease concerned in major markets (USA, Japan, Europe) and which strata of disease severity are most likely to be eligible for treatment with the new agent? If it is only the most severe stratum the numbers will be low and the price of the product will be high. If the indication is likely to extend to mild cases the price will be much lower but cost of goods (see below) may be an issue.

The commercial assessment must take into account not just the competitive situation now but, much more speculatively, what it may be like in 10 years' time when the project comes to fruition.

With a fast-follower project the commercial projections are usually quite accurate but the pharmaceutical industry is full of stories of entries into new therapeutic areas where the commercial assessment greatly underestimated the eventual size of the market, sometimes by 10-fold or more. However, the skills of those involved are increasing and the main driver of decision-making in pharmaceutical R&D is the projection of commercial value adjusted by a scientific assessment of the likelihood of success.

3. PLATFORM TECHNOLOGIES

In the third millennium most pharmaceutical targets are single human receptors or enzymes whose sequences are available in public or private genomic databases accessible to the company. It is perhaps foreseeable that once the single protein targets encoded in the genome have been thoroughly explored there will be a greater interest in using compounds, or mixtures of compounds, with multiple actions upon a control system, but that is largely for the future.

The crucial platform technologies are bioinformatics (to identify targets), high throughput screening with a validated assay, combinatorial chemistry that generates tens or hundreds of thousands of different chemical molecules and computer modelling of interactions between candidate drugs and protein targets.

3.1 The assay

The first step is to clone the DNA and express the target human protein and then to devise an assay system that can be used in high-throughput screening. Early assays were usually based on competitive binding of a labelled ligand to the target protein but it is more informative to have a functional assay. Such an assay might utilize activation of adenylate cyclase, detection of a calcium transient in a cell, inhibition of an enzyme reaction with a coloured or fluorescent product, the product of a reporter gene, etc. The guiding criteria for these assays are that they must be cheap, reliable, capable of being carried out in very small volumes of fluid and suitable for full automation in a robotic assembly that can process tens of thousands of assays per day. These assays are carried out in multi-well (256 or more) plates that are loaded, incubated and measured entirely by robots.

3.2 Combinatorial chemistry

To feed high-throughput screens very large numbers of chemicals with diverse chemical structures are needed. The numbers required substantially exceed the legacy compounds stored by chemical and pharmaceutical companies. Combinatorial chemistry is used to generate the very large numbers of molecules required.[3,4] The aim is to carry out a sequence of different reactions on a framework molecule by splitting the batch after each reaction. It is essential that the resultant molecules can be separated because the normal practice now is to use single molecules in high-throughput screens, rather than the mixtures commonly used 2–5 years ago. One way to do separate the compounds is to use tagged beads and synthetic steps similar to the amino acid by amino acid solid-state synthesis of peptides, except that in this case the derivatives may be on any available reactive group. The quantities of each chemical synthesized are tiny but they are sufficient for the small volumes of the multi-well plates of the high-throughput assay.

Although the original aim was simply to generate very large numbers of chemicals, the process is becoming more intelligent as syntheses can be directed towards structures that are, for example, likely to be protease or kinase inhibitors.

3.3 Hits and leads

The managers of a high-throughput screen will set a threshold of response in the assay that is regarded as a 'hit'. Usually the threshold is set at a concentration that is much higher than required for a drug, e.g. 10 micromolar, on the assumption that the lead optimization chemists will be able to improve the activity by 3 or 4 log units. A hit may or may not be sufficiently interesting to be regarded as a 'lead'. Medicinal chemists sometimes refer to a lead as a molecule that is drug-like. By this they mean that it is amenable to extensive chemical manipulation, it does not raise potential genotoxic alarms, looks as though it will have acceptable pharmacokinetic properties, etc. The ideal is to have leads from quite different chemical classes as this reduces the risk that a project may fail because of toxicity with all the available, closely related leads affected.

4. LEAD OPTIMIZATION

4.1 Computer modelling

Some enthusiasts dream that future drug discovery and development will be done entirely 'in silico'.[5,6] Part of this vision is being realized. An increasing number of biologically important proteins have been crystallized and their three-dimensional structure has been defined by crystallography using X-ray or synchrotron beams. This process has been greatly speeded up by the increasing availability of very 'bright' synchrotron radiation sources and advanced computing. A protein crystal formed with the natural ligand in place makes it possible to define the shape and distances of bond interactions and this knowledge can be used to design drugs that are a good fit into the active site.[7] However, these measurements are not yet sufficiently precise to be more than a useful guide in lead optimization because of the variety of properties that must be optimized to turn a 'hit' into a drug.

4.2 Objectives

Lead optimization is one of the most crucial steps in drug development. As it progresses the medicinal chemist will seek to do four things.

1. Improve the activity against the primary target.
2. Minimize activity against closely related targets. The aim is usually a minimum of 100-fold selectivity but 1000-fold is better as, for poorly understood reasons, in vivo selectivity is often less than that in vitro.
3. Optimize the pharmacokinetic properties. This in itself involves a whole series of objectives, including the avoidance of interactions with important hepatic cytochrome P450s, such as CYP450 3A4; having sufficient lipid solubility to be reasonably well absorbed from the gut (e.g. Lipinski's rule of five[8,9]); good metabolic stability to give it (in most cases) a duration of action long enough to permit once-daily dosing and avoidance of being a substrate for cellular efflux pumps, such as MDR-1.
4. Avoidance of toxicity. This is one of the

most difficult aspects, as the small quantities of chemical available at this stage limit what can be done and the number of potentially toxic mechanisms is very large. However, many companies now carry out safety testing in cell-based systems or 4-day studies in rats at this stage to reduce the cost, and time lost, if a compound fails in large-scale safety assessment done later. Even a limited rat study may require several grams of a drug, while a chemist concerned with lead optimization may be dealing in micrograms or a few milligrams. One of the most pressing needs in drug development is for better methods of weeding out potentially toxic compounds before they have incurred substantial expenditure. As formation of a reactive intermediate during drug metabolism appears to be the most common precipitating factor in toxicity, one promising approach is to screen compounds for formation of covalent adducts to drug-metabolizing enzymes in vitro.[10] Transcriptomic techniques applied to safety assessment may also increase sensitivity.[11]

5. PHARMACOLOGY

In parallel with the lead optimization programme led by the medicinal chemists a team of biologists will begin delineating the pharmacological actions of the compound. If the target is unprecedented, this may be the first opportunity to begin to understand the consequences of inhibiting a novel G-protein-coupled receptor, protease or kinase. While the team have the excitement of exploring unknown territory, they are at a disadvantage in that there is no body of existing published knowledge to draw upon. With a fast follower the situation is quite different in that there is usually extensive published and academic expertise that can be utilized.

Most of these studies will be done in isolated cells or tissues or in standard laboratory species, mainly rats and dogs. These studies will attempt to delineate dose–response relationships for the effects under study. Often the doses used in pharmacological studies are large, on a mg per kg basis, when compared with doses used in man, frequently 30–100 times greater. There are several reasons for this. Small animals often metabolize drugs much more rapidly than man and pharmacologists tend to work near the top of dose–response curves, whereas clinical pharmacologists are more often operating near the bottom of the curve. There is a problem of extrapolation, however, and it is useful to compare exposure (concentrations) across species and not just dosage.

Besides studies in normal animals, the biological programme will certainly make use of animal models of the target disease to try to build the case that the drug has therapeutic utility. Animal models vary greatly in their predictive power for man. The most reliable models are those for infection, unsurprisingly because the target is the same across species. The least reliable are those intended to model central nervous system (CNS) diseases such as schizophrenia or bipolar disorder. In between these extremes models for a number of common diseases have proved to be of value, even when the method for creating the model may not correspond very closely to the pathogenic mechanism operating in man, e.g. in inflammation, hypertension, osteoporosis, etc. But there are failures from apparently sound models. Neuroprotective agents for use in stroke are usually tested in the rat middle cerebral artery occlusion model. This produces a pathological lesion that appears very similar to human stroke but despite a number of positive results in limiting infarct size in animals using this model, all have failed in human studies.

There are special problems with protein therapeutic agents, e.g. humanized antibodies, as these may be so specific for human targets that they have little or no demonstrable effect in standard laboratory species or even in sub-human primates. In these cases the amount of whole animal pharmacology that can be done may be very small.

6. THE TRANSITION TO CLINICAL DEVELOPMENT

A stage will be reached, often after 3 or 4 years' work, when the chemists and biologists become confident that they have a molecule that has the characteristics of a candidate drug and the potential to be of value as a therapeutic agent. At this stage a series of new activities will be activated, although they will have been planned many months before. These include scaling up the synthesis to provide sufficient supplies for safety assessment and later clinical trials, consideration of the formulation of the compound to be administered to man, more extensive studies of its pharmacokinetics and metabolism and, critically, studies designed to establish that it is safe to give to man.

6.1 Chemical development

The molecule that has been studied during lead optimization has often been made by a very complex multi-stage synthesis (10–15 steps is not uncommon). It is impractical to produce kilogram quantities by such a synthesis and in any case it would be impossibly expensive. In these days of more complex molecules the cost of goods can be a substantial issue and in a very few cases it has proved so difficult to synthesize a molecule at reasonable cost that the project has been abandoned. The job of development chemists, with their pilot plants, is to simplify the synthesis, increase the yield, make sufficient of the drug at a high state of purity, to supply safety assessment and early clinical trials and, if the drug succeeds, to hand on to the mainstream manufacturing a reliable low cost synthesis. These are not always simple tasks. Often the solution is the convergent synthesis of large sections of the molecule that are ligated together at a late stage rather than the step-by-step approach that may have been used in the lead optimization process.

6.2 Pharmaceutical technology

A high proportion of modern drugs have physical properties that tax the skills of the formula-tion pharmacists. The most common problem is that they are extremely insoluble in water. Highly insoluble drugs usually have low and variable systemic bioavailability and it is difficult to produce equivalent bioavailability when formulation techniques are altered. To minimize this problem the compound must be formulated as very small particles to increase the 'surface area to mass' ratio and enhance solubility. It can be very difficult to produce a consistent formulation and prevent aggregation. The drug may turn out to have too short a half-life for once-daily dosing and pharmaceutical technology will be called upon to produce a controlled-release formulation. This often involves a degree of trial and error, as controlled-release formulations are not completely predictable. The compound may be unstable in air or moisture and may have to be given a protective coating. A filler will have to be used to make the tablet up to a standard size, etc.

To avoid these problems some companies conduct Phase I studies almost entirely with drug powder taken up into solution in water (sometimes a sizeable volume) immediately before dosing.

6.3 Safety assessment

Before a drug is given to man for the first time it must go through an extensive programme of safety assessment. The aim of these studies is to rule out genotoxicity and establish a no-effect dose, or better exposure level, in at least two different species, usually rats and dogs. The no adverse effect exposure level (NOAEL) will become one of the main pieces of evidence taken into account by the committees authorizing the doses that may be given to man. This subject is treated in more depth in Chapter 2.

6.3.1 Genotoxicity

This assessment will include an Ames test (bacterial mutagenicity) in *Salmonella typhimurium* and *Escherichia coli* with and without metabolic activation using hepatic microsomes from Aroclor-induced animals. A mouse lymphoma assay and micronucleus are used to test for genotoxicity and a chromosome aberration assay to test for clastogenicity.

6.3.2 Chronic toxicity in vivo
Before undertaking chronic studies the acute toxicity of high single doses will be studied but it is not now the practice to estimate the LD50. The duration of chronic administration will depend on the proposed duration of treatment for man. For limited human studies with single doses, dosing for 4 days may be sufficient, although 14 days is more usual. Animals normally receive daily administration of three widely spaced doses, the highest being one that approaches the dose that causes acute toxicity. The philosophy of animal safety tests is not so much to show what is safe but rather what toxicity occurs when a toxic dose is given. The animals will be closely observed by trained veterinarians, have routine biochemistry and haematology investigations, plasma concentration measurements to estimate exposure and at the end of the study will be killed and detailed histology will be undertaken. For administration of multiple doses to man, studies of longer duration, 28 days, then 3 or 6 months will be performed.

There are problems with these tests but few think that it is possible to dispense with them. Very high doses may recruit unusual pathways of metabolism, the normal routes having been swamped, and may overwhelm mechanisms for capture of chemically reactive metabolites by depleting glutathione. Often the pathology observed has no exact human counterpart or if it has, such as the very common problem of phospholipid accumulation, there is known to be a poor correlation between animal and human findings.

The clinical pharmacologist who wishes to interpret these findings may find the task difficult. At the very least he will need the guidance of a skilled veterinary pathologist who is knowledgeable about the background incidence of pathology in the chosen species and who has previous experience with compounds that have a similar type of action.

If there is a reasonably wide gap between the estimated human exposure and the NOAEL exposure (10–100-fold or more), this is reassuring, whereas if the margin is low (5-fold or less) this would be a cause for concern. But there are examples of drugs used in man where the ratio between the dose causing toxicity in animals and the dose given to man is < 1, e.g. gastrointestinal effects of some non-steroidal anti-inflammatory drugs (NSAIDs).

It is standard practice to study the reversibility of any toxic changes observed after cessation of treatment. Irreversible changes such as tissue necrosis or fibrosis will engender greater caution and mandate a wider margin of safety in most cases. However, safety assessment findings must always be interpreted with reference to the proposed use and severe toxicity may be acceptable when the disease itself has a high mortality, e.g. cytotoxic agents used in cancer.

6.3.3 Reproductive toxicology
Effects on fertility, implantation and early embryonic development are assessed by dosing rats 14–28 days before mating and for 6 days post coitus. Fetal development is assessed by dosing mated females from 6 to 15 days post coitus.

6.3.4 Toxicokinetics and exposure
The fact that an animal has been administered a certain dose in mg/kg without adverse effects and that this was many times higher than the planned dose in man was once held to represent a margin of safety. The routine application of kinetic analysis to safety assessment studies has shown how misleading this conclusion can be. At the extreme, rats given high doses of a compound have sometimes proved to have almost no systemic exposure because of the efficiency of their presystemic metabolism and/or biliary excretion. It is now routine to estimate exposure in safety assessment studies by measuring both the maximum plasma concentration (Cmax) achieved and the area under the time-concentration curve (AUC) between doses in the different species and doses. With the toxicokinetic data the apparent margins of safety based on relative doses between man and animals usually shrink, occasionally almost to

vanishing point. An example is the NSAID, phenylbutazone. When the oral dose in the dog was adjusted to give similar exposure to that achieved in man with a therapeutic dose, the animals developed very severe gastrointestinal toxicity.

Moreover, caution is needed when using exposure to assess hepatic toxicity because the liver is exposed to the whole of the enterally absorbed dose. If presystemic metabolism in the gut wall or liver is high in the chosen animal species, the systemic exposure may be low but the hepatic exposure may be very high.

6.3.5 Safety pharmacology

The main aim of safety pharmacology is to detect effects, not readily predictable from the pharmacological action, that might cause serious problems in man. Examples include hypotension, respiratory depression, seizures, coma, ataxia, etc. These studies are often done in conscious, chronically instrumented animals to look for changes in circulatory function, e.g. hypotension. Generally they are done at dose levels that are at the high end of the pharmacological dose–response curve or only a few multiples (5–10) higher.

Recently there has been a surge of interest in compounds that may blockade cardiac potassium channels, particularly I_{kr}, and predispose to the ventricular arrhythmia known as torsade de pointes. This channel has a relatively wide entry port and compounds of diverse pharmacological action (recent examples include some quinolone antibiotics) may enter it, block the channel and cause prolongation of the QT interval on the electrocardiogram. Screening of dog Purkinje tissue and cells expressing human I_{kr} has been introduced but interpretation of the findings has not yet been standardized.

7. PHARMACOKINETICS AND DRUG METABOLISM

During lead optimization the molecule will have been scrutinized for possible sites of oxidative attack by hepatic cytochrome P450s or other drug-metabolizing enzymes. As such reactions may lead to the formation of reactive epoxides it is common practice to block them, e.g. by inserting a fluorine atom at the site of oxidation. Databases will have been reviewed for possible genotoxic potential or other known toxicities. Often the chemists have considerable experience with a series of related structures and they can draw on this experience to make useful predictions.

An assay with sufficient sensitivity to measure the drug in plasma will have been developed. In the era of the LC/MS/MS mass spectrometer this is much quicker and easier than it used to be. A species of the drug labelled with carbon-14 in a metabolically stable site will have been requested. Often low water solubility is a problem and the drug may have to be solubilized in substances such as dimethyl sulphoxide (DMSO). The availability of an intravenous dosage form makes it possible to calculate the absolute bioavailability and secure an accurate assessment of half-life and metabolic clearance.

Early ex vivo metabolic studies will be undertaken with hepatic microsomes and isolated perfused rat liver. These studies will enable a preliminary estimate to be made of the rate of hepatic clearance. Later studies with isolated human hepatocytes will be used to make predictions for human kinetics. Many pharmacokineticists use allometric scaling (predictions based on relative body weight) to infer the active dose in man but this method has been criticized because it has relatively large errors in about one-fifth of cases.[12,13]

Whole animal pharmacokinetic studies are usually undertaken with doses administered by oral gavage in rats and dogs. The kinetics in dogs are often closer to man than those in rats but both species are likely to have a shorter half-life than man and metabolic routes may be significantly different, especially greater presystemic metabolism and biliary secretion in the rat. Hepatic clearance can be estimated by comparing the kinetics after intra-portal infusion against those measured during infusion into a systemic vein.

A search will be made for metabolites (easier once a C-14-labelled molecule becomes available) and, if they are found, their potential pharmacological activity will be assessed.

Knowledge of these metabolites is also very important in safety assessment as the exposure to them, as well as the parent drug, will be taken into account when considering whether the cover is adequate for man. Sometimes this issue has to be revisited when human data become available if humans produce much larger amounts of a particular metabolite than the safety assessment species. The labelled material will be used to carry out mass balance/excretion studies with bile, urine and faecal collections, the aim being to account for > 90% of the administered dose. Quantitative whole body autoradiography will also be performed with the labelled material and whole body sections prepared on a sledge microtome.

8. PULLING IT ALL TOGETHER

Before a drug can be considered for first administration to man all the preclinical evidence must be assembled, reviewed and compiled into a series of documents. The multidisciplinary team that have progressed the compound will do this and great efforts will be made to do this quickly to retain a competitive edge.

Broadly speaking, three different sets of documents will be produced, although much of the material is in common. The first set will be for internal review and is likely to be divided into three subsets. The first of these will be for scientific review when the discovery and preclinical scientists conclude that the compound is ready to progress to man. The second will concentrate on safety and will be reviewed by the company safety committee and the third will focus on commercial issues to decide whether the compound has sufficient promise to justify the substantial programme of investment once the compound enters the clinical phase.

The second set of documents is for review by the regulatory authorities that must give permission before a drug can be administered to humans. The best known of these documents is the IND (Investigational New Drug) application to the Food and Drug Administration (FDA) in the USA, although there are equivalent procedures in the European Union, Japan and many other countries (see Chapter 3).

These reviews will give particular attention to safety issues and will include the doses and routes of administration intended for the early human studies.

The third document is an Investigators' Manual, which will include a summary of all the information available about the compound that will be made available to the designated investigators who undertake clinical trials and to institutional review boards (IRBs, ethics committees). Investigators and IRBs are free to ask for additional information.

9. FIRST TIME IN HUMAN (PHASE I STUDIES)

Once all these consents have been obtained, the first studies in man can begin, although the clinical project team will have drawn up the plans for them many months in advance (see Box 1.2). In most cases the required dose and probable duration of action in man will have been modelled using pharmacokinetic predictions and measurements of pharmacodynamic activity against the target human protein (e.g. IC50). Some people have argued that in future more and more aspects of drug development will be done in silico. This may turn out to be true for precedented molecules but the time is far off for unprecedented molecules when such basic information as the degree of receptor blockade needed for a therapeutic effect (if any) is unknown.

The first administration to man is usually made either by the in-house clinical pharmacology unit of the sponsoring company, or by a contract research organization (CRO). The volunteers will be carefully screened for pre-existing health problems[14] and in the case of female volunteers, pregnancy testing and use of effective contraceptive measures. For these studies volunteers are normally resident in a specialized clinical pharmacology unit.

9.1 Dose-rising studies

These studies are often described as 'tolerance and dose-ranging' as their principal objective is assessment of safety although, where possible,

---

Box 1.2   Clinical development

Phase I

First administration to man
- Tolerability
- Pharmacological effects
- Pharmacokinetics

  20–80 patients

Phase II

IIA – developing
IIB – proving concepts
- Efficacy
- Dose-ranging
- Relative safety

  100–200 patient

Phase III

Confirmation in larger numbersconcepts
- Confirmation of dose
- Efficacy in specific subgroups
- Adverse events/safety data
- Comparative studies

  1000–3000+ patients

Phase IV

Post-marketing development
- New indications/subgroups
- Adverse effects

---

simple pharmacodynamic measurements should be included.

The first dose administered to man will be a small fraction of the dose predicted to have a therapeutic effect. The rate of dose increment for compounds that may have a narrow therapeutic index (e.g. a cardiac anti-arrhythmic agent) will be more gradual than for those where there are no such concerns. For a compound that is anticipated to have an effective dose of 50 mg the dose increments might be 2.5 mg, 5 mg, 10 mg, 25 mg and 50 mg in separate individuals. Intravenous preparations may be examined by infusion with small increasing dose increments in the same individual (see Box 1.3).

The volunteers, who are usually young adults, are paid for their time and discomfort. They are carefully screened for transmissible diseases such as hepatitis B and HIV, or consumption of addictive drugs. They will have a medical history taken, a clinical examination and a full range of haematological and biochemical tests on blood, an ECG and a urine analysis. However, the 'quality' of volunteers varies and the methods of recruitment and reward may sometimes bring in individuals who are living unhealthy lifestyles.

The subjects are generally admitted to the clinical pharmacology unit for the duration of the study to ensure protocol compliance and deal promptly with any adverse reactions. The measurements made in the single dose-rising study are simple.

The basic data collected are pharmacokinetics, vital signs, volunteered symptoms and a repeat of the initial panel of safety tests. However, if there are grounds for concern based on preclinical data, other measurements will be added. For example, if the compound was suspected of a tendency to cause renal toxicity, renal tubule-derived enzymes might be measured in urine together with more sophisticated microscopic analysis of cells in urine.

Both the mean pharmacokinetic data and their variability are useful guides to future dose increments and, once available, ought to supersede predictions made from preclinical

Box 1.3   Phase I: dose-rising study

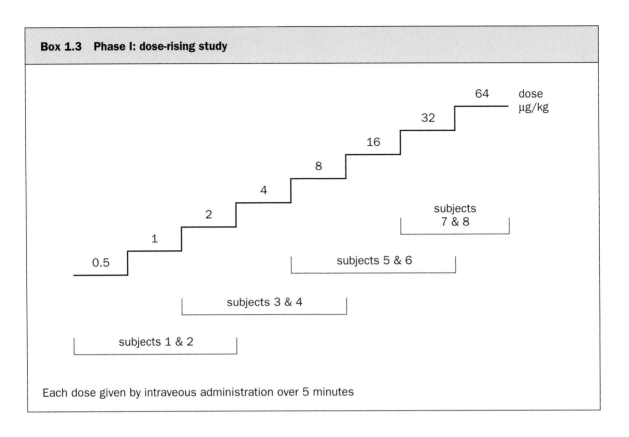

Each dose given by intraveous administration over 5 minutes

data. For that reason it is highly desirable that samples are analysed promptly and that plasma concentration values are available before the next increment in dose is made.

This methodology has some problems. The most common volunteered complaints are headache, usually triggered by caffeine withdrawal, and nausea caused by the combination of fasting and the procedure. There is evidence that a prolonged sojourn (> 1 week) in a residential clinical pharmacology unit may be accompanied by a moderate rise (2–3 times normal) in liver-derived enzymes such as alanine transaminase.[15] The liver function changes have been ascribed to diet changes and lack of exercise but can cause considerable difficulties of interpretation as it may be impractical to decide whether or not they are drug-related. Healthy normal volunteers at rest may also approach or pass the 'lower limit of normal' for blood neutrophil counts defined by pathology laborato-

ries that use more diverse populations to establish their normal range.

There is also the possibility that dosing may be taken unnecessarily high if there are no dose-limiting adverse effects or that high doses may be given that do cause adverse effects that could have been avoided. For this reason it is highly desirable to incorporate an indication of the pharmacodynamic response such as measurements of biomarkers or physiological responses into these early studies. However, this is often easier said than done.

For highly toxic drugs, mainly cytotoxic agents used in oncology, a different approach is adopted. The studies are done in patients and the objective is usually to find the maximum tolerated dose (MTD) in as small a number of patients as possible, often groups of only 3–6 at each dose level. The endpoint is usually either gastrointestinal side-effects, mainly diarrhoea, or fall in blood count with neutropenia with or without thrombocytopenia. However, as drugs used in oncology become more specific and survival improves there is a need to move away from MTD towards more conventional and safer approaches to establishing dose-response.

9.2 Repeated dosing studies

If there are no serious safety issues from the dose-rising study, this will be followed by a repeat dose study, often of 14 days' duration, and also undertaken in normal volunteers housed in an in-patient clinical pharmacology unit. A frequent design is to use three dose levels, the highest one close to the maximum safe dose in the single-dose study. If the drug is known to have a half-life that substantially exceeds 24 hours, the dosage schedule may have to be modified. The main aims are to obtain pharmacokinetic information at steady-state and safety data during more prolonged administration. Special attention will be given to compounds that have non-linear kinetics or active metabolites. A very different metabolic profile in man from those seen in animals may require further animal studies to establish safe exposure limits for the metabolites. Here again it is desirable to incorporate pharmacodynamic or biomarker measurements into the study design as a first step in relating dose and/or concentration to an indication of biological activity in man.

9.3 Interaction studies

9.3.1 Food
It is standard practice to meet regulatory requirements to investigate the effect of an FDA standard greasy North American breakfast on the absorption of oral doses of the drug. With drugs that have a low bioavailability or with those largely absorbed high in the gastrointestinal tract, the effect of food upon absorption can be substantial. In the latter case food may increase the fraction absorbed because it prolongs gastric emptying.

9.3.2 Drug interactions
Knowledge of a new drug's interaction with drug-metabolizing enzymes and excretory

pathways often makes it possible to make reasonably accurate predictions about likely interactions with other drugs. For example, a new drug that was a potent inhibitor of CYP450 3A4 would probably not be progressed these days because of the very long list of likely drug interactions. A drug that is almost exclusively metabolized by CYP450 3A4 is likely to show large inter-individual differences because the activity of this enzyme in the gut wall and liver can vary 40-fold between individuals.[16] Interactions with membrane pumps of the ATP-binding cassette class (ABC), e.g. multi-drug resistance gene (MDR-1), are an increasing subject of study. For example, most of the reported interactions with digoxin are due to effects at membrane transporters.[17] These interactions can overlap one another.[18]

Among drugs that are commonly the subject of interaction studies, warfarin and digoxin stand out but additions to the list depend upon therapeutic utility, likely concomitant use and potential to cause inhibition or induction of drug-metabolizing enzymes. Most of these studies are confined to pharmacokinetic interactions.

10. PHASE IIA

The most important question about a new drug is, does it have therapeutic activity? However, this is a much more complex question than appears on the surface. What does proof of therapeutic activity (sometimes termed 'proof of concept') mean? Does it mean demonstrating that the new drug has the anticipated pharmacological action in man? This question might be answered by a receptor occupancy study using positron emission tomography (PET), if a suitable labelled ligand is available (see Chapter 8), or by a pharmacological challenge if there is a suitable agonist for use in man. An example is the use of an isoprenaline (isoproterenol) challenge upon heart rate and diastolic blood pressure to study the efficacy of propranolol in blocking beta-adrenergic receptors. As there is often a relatively indirect link between the pharmacological action and therapeutic effect, to demonstrate only the former is clearly insufficient. An effect upon the disease process is required unless there is a precedent. For example, when cimetidine was developed there were initial doubts about how effective antagonism of histamine-2 receptors would be in suppressing gastric acid secretion. By the time ranitidine and famotidine were developed those issues had been resolved and those compounds were able to pursue a fast-track development. But even with cimetidine there was already a large body of knowledge about histamine and acid secretion in the stomach.

The difficulties are much greater with new targets picked out of the genome. There may be several possible disease targets in different therapeutic areas. For example, a new drug that inhibited fibrosis might have applications in the lung, kidney, skin, liver, or postoperative peritoneum, to name only a few. The complexity and time (and therefore cost) taken to explore all these possibilities with conventional large Phase II trials would be considerable. This type of problem has led to a revival of interest in 'experimental medicine' (see below). In some instances it may be relatively easy to demonstrate the desired action of the drug, for example, a fall in blood pressure in mild hypertension or an increase in forced expiratory volume in 1 minute (FEV1) or peak expiratory flow in mild asthma. In others, it may involve sizeable, lengthy, complex and expensive studies, as with, for example, the relief of negative features of schizophrenia or the prevention of fractures in osteoporosis. This has prompted a search for early indicators of drug response, sometimes called 'surrogate indicators' or biomarkers.

10.1 Use of biomarkers

The expense and time involved in conducting medium-scale clinical trials to gain an early insight into therapeutic activity has fuelled an intense search for biomarkers of therapeutic activity that may give a faster readout (see Chapter 7). Investigation of the action of drugs in patients with osteoporosis provides a good illustration of the use of different levels of biomarkers such as the C-terminal telopeptides of type I collagen and urinary N-terminal telopeptides of type I collagen.[19] Plasma or urine concentrations of bone collagen degradation products give a quick (days) readout of changes in bone turnover. Changes in bone mineral density take much longer to detect (3–12 months). Clinical trials to demonstrate reduction in vertebral or femoral neck fracture take even longer (3+ years). In this case there is strong scientific evidence to connect the biomarkers with the disease process but even here interpretation of the results is not straightforward. The selective oestrogen receptor modifier, raloxifene, has less effect on bone mineral density in osteoporosis than the bisphosphonate, alendronate, but has a similar effect in preventing vertebral fractures. However, later trials showed that alendronate is effective in preventing fractures of the femoral neck but raloxifene may not be effective. Biomarkers have been used extensively in HIV infections but measurement of viral envelope proteins in plasma proved somewhat misleading and it is current practice to measure plasma viral RNA levels. Even here the measurement is indirect in that it may not be a reliable indicator of virus in reservoirs like follicular dendritic cells.

Many new biomarkers are being explored that have a less direct or more problematic association with therapeutic response. Among these, changes in gene expression using RNA chips and changes in protein composition investigated by use of 2-D gels and mass spectrometry (proteomics) are particularly active areas of research. This field is sometime referred to as the *omics (transcriptomics, proteomics, metabonomics, etc.). Substantial investment will be required to validate proposed new biomarkers. In a tumour or during an inflammatory response it is commonplace for the expression of several hundred genes to change.[20] One great advantage of the transcriptomic chip technology is that it can be used to make a sequence of measurements as a disease process evolves, if tissue is available for study. This makes it much easier to distinguish cause from effect. The use of proteomics has been facilitated by the use of automated spot samplers that feed directly into a mass spectrometer to identify the protein concerned. The advocates of proteomics hope that characteristic patterns of changes in plasma or tissue proteins will be identified that can be used to track disease response. For example, an assay for the acute phase reactant C-reactive protein (CRP) has been available for many years but it is only comparatively recently that it has been adopted widely as a marker of systemic inflammation in conditions as wide ranging as infection and atherosclerosis.[21] The difficulty with proteomics[22] is likely to be low specificity until much more is known about the biology of secreted proteins. Profiling of metabolites (metabonomics) by techniques such as biofluid nuclear magnetic resonance (NMR) on urine and plasma is also an area of growing interest.[23]

At present most biomarkers are of greatest value in guiding management decisions in drug development but are not sufficiently reliable to obviate the need for clinical trials with hard clinical endpoints such as fracture.

10.2 Planning for success

For a drug to repay its very high development costs, plans will be made to make it available throughout the world. This process has been facilitated by the efforts made to harmonize the requirements of international regulatory agencies. This is a vast topic and the detail is beyond the scope of this chapter but excellent information can be found on the web-site of the International Federation of Pharmaceutical Manufacturers Associations (IFPMA) and that of the Center for Drug Evaluation and Research (CDER) at the US Food & Drug Administration (FDA) (see below for details).

The conventional fast-track development process in the pharmaceutical industry is based on planning for success, so Phase II and III studies are designed at least in concept and often in detail before Phase I begins. The incentives of industrial clinical development staff often depend upon achievement of demanding time lines that assume that development will proceed as a through-train to the regulatory submission or marketing. When it works the outcome is excellent but many pharmaceutical companies are experiencing increasing numbers of expensive failures in Phase III, some of which can be traced back to inadequate preparatory work in Phase II. Much effort is now being focused on means of reducing the risk of Phase III failure. There are numerous reasons for such failures but two stand out above the others.

10.2.1 The wrong choice of dose

It is a truism that the most likely thing to get wrong in drug development is the dose. There are several reasons for this. One is the desire to find one dose that suits most patients, on the (probably correct) assumption that many doctors are too busy to take the time to undertake individual dose titration. A single (or very limited range) of recommended dose presupposes a narrower range of dose–response than is usually realized in practice. The consequence is that a cautious choice of the average dose may be too low for some patients.

A second problem is inadequate clinical trial design. If the dose–response data from Phase II are inadequate the temptation to press ahead with the best of those doses in Phase III is strong because of time pressure. A better approach is to use a pure dose–response design in Phase IIA with a wide range of doses and collect good quality data about both therapeutic response and adverse effects. Such a design will give useful information about the shape of the dose–response curve and does not require a placebo.[24,25] The optimum dose(s) can then be chosen, taking both efficacy and adverse effects into account. Another possibility is to start a parallel group trial with, for example, six dosage groups and drop some at a pre-scheduled interim review once the shape of the dose–response curve has emerged. This is sometimes referred to as an 'adaptive design'.[26,27]

A third problem is that the desire to demonstrate an effect with small numbers of patients in Phase IIA may lead the investigators to progress high up the dose–response curve, motivated by the desire to demonstrate an unequivocal effect. The patients who take part in these studies will be in protocols with long lists of inclusion and exclusion criteria. Such studies may yield good results in small numbers of closely monitored, highly selected patients but the dose may prove to be too high for less tightly selected or supervised patients on the open market.

A particular problem arises with dose-ranging for drugs that act upon the CNS. In the past some drugs have been taken into late phase trials that, in retrospect, failed because of poor penetration into the CNS. Even if the drug enters the brain it may require relatively large-scale, placebo-controlled Phase II studies to demonstrate a response, let alone define a dose–response curve.

The use of cyclotron-produced, short half-life, positron-emitting isotopes to label ligands for specific brain receptors has gone far towards solving this problem, at least in terms of brain penetration and receptor occupancy (see Chapter 8). A range of doses of the new drug are used as a cold ligand to displace a specific receptor ligand labelled with a positron-emitting isotope (usually Carbon-11). This technique has the advantage of answering two questions at once. First it shows how well the drug penetrates the human brain and secondly it identifies doses that cause high enough receptor occupancy to be plausible in therapy. PET with [11]C- or ^{18}F-labelled compounds has applications in many other tissues but there are few alternatives in the brain.[28,29]

10.2.2 The wrong choice of disease or disease severity

Drugs of proven efficacy and safety are rarely suitable for all grades of disease severity. One of the challenges in drug development is to identify the therapeutic niche that a new drug is likely to occupy. This is obviously important from the standpoint of late phase trial design but it also has great commercial importance because it affects pricing. Serious errors of this kind are unlikely with a compound that has a precedented action but can be a major problem with drugs that have a novel action with potential applications in several different therapeutic areas.

Basically there are two options. One is to choose the most promising disease target and proceed quickly with large Phase II studies in the conventional manner. The second is to deploy modern techniques of clinical investigation in smaller, intensively investigated groups of patients to increase the likelihood of making the best choice. This approach is often termed 'experimental medicine' and its espousal by industry has coincided with a realization in academic medical circles that the skills of the clinical investigator working directly with patients have been neglected in an era filled with the fascination of laboratory studies of genomics.

A very wide range of techniques are at the disposal of the clinical investigator undertaking experimental medicine studies with new drugs. These range from the well-established methods of pharmacological challenge, epitomized by recording the effect of beta-blockers on an iso-proterenol dose–response curve, using heart rate and diastolic blood pressure as the responses, to sophisticated modern methods using genomics, proteomics and imaging. Old methods combined with new can be used as a read-out in challenge studies, e.g. ex vivo challenge of human white cells with lipopolysaccharide in the investigation of cyclo-oxygenase 2 (COX 2) inhibitors.[30]

The extraordinary development of imaging and endoscopic techniques has provided very powerful new tools for experimental medicine. PET has already been mentioned. It can provide information about receptor occupancy in otherwise inaccessible tissues such as the human brain. Functional magnetic resonance imaging (fMRI) of the brain has many applications to investigate brain pathways and their response to drug administration.[31] Local magnetic resonance coils have enabled high-resolution images of smaller lesions such as atheromatous plaques to be recorded. Labelling of neutrophils can be used to study the effects of drugs upon cell adhesion and migration into areas of inflammation. In oncology, imaging techniques can be used to study drug penetration into the tumour, changes in tumour volume and effects of treatment upon cell viability (using ^{18}F-labelled fluoro-deoxyglucose).

11. PHASE IIB AND PHASE III

11.1 General considerations

In an ideal drug development world, Phase IIA is for developing concepts, Phase IIB is for proving them and Phase III is for confirming them in larger numbers of patients. Not all drugs fall into this pattern. For example, an anti-infective agent may go straight into Phase IIB or III if it shows appropriate pharmacokinetic properties in Phase I.

By the time of entry into Phase IIB a number of issues should have been settled. There should be data about the dose–response relationship and preliminary indications of therapeutic efficacy in one or more disease entities. Single and multiple dose pharmacokinetics should have been defined and modelled and correlations between pharmacokinetic and pharmacodynamic data (PK-PD) should have been investigated. There should be a reasonable volume of safety data in man, both from laboratory safety tests and patients' and healthy volunteers' symptoms. Outstanding issues should have been identified. Few drugs are free of some warts. If the new agent causes an appreciable burden of side-effects it may not be suitable for mild forms of a chronic disease. Conversely if the drug promises substantial benefits in a disabling or deadly disease, some quite marked adverse effects may be acceptable. In the latter case every effort must be made to understand the circumstances in which such adverse effects arise and to minimize their impact.

In Phase IIB the skills of the clinical specialist and statistician in trial design, and the great logistic machine of the major international pharmaceutical companies that run trials, come into their own. That is not to imply that excellent large clinical trials are not run by non-commercial organizations such as the National Institutes of Health (NIH) and the Medical Research Council (MRC) but the majority of such trials are now industry-sponsored. This arrangement is not entirely free from controversy. Some critics are uneasy that the organization with the greatest financial interest in the outcome also designs, manages and interprets the trial results. There are, however, several important safeguards. If the trial is to be used to register a therapeutic claim, the US FDA will almost certainly have reviewed it. Furthermore, major companies have a great incentive to ensure that their trials are designed to a high standard so that a critical audience will accept the results, and internal review processes are strict. Steering committees for Phase III outcome trials frequently include independent members and safety monitoring boards and such trials usually exclude company employees from decision-making.

The trial designers have to answer a number of critical questions about Phase IIB and III trials. The first is the disease target and the second is its therapeutic niche within the spectrum of severity of that disease. A drug that will cover almost the whole range of disease severity is more attractive commercially but, if patient groups that are less likely to respond are included, the whole trial may fail. A very good and up-to-date knowledge of the disease process and its current treatment is essential. This is where the therapeutic area specialists in industry, with the help of outside opinion leaders, come into their own. Epidemiological advice is crucial to get a precise idea of the prevalence of the disease. Thought must be given to how and where the patients will be recruited.

The next question is the measuring technique(s) to be used to assess the trial outcome. The assay may be a physiological or biochemical measurement or a complex questionnaire, such as is used to assess antidepressants. These measuring instruments must have been validated previously and their accuracy must be known, otherwise a regulatory body may not accept the data. This apparently sensible policy has its limitations. The FDA requires demonstration of improvement in lung physiology in trials in chronic obstructive pulmonary disease (COPD). As a result, most trials incorporate measurement of FEV1, although this is a poor indicator of improvement in COPD. However, besides the more obviously clinical endpoints, other factors must be assessed. For many diseases the effect upon improving the quality of life is a very important factor. For example, in Parkinson's disease rating scales are used to assess the patient's ability to manage tasks of daily living. Increasingly, those who pay for drugs are asking pharmacoeconomic questions. How quickly will the drug help the patient to get back to work, will it shorten an expensive hospital stay, or reduce suffering by a worthwhile amount? Last but not least a very thorough assessment must be made of safety with special attention paid to any concerns that have arisen in Phase I or IIA or may be predictable from preclinical data. For example, if liver enzymes (such as alanine transaminase) have been elevated to more than three times normal in several patients in Phase IIA, intensive monitoring of liver function may be required in later phases.

Great care is needed in the precise specification of the primary and secondary efficacy criteria and the inclusion and exclusion criteria. The best available epidemiological data will be used to estimate event rates, as these are crucial to the calculation of patient numbers. Often the estimates of event rates prove to be too high, as multiple exclusion criteria lead to selection of patients who are exceptionally healthy in other respects.

The clinical pharmacologist has a very important role in relation to the choice of dose(s). The ideal is to use at least three doses so that a therapeutic dose–response curve can be constructed. Cost and commercial pressures may lead to choice of only a single dose or perhaps two.

All these data will be taken into account when calculating the number of patients and the duration of treatment required in the trial. It is usual for the power calculations to require a 90% probability that a negative trial result is true and the significance level for a positive result is usually set at 1%.

Another very important aspect of trial design is safety monitoring. It is routine for blood biochemistry and haematology to be monitored at intervals and all adverse events (AEs) must be reported promptly to the sponsors and by them to the regulatory authorities. ECG monitoring to detect QT prolongation is becoming a very common requirement. Concern about abnormalities detected in animal safety tests may mandate specific safety monitoring that is designed to detect those abnormalties in patients.

Investigators conducting trials have a very important responsibility when potentially serious AEs occur. Prompt investigation of all the circumstances immediately an AE is recognized greatly increases the chance of understanding the mechanism and its relationship, if any, to the investigational drug. Regrettably, this is often not done as thoroughly as it might be. The front-line investigator must bear in mind that a serious AE is an emergency not just for the patient concerned but for every other patient on the drug, now and in the future. Sometimes an apparently drug-related effect may prove to have another explanation – the patient who resumes heavy exercise and has a greatly elevated CPK or the patient who develops jaundice but has contracted an intercurrent hepatitis A infection.

11.2 Use of placebos, equivalence and non-inferiority trials

The world of clinical trials is becoming more complex because it is a victim of past success. Once an effective form of treatment has been established it becomes difficult to justify the use of a placebo control group in later trials for conditions that have potentially serious outcomes. Indeed the latest version of the Declaration of Helsinki by the World Medical Association is quite negative on the use of placebos (www.wma.net). The FDA position appears to be that it still regards the use of placebos as necessary in a range of conditions with a relatively good prognosis over the likely trial duration, such as mild hypertension, asthma, anxiety, depression, etc.

Sample size calculations for a superiority trial of a new medicine against an active comparator are often impractically large. In consequence trials are often designed not to show that the new treatment is better but that it is at least as good (equivalence or non-inferiority) – usually interpreted as not more than 10% worse.[32–34] This is already a long-established practice in antibiotic trials. These issues are considered in the ICH report E9.[35] One of the most basic problems is that the poorer the technical design or execution of an equivalence trial, the more likely it is to fail to detect a difference, even if there is one. This problem places a substantial responsibility on trial designers and reviewers to demonstrate that the trial would have been capable of detecting a difference if there was one.

11.3 The regulatory submission

Most clinical trials are intended to support a therapeutic claim for the product under study and the final conclusion of this process is a formal submission to the FDA (a New Drug Application or NDA) or the EMEA requesting approval of a new drug or addition of a new claim to the label of an existing one. These documents are massive and, for a new chemical entity, will include data from every stage of the process, from chemical synthesis to Phase III trial outcome. The detailed requirements are dealt with in Chapter 3. Investigators should understand that their findings will be subject to the most meticulous review and relatively minor errors and omissions may cause regulatory reviewers to downgrade their assessment of data quality.

12. CONCLUSIONS AND FUTURE CONSIDERATIONS

The history of drug discovery and development over the past 50 years has become progressively more complex and expensive. The sums expended on pharmaceutical industry R&D have expanded much faster than inflation but productivity in terms of new chemical entities registered has not kept pace. In part, but only in part, this is because of the regulatory environment. New requirements are added to regulations far more often than older ones are deleted. Another major factor is the need to jump higher each time the hurdle is raised. If there is already a moderately effective drug available to treat a disease a new drug must be more effective or safer and preferably both, and the cost of demonstrating a marginal improvement is very high. Yet most therapeutic progress is incremental rather than quantal.

However, the population of the developing world is ageing and individual expectation of a healthy and active old age is rising. Medicine and therapeutic drugs have a large part to play in meeting those expectations. Existing therapeutic agents for a whole range of human diseases, but most obviously for cancer and dementia, are often only marginally effective. Biological and medical science has scarcely passed the threshold of the revolution in molecular genetics that will eventually deliver a far more detailed understanding of disease mechanisms and the biological control systems that will form the targets for new kinds of treatment. The probability of great therapeutic advances in the future is high, the timescale is unpredictable and cost is likely to be enormous; but it will be met because life and health are the most valuable assets that anyone possesses.

New technology will help. Is it fanciful to imagine that when a new chemical entity is submitted for regulatory approval there will be a short paragraph saying that it has been tested against every other human kinase, protease and GPCR and has been found to be free of biologically significant activity against any of them? That safety screens in a non-human primate have looked at transcripts of every gene in its genome and only those with a known relationship to the desired pharmacological activity have shown material changes? Will the tablet of the future include 8 or 10 different compounds, the mixture of properties designed to fine-tune a deranged control system back to as close to normal as can be achieved? Will the predictions about factors like metabolic activation, protective mechanisms, hapten formation and immunological response become so precise, based on genomics, that serious adverse drug reactions will be almost eliminated? Will physicians, at last, start to individualize drug therapy?

The future is always hard to see, that is why it is fun. But some of these things will happen, although perhaps not in the way we expect.

REFERENCES

Web-sites

■ http://www.fda.gov/cder/handbook/
The *Center for Drug Evaluation and Research (CDER) Handbook* was developed to provide a user-friendly resource on the worldwide web for obtaining information on the Center's processes and activities of interest to regulated industry, health professionals, academia and the general public.

■ http://www.emea.eu.int/
The European Agency for the Evaluation of Medical Products.

■ http://www.ifpma.org/ich1.html
The International Conference on Harmonisation of Technical Requirements for Registration of Pharmaceuticals for Human Use (ICH) is a unique project that brings together the regulatory authorities of Europe, Japan and the USA and experts from the pharmaceutical industry in the three regions to discuss scientific and technical aspects of product registration.

■ http://www.wma.net
The WMA provides a forum for its member associations to communicate freely, to cooperate actively, to achieve consensus on high standards of medical ethics and professional competence, and to promote the professional freedom of physicians worldwide.

Scientific papers

1. Sakurai T, Amemiya A, Ishii M et al. Orexins and orexin receptors: a family of hypothalamic neuropeptides and G protein-coupled receptors that regulate feeding behavior. *Cell* 1998; **92:** 573–85.
2. Hoess RH, Abremski K. Mechanism of strand cleavage and exchange in the Cre-lox site-specific recombination system. *J Mol Biol* 1985; **181:** 351–62.
3. Kirkpatrick DL, Watson S, Ulhaq S. Structure-based drug design: combinatorial chemistry and molecular modelling. *Comb Chem High Throughput Screen* 1999; **2:** 211–21.
4. Lam KS. Application of combinatorial library methods in cancer research and drug discovery. *Anticancer Drug Des* 1997; **12:** 145–67.
5. Sanseau P. Impact of human genome sequencing for in silico target discovery. *Drug Discov Today* 2001; **6:** 316–23.
6. van de Waterbeemd H. High-throughput and in silico techniques in drug metabolism and pharmacokinetics. *Curr Opin Drug Discov Devel* 2002; **5:** 33–43.
7. Oakley AJ, Wilce MC. Macromolecular crystallography as a tool for investigating drug, enzyme and receptor interactions. *Clin Exper Pharmacol Physiol* 2000; **27:** 145–51.
8. Oprea TI, Gottfries J. Toward minimalistic modeling of oral drug absorption. *J Mol Graph Model* 1999; **17:** 261–74.
9. Lipinski CA, Lombardo F, Dominy BW, Feeney PJ. Experimental and computational approaches to estimate solubility and permeability in drug discovery and development settings. *Adv Drug Deliv Rev* 2001; **46:** 3–26.
10. Baillie TA, Kassahun K. Biological reactive intermediates in drug discovery and development: a perspective from the pharmaceutical industry. *Adv Exper Med Biol* 2001; **500:** 45–51.
11. Waring JF, Jolly RA, Ciurlionis R et al. Clustering of hepatotoxins based on mechanism of toxicity using gene expression profiles. *Toxicol Appl Pharmacol* 2001; **175:** 28–42.
12. Bonate PL, Howard D. Prospective allometric scaling: does the Emperor have clothes? *J Clin Pharmacol* 2000; **40:** 665–70.
13. Hu Teh-Min, Hayton WL. Allometric scaling of xenobiotic clearance: uncertainty versus universality. *AAPS Pharm Sci* 2001; **3:** 1–14.
14. Singh SD, Williams AJ. The prevalence and incidence of medical conditions in healthy pharmaceutical company employees who volunteer to participate in medical research. *Br J Clin Pharmacol* 1999; **48:** 25–31.
15. Merz M, Seiberling M, Hoxter G, Holting M, Wortha HP. Elevation of liver enzymes in multiple dose trials during placebo treatment: are they predictable? *J Clin Pharmacol* 1997; **37:** 791–8.
16. Dai D, Tang J, Rose R et al. Identification of variants of CYP3A4 and characterization of their abilities to metabolize testosterone and chlorpyrifos. *J Pharmacol Exper Therap* 2001; **299:** 825–31.
17. Hoffmeyer S, Burk O, von Richter O et al. Functional polymorphisms of the human multidrug-resistance gene: multiple sequence variations and correlation of one allele with P-glycoprotein expression and activity in vivo. *Proc Natl Acad Sci USA* 2000; **97:** 3473–78.

18. Katoh M, Nakajima M, Yamazaki H, Yokoi T. Inhibitory effects of CYP3A4 substrates and their metabolites on P-glycoprotein-mediated transport. *Eur J Pharmaceut Sci* 2001; **12:** 505–13.
19. Woitge HW, Pecherstorfer M, Li YM et al. Novel serum markers of bone resorption: clinical assessment and comparison with established urinary indices. *J Bone Miner Res* 1999; **14:** 792–801.
20. Petricoin EF, Ardekani AM, Hitt BA et al. Use of proteomic patterns in serum to identify ovarian cancer. *Lancet* 2002; **359:** 572–7.
21. Blake GJ, Ridker PM. Novel clinical markers of vascular wall inflammation. *Circ Res* 2001; **89:** 763–71.
22. Ong SE, Pandey A. An evaluation of the use of two-dimensional gel electrophoresis in proteomics. *Biomol Engin* 2001; **18:** 195–205.
23. Cascante M, Boros LG, Comin-Anduix B, de Atauri P, Centelles JJ, Lee PWN. Metabolic control analysis in drug discovery and disease. *Nat Biotechnol* 2002; **20** 243–9.
24. Emilien G, van Meurs W, Maloteaux JM. The dose-response relationship in Phase I clinical trials and beyond: use, meaning, and assessment. *Pharmacol Ther* 2000; **88:** 33–58.
25. Greenland S, Michels KB, Robins JM, Poole C, Willett WC. Presenting statistical uncertainty in trends and dose-response relations. *Am J Epidemiol* 1999; **149:** 1077–86.
26. Muller HH, Schafer H. Adaptive group sequential designs for clinical trials: combining the advantages of adaptive and of classical group sequential approaches. *Biometrics* 2001; **57:** 886–91.
27. Heyd JM, Carlin BP. Adaptive design improvements in the continual reassessment method for phase I studies. *Stat Med* 1999; **18:** 1307–21.
28. Meyer JH, Ichise M. Modeling of receptor ligand data in PET and SPECT imaging: a review of major approaches. *J Neuroimag* 2001; **11:** 30–9.
29. Halldin C, Gulyas B, Langer O, Farde L. Brain radioligands – state of the art and new trends. *Q Nucl Med* 2001; **45:** 139–52.
30. Santini G, Patrignani P, Sciulli MG et al. The human pharmacology of monocyte cyclooxygenase 2 inhibition by cortisol and synthetic glucocorticoids. *Clin Pharmacol Ther* 2001; **70:** 475–83.
31. Tracey I. Prospects for human pharmacological functional magnetic resonance imaging (phMRI). *J Clin Pharmacol* 2001; **41**(July Suppl.): 21S–28S.
32. Rohmel J. Statistical considerations of FDA and CPMP rules for the investigation of new antibacterial products. *Stat Med* **20:** 2561–71.
33. Committee for Proprietary Medicinal Products. Points to consider on switching between superiority and non-inferiority. *Br J Clin Pharmacol* 2001; **52:** 223–8.
34. Steinijans VW, Neuhauser M, Bretz F. Equivalence concepts in clinical trials. *Eur J Drug Metabol Pharmacokinet* 2000; **25:** 38–40.
35. Lewis J, Louv W, Rockhold F, Sato T. The impact of the international guideline entitled Statistical Principles for Clinical Trials (ICH E9). *Stat Med* 2001; **20:** 2549–60.

2

The toxicologist's view: non-clinical safety assessment

Anthony Lynch, John Connelly

Summary • Introduction • Safety assessment • Risk assessment • Future challenges and new technologies • Conclusions • References

SUMMARY

This chapter provides an overview of the role of non-clinical safety assessment (also known as non-clinical or 'preclinical' toxicology) in drug development. It outlines the challenges faced by non-clinical safety assessment in the new millennium and describes developments within the discipline to meet these challenges.

1. INTRODUCTION

Characterization of hazard (qualitative) and assessment of risk (quantitative) potentially associated with human exposure to a new substance are important elements of drug development. There is a regulatory and ethical requirement that evidence of acceptable risk must be obtained in non-human systems before first administration of a drug candidate to volunteers or patients. Further non-clinical safety data are generated thereafter in phase with clinical trials, and to support post-marketing use. Provision of such safety information from in vivo and in vitro studies is the responsibility of

a department known as Non- (or Pre)-clinical Safety Assessment, 'Toxicology', or a related term. However, it should be recognized that the administration of pharmacologically active materials to humans will always carry some element of risk, which must be weighed carefully against the severity of the targeted indication, the nature of the patient population and the availability of other effective therapies. That is, a rigorous and favourable risk-benefit assessment must be demonstrated before a new product can successfully be brought to the market.

The strategies, study designs and terms described largely reflect the custom and practice in those laboratories of which the authors have experience. However, similar approaches are used throughout the pharmaceutical industry. By default, development of a drug intended for oral administration in the clinic is assumed. This is by far the predominant route in clinical practice, although drugs may also be delivered intravenously, intramuscularly, subcutaneously, topically, transdermally, intranasally, by inhalation, intravaginally, rectally and even intrathecally or intraventricularly. Non-clinical evaluation of the toxicity of a compound given by non-oral routes requires some specialized studies, but the principles of testing remain the same.

2. SAFETY ASSESSMENT

2.1 Overview

The principal aim of the non-clinical safety studies is provision of sufficient information to estimate an acceptably low-risk first dose of the new drug substance to humans, and to support its administration thereafter in clinical trials of increasing length in the appropriate patient populations, including, for example, women of child-bearing potential or children. (Note that the active substance, not the formulated product, generally is dosed throughout the non-clinical studies.) The studies seek characterization of target organs for toxicity, dose- or systemic exposure-dependence, including a no-effect dose (NED), progression of toxicity or new targets with increasing duration of dosing, and reversibility of adverse effects. Many potential target organs, particularly portals of entry to the body and subject to first exposure (e.g. liver) and those of excretion (e.g. kidney), are common sites of toxicity in both animals and man, and the non-clinical studies may provide biomarkers of effect that are valuable in clinical trials. Often, the first dose in humans is calculated to be a fraction of the NED in animal studies, or more usually now, to provide a fraction of the systemic (plasma) exposure at the NED. Plasma concentrations of drug substance, and possibly of its metabolites, are generally measured in both animal and human studies, and exposure is calculated typically in terms of the maximum concentration achieved (Cmax) and area under the curve over a defined period (AUC_{0-t}). Increasingly, in vitro studies are also employed in providing information to support first administration to humans, or to solve problems in development via understanding of toxic mechanisms.

The pivotal studies intended to support marketing authorization for a new drug substance are conducted to Good Laboratory Practice (GLP) standards (Box 2.1). Supporting or screening studies may not comply fully with

---

Box 2.1   Principles of Good Laboratory Practice

Under the auspices of the Organisation for Economic Co-operation and Development (OECD) the Principles of Good Laboratory Practice (GLP) were established in 1978 and formally recommended for use by member countries by the OECD Council in 1981. The Principles form a legislative framework for the conduct of laboratory studies submitted to regulatory authorities for the purposes of assessment, and are mainly concerned with the process of effective organization and the conditions under which studies are planned, performed, monitored, recorded and reported. Thus they promote the quality and validity of test data used for determining the safety of chemicals and chemical products to humans and the environment. The Principles are reviewed from time to time in the light of scientific progress and understanding, and revised OECD Principles of GLP have been published (1997). For additional information visit: http://www.oecd.org/ehs or http:/www.open.gov.uk/mca/glpguide.htm

---

the letter of GLP, but are expected to be of comparable scientific quality.

Most pivotal regulatory studies are performed in free-living animals, whose welfare is of paramount importance for ethical, legal and experimental quality reasons (see Box 2.2). Claims of the ability of animal studies to predict risk in man are subject to bias or exaggeration in either direction. However, there are as yet no in vitro models that adequately reflect the cellular, organ and systemic interdependencies of living mammals, or therefore the impact of exposure of the latter to potential toxins. It goes without saying that the comparative (versus humans) biochemistry, physiology and natural pathology of the laboratory species

---

Box 2.2   Animal welfare

Proper care and humane treatment of laboratory animals are mandated by ethical practice, by good experimental conduct and by the law. The moral imperative to avoid unnecessary suffering is obvious, and any stress should not exceed the minimum consistent with achieving the goals of studies supporting human safety. Good science also dictates that variables other than those introduced deliberately (the principal one usually being the dose of active substance in the case of safety studies) are minimized. Undue stress of animals leads to wrong or uninterpretable results. Finally, most nations or regions have enacted laws to safeguard welfare. In the UK, animal studies during drug discovery and development are governed by the Animals (Scientific Procedures) Act, 1986. The Act requires studies to be conducted under personal and project licences, and for facilities to possess a certificate of designation. Compliance is monitored by an Inspectorate, and penalties for failure to adhere to the law include loss of licences, fines or imprisonment. European Union legislation is represented by Directive 86/609. In the USA, there is the Animal Welfare Act of 1966 and its amendments, and the Health Research Extension Act (passed in 1985), from which stems the Public Health Service Policy on Humane Care and Use of Laboratory Animals. For further information see http://www.homeoffice.gov.uk/leg.htm#research.

---

portal, and so on. Sound study design is critical. All relevant factors, especially statistical considerations, have to be taken into account. Use of too many animals to meet the study's aim is indefensible, but so is the use of too few, because more will have to be dosed later to salvage the flawed experiment. The '3Rs' – **reduction** of animal numbers, **refinement** of design (e.g. non-invasive models to monitor basal state, toxicity and recovery in the same individuals; see section 4.0 and subsections) and **replacement** of animals with in vitro systems where possible – may be used as guiding principles.[1] Species used in studies suggested by ICH guidelines – predominantly mice, rats, rabbits and dogs – are all purpose-bred; and a large database of growth, appearance, behaviour and pathology parameters in normals assists sound interpretation and supports minimization of numbers needed.

Non-clinical safety studies are targeted in part at establishing a drug candidate's toxic *potential*, in susceptible individuals, with prolonged administration, or possibly in overdose. Additionally, even in well-designed studies relatively small numbers of animals are used compared with human patient populations. For these reasons, the highest non-clinical doses used often considerably exceed the therapeutic dose. Primary effects should be produced that increase understanding of the toxicity of the compound given, but not secondary consequences or debility that confound interpretation or cause suffering. The first dose in humans is selected on the basis of these boundaries, i.e. of site, nature and severity of toxicity, insight into mechanism given by the compound's pharmacology, toxic and no-effect doses, and ADME (absorption, distribution, metabolism and excretion) data. At present, an adequate risk assessment can be built on these complexities only by in vivo studies. In addition, the shorter life cycle of rodents, in particular, also permits information to be gained about the outcome of lifetime exposure to the drug, about toxicities such as carcinogenesis with long latency periods, and about potential effects on reproduction.

That said, huge strides have been made in developing in vitro systems for the study of

employed must be understood as fully as possible. In practice, choice of test species may be limited by the availability of this detailed background knowledge, but must always recognize relevance to human risk estimation in terms of, for example, appropriate exposure, metabolism, receptor population, characteristics of dosing toxicity, replacing animal use altogether (or replacing mammals with lower vertebrates), or reducing numbers required (see http://www.frame.org.uk). Perhaps the largest impact lies in improvement of screening strategies for drug candidates, limiting the number that progress into animal studies only to fail for reasons of marked toxicity or poor bioavailability. Economic pressures on the industry have contributed to strenuous efforts to identify failures early, and new in vitro and in silico screening procedures are rapidly being adopted (see section 4.1). In vitro techniques also have a role in solving issues of toxicity recognized later in the development process, when the ability to focus on a single organ or cell type may be a real advantage.

The development of a new active substance involves a multidisciplinary and multilayered effort (Fig. 2.1). In many instances, the non-clinical safety assessment will broadly follow a 'standard' or 'default' path. However, there are circumstances in which specific additional tests may need to be adopted, and others in which certain studies may be excluded as irrelevant. The target indication, patient population and route and duration of treatment will all influence the type, sequence and timing of studies conducted, in addition to the results of early non-clinical or clinical studies. For example, drugs for terminal diseases may be 'fast tracked' on the basis of promising results in early clinical trials when there is no existing therapy. Alternatively, drug development may be continued despite adverse results in non-clinical tests if the perceived risks are outweighed by clinical need, e.g. many cancer chemotherapeutics are genotoxic and carcinogenic in laboratory tests, but maintain a favourable risk-benefit profile. The need to address issues may provoke an investigative programme that temporarily halts routine development or runs in parallel with it. Altered clinical plans or particularly short clinical time

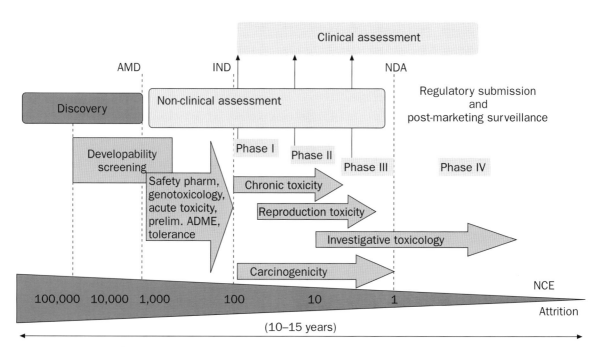

Fig. 2.1 The position of non-clinical assessment in the drug development process.
ADME, absorption, distribution, metabolism, excretion; AMD, asset management decision; IND, investigational new drug; NDA, new drug application; NCE, new chemical entity.

lines may cause non-clinical studies to be conducted out of their 'normal' phasing. Nevertheless, in the main it is fair to say that toxicology studies progress from the shorter to the longer, and from the default to the knowledge-based, during the course of that rarity, an 'uncomplicated' development.

Early non-clinical studies are relatively short, but aim to be rich in information. They are intended to support the first single and limited repeat-dose clinical trials in humans, in which the principal goals usually are measures of pharmacokinetics (PK) and tolerance. They differ from later studies in that they have to provide sufficient risk information to warrant administration of the drug candidate to people in the absence of any pre-existing clinical safety information. Accordingly, these non-clinical studies concentrate on genotoxicity, acute major organ system effects, and an evaluation of general toxicology after a number of doses exceeding those proposed for human exposure.

A typical package to support first-time dosing in humans is shown in Box 2.3. There are exceptions to this approach. For instance, in the USA it may be possible to administer low doses of one or several pharmacologically related molecules in order to obtain PK values, based on a programme in which the general toxicology component consists of short (1–4 dose) studies that are very data-intensive.

Poor bioavailability is a common reason for non-progression of molecules; it is now more recognized that low-dose, safe measurement of exposure in humans supporting rapid go/no-go decisions may favour overall speed of marketing effective therapies and avoid wastage of drug substance, animals and effort. Providing early compound supplies for safety testing consumes much resource and can be fantastically expensive. Given this, it is in no one's interest to pursue a lost cause.

Safety studies are planned and conducted in parallel with clinical trials (Phases I–III). The studies may be modified in the light of findings in humans or animals, or additional studies may be conducted, particularly to investigate the mechanism underlying an adverse effect. Major human metabolites not formed by the non-clinical species, and impurities formed during synthesis or breakdown of the active substance may require testing. Post-launch non-clinical studies may be requested by regulatory agencies ('Phase IV commitments'), or rare adverse events identified only in large patient populations after marketing may trigger further laboratory investigation.

Protection of the workforce involved in large-scale drug synthesis is also important; data acquired in laboratory animals and patients are used to evaluate occupational safety, and synthetic intermediates are studied, particularly for genotoxicity, irritancy and contact sensitization potential. A risk assessment for adverse impact of the new drug on the environment, which may involve extensive experimental work, is required additionally at filing.

2.2 Development of the toxicity profile of a new active substance

The first pointers to the toxicity of a new active substance will probably have been gained

---

Box 2.3 A typical package to support 'first time in humans' includes the following components

- Tests for acute effects on major organ systems, generally cardiovascular, respiratory, renal and neurobehavioural ('safety pharmacology').
- General toxicology studies (generally 14–28 days) in one rodent and one non-rodent species.
- In vitro genotoxicity tests, commonly an Ames bacterial mutation test and a test for gene mutation and/or cytogenetic damage in mammalian cells (such as the mouse lymphoma assay); some laboratories may also conduct an in vivo test for cytogenetic damage at this stage.

during screening for pharmacological profile. At high doses 'excessive pharmacology' may result in a potentially very damaging or even fatal outcome; occasionally, the target receptor may also have a critical role in embryonic or fetal development, and its interaction with an agonist or antagonist during gestation may have profound consequences. Although the lead molecule will have perhaps 100-fold or greater selectivity for the intended receptor versus others, responses related to undesired pharmacological responses may be seen at the relatively high doses used in toxicity studies. Thus, some effects are predictable if the characteristics of the receptor(s) involved are known.

Short-term screening studies are also likely to have been carried out to eliminate the most toxic compounds during the discovery phase. A lead candidate selected from the ones that remain is by no means fully characterized by these tests – nor is there any prescriptive answer to the question of what constitutes 'sufficient toxicity' to preclude development – but the results provide something of a foundation on which to build. The physicochemical properties of the compound or structure–activity relationship analysis (see later) may also provide indicators.

The key non-clinical 'regulatory' studies conducted in pursuit of a toxicity profile fall broadly into the categories shown in Box 2.4. The brief outlines below of the studies carried out within these areas are based on current guidelines produced under the auspices of The International Conference on Harmonisation of Technical Requirements for the Registration of Pharmaceuticals for Human Use (ICH). However, it should be noted that variations in strategy, design and procedure occur – some still because of regional practices – without invalidating the investigations.

2.2.1 Safety pharmacology

Safety pharmacology studies address the potential for undesirable pharmacodynamic responses to doses in the anticipated therapeutic range and above. (You may see them referred to occasionally as 'high dose pharma-

cology' or 'major organ system toxicology' studies, reflecting that they are intended to evoke any significant responses in key systems in, for example, highly susceptible individuals, or overdose.) The effects considered arise from lack of selectivity for the intended receptor, or are the result of an 'excessive' response at that receptor at high doses. Historically, there has been much variation in the nature and extent of studies carried out. The relevant ICH guideline, Topic S7A *Safety pharmacology studies for human pharmaceuticals,* is an attempt to establish objectives and recommended designs.

For obvious reasons, potential effects of a new active substance on systems immediately critical for life have to be characterized before first administration of the compound to humans. The cardiovascular, respiratory and central nervous systems are generally regarded as the most important, although effects on renal function are also often investigated. Animal models, and ex vivo or in vitro preparations, may be used. Examples of the latter systems include cells expressing human cardiac ion channels, or isolated purkinje fibres; both are useful in testing for cause of prolongation of the

---

Box 2.4   The key non-clinical 'regulatory' studies conducted in pursuit of a toxicity profile fall broadly into the following categories

- Safety pharmacology
- General toxicology
- Genetic toxicology
- Carcinogenicity
- Reproductive toxicology
- Other toxicology (e.g. irritancy, skin sensitization, antigenicity, phototoxicity, drug dependence and many others; the choice of studies that are actually conducted is guided by indication, pharmacology, therapeutic route and other findings)

QT interval, which has been perceived as an important issue with several developmental or marketed drugs in recent years. Where in vivo studies are done, typically a range of single doses is given to small groups of, preferably, conscious animals by the therapeutic route, and the time course of any effects is monitored. Other elements of study design should comply with accepted standards of scientific practice.

Commonly measured parameters include, but are not limited to, blood pressure, heart rate and ECG waveform, and further investigation of cardiac repolarization and conductance if indicated (cardiovascular); motor activity, sensory/motor reflex responses, behaviour and coordination and body temperature (CNS); breathing rate, tidal volume and airway compliance and resistance (respiratory); urine volume, pH and osmolality, electrolyte excretion and glomerular filtration rate (renal).

Studies to extend understanding of effects on specific aspects of cardiovascular, CNS, respiratory and renal function are carried out later in development, as are tests of impact on, for example, gastrointestinal, immune and endocrine function, as appropriate. What is done at any stage depends on the drug, the route of administration and the target population. For example, cancer chemotherapeutic agents may not need to be characterized in safety pharmacology studies before first administration to man. Topical drugs may not require testing if there is minimal systemic exposure and the pharmacology is not novel. In all cases, a decision not to carry out studies has to be justified.

2.2.2 General toxicology

The term 'general toxicology' as used in the pharmaceutical industry may be taken to cover by exclusion non-clinical safety studies other than those aimed at specific systems (e.g. reproductive toxicity, safety pharmacology) or at investigation of specific endpoints (e.g. genotoxicity, carcinogenesis). More positively, it can be seen as central to addressing the safety of patients exposed to drugs at therapeutic doses on a daily basis for periods of from a few days to a lifetime. For the majority of the patient population, and for most of the time during which even long-term administration of drugs is pursued, those treated will not be pregnant, not unduly or idiosyncratically susceptible to adverse effects, not overdosed, and not exposed to significant genotoxic or carcinogenic hazards. However, all patients are at least theoretically at risk of functional or morphological damage to multiple, often interdependent, organs and tissues while receiving treatment. Many factors influence risk, but one of the key factors is period of exposure to a chemical. Studies of increasing length in animals are required to support longer clinical trials as development progresses. The recommended duration of non-clinical studies supporting clinical trials is given in an ICH guideline, Topic M3(M) *Maintenance of the ICH guideline on non-clinical safety studies for the conduct of human clinical trials for pharmaceuticals*, as shown in Table 2.1.

Requirements for marketing vary somewhat, but depend essentially on the duration of therapy. Drugs given for <1 month, e.g. antibiotics, may be supported by 3-month non-clinical studies. Longer (6–12-month) studies, and usually carcinogenicity studies, are needed for drugs given for the remainder of the patient's lifetime, e.g. for asthma or arthritis. The terminology describing studies in laboratory species – 'acute' (single dose), 'subchronic' (multiple dose, <6 months' duration) and 'chronic' (multiple dose, >6 months in length) – is rather arbitrary, contrived and imprecise, but it is widely used. (The term 'subacute', used variously for relatively short-term studies, is still sometimes seen, but is an absurdity and should be avoided.)

ICH guidelines suggest that single-dose studies in two mammalian species precede administration of the first dose to humans. These are carried out by the intended therapeutic route, and most commonly in rodents (rats and mice), although a stepwise, rising single-dose study in a non-rodent species may also be performed to establish a maximum tolerated dose (MTD) for subsequent investigations. In the case of orally administered compounds, a second route (e.g. intravenous) may be used to

Table 2.1 Duration of repeated dose toxicity studies to support Phase I and II trials in the EU[a] and Phase I, II and III trials in the USA and Japan

Duration of clinical trials	Minimum duration of repeated-dose toxicity studies	
	Rodents	**Non-rodents**
Single dose	2 weeks[b]	2 weeks
Up to 2 weeks	2 weeks	2 weeks
Up to 1 month	1 month	1 month
Up to 3 months	3 months	3 months
Up to 6 months	6 months	6 months[c]
> 6 months	6 months	'Chronic'[c]

[a]Requirements to support Phase III clinical trials are slightly different in the EU.
[b]As described in section 2.1, in the USA single-dose studies with extended examinations may support single-dose human trials.
[c]Data from 6-month studies in non-rodents should be available before the initiation of clinical trials longer than 3 months. Alternatively, if applicable, data from a 9-month non-rodent study should be available before treatment duration exceeds that supported by the available toxicity studies. Non-rodent studies exceeding 9 months in duration are not usually required even for marketing; in the EU, studies of 6 months' duration are acceptable (75/318/EC). In certain cases the USA may require a 12-month study in a non-rodent species.

ensure systemic exposure. Extensive monitoring is rarely carried out, but single-dose studies with a period of observation of up to 14 days provide information about overdose and delayed toxicity, and evocation of a response is evidence of systemic exposure at a time when toxicokinetic data (see below) may not be available. The results also provide dose range-finding data for early multiple dose studies. The endpoint sought should be the MTD, and *not* lethality; supposedly quantitatively comparative concepts such as the LD50 are of no value here, and are explicitly not required by ICH guidelines. Establishing a tolerable dose in a few animals at this stage minimizes the possibility of unacceptably marked reactions in larger numbers later.

Typically, the regulatory studies conducted in two species (one rodent, one non-rodent) before humans are exposed to a new active substance involve daily dosing for 28–30 days. The doses used are guided by range-finding repeat-dose studies, usually of 7–14 days in duration, in small groups of animals, and with a relatively limited number of measured endpoints. In most cases, the results of the 28-day study determine doses in the subsequent 3- or 6-month study in the same species, the results of which in turn assist in the design of a 9- or 12-month study, if appropriate. Occasionally, changes in route of administration for longer-term studies, most often from oral bolus dosing to intake via the diet (the compound being mixed with powdered rodent chow), necessitates additional range-finding later in development. Rarely, findings in animals or man may cause one laboratory species to be substituted for another, which may also lead to more dose-ranging efforts. Such a switch is invariably avoided if at all possible, and clinical trials typically will be supported by studies of increasing length in the same rodent and non-rodent species throughout development.

Studies of from several days' to several

months' duration are designed to evaluate the adverse effects occasioned by repeated exposure to a new active substance. Accumulation of the compound in tissues, altered clearance because of enzyme induction or inhibition, cumulative effects of low-grade damage, acquired tolerance and irreversible changes that are evident only after a period of latency, may produce markedly different effects from those observed in single-dose studies. Studies that are conducted throughout most or all of a rodent species' lifetime will also be subject to changes in response produced by the natural pathology of ageing.

Selection of appropriate doses is critical in all studies involving repeated administration. A dose–response relationship is a fundamental principle of toxicology. Commonly, three dose levels and a vehicle control are used in non-clinical pharmaceutical investigations. Additional test and control animals may be treated and then left off dose to monitor recovery from any adverse effects. The low dose should be non-toxic (NED), but result in exposure (see below) that is a small multiple of the anticipated therapeutic exposure. The high dose should be sufficient to identify target organs for toxicity, but ideally not produce death or the confounding secondary outcomes of gross ill health. At least one intermediate dose should be included to allow an exposure–response relationship to be determined with a degree of confidence. A similar principle of dose or concentration relationship is also used in much other toxicological testing.

To a considerable extent similar adverse event monitoring is included in repeat-dose toxicity studies whether they are of 28 days' or 12 months' duration. Detailed observations of physical condition, behaviour, growth (body weight) and food consumption are made in rodents and non-rodents, and water intake is often recorded in the former. Effects on ophthalmic health, haematology, haemostasis, clinical chemistry, urine characteristics, macroscopic appearance at necropsy, organ weights and tissue morphology are also routinely recorded in both species. Electrocardiographic monitoring is undertaken in non-rodents. Other markers or functional tests may be included if the pharmacology of the compound or previous observations warrant them. Findings in compound-treated animals are compared with those in the vehicle-dosed controls, and when periodic measurements are made during the study, with results at earlier time-points. On rare occasions comparator compounds with pharmacology or chemistry related to that of the new active substance are dosed in parallel in a separate group of animals.

As noted above, dose–relationship is a key concept. Likewise the concept of 'safety margin' is important in determining what dose in man is justified by animal data, especially in early clinical trials when human experience is very limited. In effect, the 'safety margin' (in some respects an overly simplistic and inaccurate term as applied, but widely used) is the result of dividing the lowest NED in animals by the desired dose in humans, or may be set in advance at a value considered to be reasonable, in which case the animal NED defines the acceptable clinical trial dose. The problem is that an orally administered drug may be absorbed, distributed or cleared to widely varying extents in laboratory species and people. This means that a NED of 100 mg/kg per day in, for example, the rat, may appear to provide a safety margin of 5 versus a human dose of 20 mg/kg per day, but is perhaps dangerously misleading if systemic exposure in the two species is the result of a bioavailability of 10% in the animal, compared with 50% in the patient. This is one reason why measurement of toxicokinetics, which relates to concentrations of compound in (usually) plasma after toxic or supra-pharmacological doses, is now included in practically all repeat-dose studies during development of a new active substance. Plasma Cmax and AUC values (see section 2.1) are used to provide exposure-based safety margins that in most cases are considered to be a better foundation for determination of a safe dose in humans than the amount of drug given to the animal.

Toxicokinetic analysis provides much other useful information, such as explanation of species differences in toxicity, and evidence of non-linear kinetics at high doses in animals compared with linear relationships at therapeutic doses in humans, accumulation of compound and altered clearance on prolonged administration. Data on metabolism in animals compared with humans, although generally obtained in separate non-clinical studies, also may explain differences in toxicity, and assist in validating the choice of model species for toxicity testing.

Special groups of patients have to be considered in clinical trials; examples are those individuals with compromised hepatic or renal function, those with multiple health problems receiving polytherapy, the old and the young, especially the very young. The impact of reduced organ function on risk is relatively rarely investigated in non-clinical toxicity studies. Pharmacokinetic and pharmacodynamic consequences of drug–drug interactions are also usually tested in humans, although indicators of the likelihood of one compound affecting another's pharmacokinetics come from in vitro and in vivo non-clinical studies of enzyme inhibition and induction. Development of appropriate drugs for use in children as well as in adults, which has often been somewhat neglected, is now the focus of more vigorous regulatory encouragement. Although ICH guidelines indicate that prior safety data in human adults (plus non-clinical reproductive and genetic toxicity testing) provide an appropriate foundation for clinical trials in children, there are occasions when 'general toxicology' studies in juvenile animals are warranted. These include development of drugs of classes known to have specific toxic actions in immature subjects (e.g. quinolone antibiotics), and of course, some agents are developed for indications wholly or predominantly occurring in children.

Finally, the existence of regulatory guidelines and convergent custom and practice mean that there is a danger of toxicology study design in drug development becoming stereotyped, unquestioning and unchallenged. However, these studies are no different in objective from other scientific investigations, and if alternative approaches (including the use of in vitro assays, new methodologies, different strategies, etc.) are logical, their use should be proposed, debated, and – if valid – accepted.

2.2.3 Genetic toxicology

The integrity of human DNA is essential for the future of the species and the health of its individuals. The fidelity of DNA replication is not perfect, however, and neither is repair of the errors induced in this way or by environmental factors. Novel drugs represent an additional potential source of damage to DNA or its repair mechanisms, and so appropriate testing is required to minimize the risk of genotoxicity. The discipline of genetic toxicology as applied to drug development exists to achieve this aim.

There is overwhelming evidence that inherited mutational changes in humans are responsible for a significant proportion of genetically determined diseases and congenital (heritable) malformations. In addition, the accumulation of somatic cell mutations is known to be implicated in cancer, and to some extent in other multifactorial diseases, e.g. heart disease. Thus an additional role of genetic toxicology is the assessment of the relative risk arising from exposure to carcinogens, particularly those which are DNA-reactive.

Genetic toxicology is one area in which the strength of in vitro testing is particularly apparent. Many genotoxins require metabolic activation, and in vitro assays facilitate control over the provision of a bioactivating system, usually a microsomal enzyme-containing preparation from the liver of rats treated with a wide-spectrum cytochrome P450 inducer. Microbial or cellular systems often also permit concentrations to be used that could not be achieved in the plasma of animals or humans. This is important in evaluating a compound's *potential* for genotoxicity, which is relevant to particularly susceptible individuals, or to tissues in which the compound accumulates to very high local concentrations. In vitro studies are also useful in investigating mechanisms of genotoxic action that would be extremely difficult to pursue in animals.

Compounds shown to be potent genotoxins in in vitro assays can be – and generally are –

eliminated from further development at that point. Those that are negative, or in which a risk-benefit estimate remains favourable, still require in vivo assessment, which is mandatory for drug registration. A tiered strategy towards testing is usually adopted (see Fig. 2.2). The ICH guidelines for genotoxicity (ICH Topic S2A *Guidance on specific aspects of regulatory genotoxicity tests for pharmaceuticals* and Topic S2B *A standard battery of genotoxicity testing of pharmaceuticals*) describe both the philosophy and types of assays that comprise the testing regimen recommended by regulatory agencies for the assessment of a new active substance's

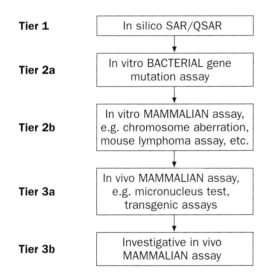

Tier 1	In silico SAR/QSAR
Tier 2a	In vitro BACTERIAL gene mutation assay
Tier 2b	In vitro MAMMALIAN assay, e.g. chromosome aberration, mouse lymphoma assay, etc.
Tier 3a	In vivo MAMMALIAN assay, e.g. micronucleus test, transgenic assays
Tier 3b	Investigative in vivo MAMMALIAN assay

Fig. 2.2 Tiered approach to genotoxicity testing. The tiered approach involves an initial evaluation of potential drug candidates without any biological experimentation whatsoever using (quantitative) structural activity relationships, (Q)SAR (tier 1). Selected compounds are then evaluated for genotoxicity using a simple in vitro bacterial system (tier 2a), usually the Ames test. This is followed by further testing using an in vitro mammalian cell system (tier 2b), e.g. a chromosome aberration or mouse lymphoma test. The use of these assays permits highly genotoxic compounds to be filtered and thereby reduces potential toxicity issues in later development (tier 3). The tiered approach promotes the 'clean development' of drug candidates, which reduces the need for additional in vivo investigative studies (tier 3b) and therefore animal usage.

potential to induce genetic damage, directly or indirectly, by various mechanisms.

A comprehensive description of all the test systems may be found in Kirkland (1990; Further reading). The in vitro studies should be completed before commencing Phase I clinical trials and the whole battery of tests should be completed by the time Phase II begins. The minimum genotoxicity package consists of (a) an in vitro bacterial assay for gene mutation, (b) an in vitro mammalian cell assay for gene mutation and/or cytogenetic damage, and (c) an in vivo mammalian assay for cytogenetic damage. A negative result in all three assays is usually sufficient to provide evidence for a lack of genotoxic potential, although additional testing may be required for substances with structural chemical alerts, or when there is evidence of the carcinogenicity of structurally similar compounds. More testing is also needed if one or more of the assays produces a positive result, but the nature of the findings is insufficient to drive immediate termination of development.

A risk assessment is made using the results of the complete package, taking into account the significance and limitations of each test. Thus a single positive result may reveal a theoretical hazard, but cannot automatically be interpreted as an unacceptable genotoxic risk to patients, especially if in vivo studies are negative. One option is to consider whether the test compound induces tumours in animal models (see section 2.2.4).

2.2.4 Carcinogenesis (oncogenesis)

Carcinogenicity studies are intended to provide an assessment of risk of a new active substance producing tumours in humans, based on its tumorigenic potential in laboratory species. Insofar as the majority of potent genotoxins will have been eliminated from development by the genotoxicity assays described above, lifetime studies in animals may be regarded most commonly as a means of identifying 'non-genotoxic' carcinogens, i.e. those drug candidates which prescribed testing has not detected as interacting directly with DNA to produce an adverse effect. Clearly, this is a pragmatic rather than an exhaustive definition, as it is not feasible to apply all possible genotoxicity assays to any compound. However, if it is accepted that 'non-genotoxic' carcinogens exist, the task of human risk evaluation, given practicable non-clinical study design (see below), is among the most challenging of all.

ICH Topic S1A *Guideline on the need for carcinogenicity studies of pharmaceuticals* states that carcinogenicity studies should be performed on any new pharmaceutical that is expected to be used therapeutically for a continuous period of at least 6 months. The status of repeated intermittent use remains vague. Testing of agents given frequently in a discontinuous manner to treat chronic or recurrent conditions (such as allergic rhinitis, depression or anxiety) generally is needed. It is also not uncommon for carcinogenicity studies to be carried out on other compounds anticipated to be used intermittently for 6 months or more in total, if only to be 'on the safe side', considering the difficulty of predicting use patterns precisely. Cause for concern arising from previous product class liability, structure–activity alerts, evidence of preneoplastic change in repeat-dose toxicity studies, weak positive results in genotoxicity studies, or prolonged tissue retention of compound-derived material may drive studies in appropriate circumstances. Reported results are usually required for a new drug application (NDA) or MAA, rather than to support large clinical trials, unless there is specific reason for concern for the patient population.

Probably no other non-clinical protocols have come under as close scrutiny recently as those for carcinogenicity testing. The current and practically invariable approach, established over many years, involves 'lifetime' studies in two species, almost always rats and mice. There are a number of advantages to using such species. In humans, cancer is largely a disease of middle-to-old age, and in rodents even tumours driven by chemical agents (both genotoxic and non-genotoxic) require a substantial time to develop. As the lifespan of rats and mice is approximately 2 years, use of these species keeps study length within acceptable bounds. Secondly, their size facilitates handling and husbandry. Certain strains of both species

have also been the mainstay of carcinogenicity screening for many years, during which time a wealth of data on spontaneous tumour incidence have been accumulated, which aids interpretation of results.

Nonetheless, there are several significant issues to contend with. The proportion of compounds of *all* types, not only drugs, that produce apparently positive results in 2-year studies is far above that supported by common-sense observation of human disease patterns (note that almost all confirmed human carcinogens have been shown to be genotoxins). In addition, there is often inconsistency in results between species, strains and sexes, and dose–relationships may be far from coherent. However, concern over the carcinogenic potential of pharmaceuticals in humans is justified and, for the present, risk must be evaluated against this background of limitations.

Logical rationales for dose selection have long been a subject of debate. Conventionally, animals have been treated at up to the MTD; this is routinely understood to be a dose that causes no more than a 10% decrease in body weight gain compared with controls, nor shortens lifespan other than by induction of tumours. In some cases the MTD in animals grossly exceeds the therapeutic dose, and in other cases laboratory rodents tolerate a regimen that provides only parity with, or a fraction of, human exposure. Both circumstances pose difficulties. Non-genotoxic carcinogens would be expected to have a mechanism-dependent threshold for effect, and tumorigenicity anticipated to be a consequence of altered physiology. As such, linear back-extrapolation from effects at very high multiples of the human dose is suspect. For example, doses high enough to produce cell death encourage chronic cell proliferation that may result in tumours, but have no relevance to clinical use in humans. Equally, saturation of clearance routes may lead to exposure to metabolites, or colossal levels of parent compound, and an outcome that is largely uninterpretable in terms of human risk. Conversely, if lifetime rodent studies are considered to be valid at all, concerns attending exposure at less than human levels are obvious.

Two ICH guidelines – Topic S1B *Testing for carcinogenicity of pharmaceuticals* and Topic S1C *Dose selection for carcinogenicity studies of pharmaceuticals*/S1C(R) *Addendum to the dose selection for carcinogenicity studies of pharmaceuticals: addition of a dose limit and related notes* – have attempted to at least rationalize study strategy across the member regions, provide a consistent basis for dose selection, and offer alternatives to the 2-year test in mice.

Two-year carcinogenicity studies are expensive in terms of time, animal use, total resource and monetary cost. It would be wholly impractical to conduct these studies at therapeutic exposures using numbers of rodents capable of detecting an increase in cancer occurrence of, say, 1 in 10 000. High doses and minimum group sizes are employed to at least partly address this situation – and are sources of some of the difficulties with interpretation mentioned above – but it would be desirable to reduce animal usage still further. ICH guideline S1B seeks to promote a 'weight of evidence' approach to enhance estimation of carcinogenic risk, based on a lifetime assay in one species supported by other experimental investigations. These additional studies include various recommended short- or medium-term 'alternative' in vivo carcinogenicity models, which use fewer animals, and are described in section 4.3.3. Note that a lifetime study in a second rodent species is still considered acceptable, if scientific judgement shows it to be the preferable option.

The test compound's pharmacological, toxic, toxicokinetic and metabolic characteristics should provide the basis for selecting a single species for a 2-year study. However, the rat is recommended if obvious cause to favour one species is lacking. This arises from the observation that more compounds are carcinogenic in 'rat only' than in 'mouse only'; the doubtful relevance to human risk of the marked susceptibility of mice to liver tumours; and on the whole more data on mechanism and biotransformation enzymes in rats. If the mouse is used, an additional range-finding study may be required, as no substantial evaluation of general toxicity in mice is likely to have been car-

ried out. Finally, several of the alternative models involve mice, and conducting the long-term study in rats maintains trans-species assessment of carcinogenic potential.

ICH guideline S1C and addendum seek to broaden and clarify the principles on which dose selection should be based. In ideal circumstances, exposures at the doses used should (1) provide adequate multiples of human therapeutic exposure; (2) be tolerated without a degree of chronic physiological dysfunction or ill health incompatible with attainment of a normal lifespan; (3) be based on thorough understanding of comprehensive human and animal data; and (4) allow interpretation of risk, including the nature of response in relation to dose, in the context of clinical use.

Selecting the high dose for a carcinogenicity study is a critical decision, and various alternative criteria are considered to be applicable (Box 2.5).

Additional rationales for high-dose selection will be considered by the regulatory agencies, if scientifically justified. Middle and low doses should provide information that supports estimation of human risk, and should take pharmacodynamics, pharmacokinetics and profile of toxicity into account. Ideally, the overall dosing strategy should seek to span a range that detects carcinogenic potential, but also facilitates understanding of dose–response or threshold-dependent effects.

2.2.5 Reproductive toxicology

Reproductive toxicology is concerned with detecting any adverse effect of drug candidates on sexual organ structure and function, fertilization, implantation, embryonic and fetal development, lactation and postnatal development until sexual maturation and conception. Although the whole process comprises an integrated sequence, toxicological assessment is generally regarded as divided broadly into tests of male and female sexual behaviour and fertility, and of developmental toxicity through intrauterine stages and postnatally.

The ICH harmonized guidelines, Topic S5A *Detection of toxicity to reproduction for medicinal products* and Topic S5B *Maintenance of the ICH*

> **Box 2.5 Criteria for highest dose selection in carcinogenicity studies**
>
> 1. The MTD as a toxicity endpoint continues to be recognized, but use of as broad a range as possible for biological information is encouraged.
> 2. A rodent:human exposure ratio of at least 25:1 is sufficient, based on plasma AUC because it contains elements of both concentration and residence time of the agent.
> 3. Pharmacodynamic effects, which will be highly compound-specific, may preclude dose increase.
> 4. Saturation of absorption may be observed, i.e. further dose increments do not result in an increase in systemic exposure.
> 5. Practicality or avoidance of adverse effects of the formulation itself may intervene. For example, 5% compound in diet is considered to be the maximum compatible with unimpaired nutrition, and the volume or viscosity of liquids that can be given orally is limited.
> 6. In certain circumstances, if the human dose does not exceed 500 mg/day and there is no evidence of genotoxicity, a 'limit dose' of 1500 mg/kg per day in rodents may be acceptable.

guideline on toxicity to male fertility, emphasize the need for flexibility and scientific thought in designing studies to reveal effects of new active substances at any stage of reproduction. All relevant available pharmacological and toxicological information should be taken into account. In most cases, a three-study design is sufficient (see following), although various combinations of studies may be more appropriate in certain circumstances. The important consideration is that they leave no gaps unevaluated.

A three-study design addresses fertility and early embryonic development, pre- and postnatal development including maternal function, and embryofetal development. Selection of species is a critical decision at all stages of testing. No species is ideal, for reasons of physiology, size, inappropriate sensitivity to chemicals, compound handling or sparse background data, and their limitations have to be understood in rational study design. Rats have the most fully characterized reproductive parameters, and are frequently used in all phases. However, poor compound absorption, grossly inappropriate metabolism or specific physiological aspects of the rat may direct other choices. For example, because of the primary role of prolactin in early pregnancy in rats, they are not suitable for reproductive toxicity testing of dopamine agonists, which reduce circulating dopamine levels. Despite several limitations, including size of fetus, mice are common alternatives. Two species are required for evaluation of embryofetal development, one being a non-rodent, and the rabbit is overwhelmingly the first additional selection.

The dose route is usually that intended in humans, and the doses chosen are based on a combination of data from general toxicology studies in the same species and specific range-finding where necessary. Alternative or supplemental routes of exposure may be used to circumvent problems of low oral bioavailability.

The following illustrates the three-study design, with each component covering various stages of development.

1. *Fertility and early embryonic development to implantation.* If no effects on spermatogenesis have been observed in repeat-dose studies, pre-mating treatment for 2–4 weeks in males and 2 weeks in females is sufficient. Treatment of males is continued through mating, and of females at least through implantation. Young mature males and virgin females are allowed 2–3 weeks of cohabitation for conception to occur. Maintaining females until days 13–15 of pregnancy generally is adequate to differentiate between implantation and resorption sites. Toxicity at the following key

phases is investigated in one species, preferably rats.

- ICH guideline stage A. Pre-mating to conception – effects on the development and maturation of gametes, mating behaviour, fertility and fertilization are evaluated.
- ICH guideline stage B. Conception to implantation – effects on adult female reproductive function, pre-implantation stages and implantation are assessed.

2. *Embryofetal development*. Pregnant females are dosed with the compound during the period from implantation to closure of the hard palate. Litters are delivered by caesarean section shortly before normal parturition and fetuses are examined for adverse effects on skeletal and soft tissues. The following key stages are evaluated in two species, one a rodent (preferably the rat) and one non-rodent (preferably the rabbit).

- ICH guideline stage C. Implantation to closure of hard palate – adult male and female reproductive functions, embryonic development and major organ formation are studied.
- ICH guideline stage D. Closure of hard palate to the end of pregnancy – adult female reproductive function, fetal development and growth, and organ development and growth, are evaluated.

3. *Pre- and postnatal development, including maternal function*. Females of at least one species, preferably rats, are dosed from implantation to the end of lactation. Females are allowed to litter and rear their offspring to weaning, and a proportion of offspring at maturity are mated to assess reproductive function.

- ICH guideline stage C, as above.
- ICH guideline stage D, as above.
- ICH guideline stage E. Birth to weaning – adult female reproductive functions, neonatal adaptation to extrauterine life and pre-weaning development and growth are assessed.
- ICH guideline stage F. Weaning to sexual maturity – post-weaning development and growth, adaptation to

independent life, and attainment of full sexual function are evaluated.

If an adverse effect is detected in any one of the studies described above, further effort is usually required to fully characterize the response using the most appropriate methods available. Cell systems, such as embryo culture, may be employed to investigate the mechanism. In vitro systems are also being used increasingly during early drug candidate screening in an attempt to eliminate reproductive toxicants at that stage. Greater understanding of the effects of pharmacological disturbance (receptor agonism and antagonism) during embryofetal development is also being applied to risk assessment for humans.

Reproductive toxicology studies are phased through compound development. Microscopic evaluation of sex organs in early repeat-dose general toxicology studies, and especially of stages of testicular development, can provide important information about effects on male fertility. Hence, male human volunteers are usually first dosed with a new active substance. If females are exposed in early trials, they must be post-menopausal, or great care must be taken to ensure effective contraception. There has been much pressure, especially in the USA, to include women of child-bearing potential in clinical trials as early as practicable. Non-clinical studies of effects on embryofetal development are usually conducted before these women are treated, and an assessment of female fertility is completed before significant numbers are included in larger trials. Specific animal studies of male fertility may not be required until clinical Phase III, although fertility in both sexes will frequently have been assessed in the same study. Full evaluation of postnatal development often is not carried out until Phase III unless there are concerns associated with the compound's chemistry or pharmacology, or with other toxic findings.

2.2.6 Other toxicology

Toxic effects discovered at any stage during the 'regulatory' testing of a new active substance may lead to investigative work being carried out to determine mechanism, relevance to man, reversibility and so on, to allow a risk assessment to be made. These case-by-case studies can be of literally almost any strategy and design, and conducted in animals or in vitro models. There are other studies which, while not readily falling into any of the main types described above, are of relatively standard design and can be anticipated to be required in the development of a greater or lesser proportion of new drugs. Again, there are many possibilities, and the following examples are not exhaustive.

The potential for topically applied agents to markedly irritate or corrode the eyes or skin is assessed in animals (or where possible, in in vitro models). Skin sensitization testing, i.e. for topically induced allergenicity, is also appropriate for these materials. Many chemical intermediates used in drug synthesis facilities are evaluated in the same manner to protect against occupational adverse effects.

Furthermore, a chemical coming into direct dermal contact may cause photosensitization if it reacts in the right manner with ultraviolet light. Transient excitation by light energy leads to free-radical generation as the molecule returns to the lower energy state. Adverse effects caused directly by these free radicals are termed phototoxicity. If the reactive species bind to proteins to produce antigens, photoallergy may result. Some drugs produce photosensitization after systemic administration; in particular, some orally active quinolone antibiotics have been terminated during development or withdrawn from the market. New members of this class of drugs are now commonly evaluated non-clinically for photosensitizing and photocarcinogenic potential. Quinolone antibiotics also provide an example of a class-specific toxicity being recognized and routinely investigated. Many of these compounds have been shown to produce arthropathy in juvenile animals, and are used with caution in children.

Some assessment of the interaction of new active substances with the immune system is required. Potential for systemic antigenicity, which involves covalent coupling of the agent (a hapten) with body proteins to elicit an anti-body response, is usually carried out in mice and guinea pigs. Testing for immunotoxicity (i.e. adverse effect on the immune system, as opposed to immune involvement in the toxic response) may be carried out to an extent as part of a general toxicology study. However, if there is evidence of a reaction, specific studies are performed. These generally involve in vivo antigenic challenge, but in vitro systems can be applied to some aspects of immunotoxicity by considering the immune system as a series of targets for toxicity, and modelling the individual elements. The in vivo approach is tiered, such that evaluation of haematology and pathology (tier 1) may be added on to an existing study. Tier 2 involves host defence studies, quantitation of several appropriate cell types and functional assessment of cell populations.

New active substances with potential for abuse, e.g. those designed to act at certain central nervous system receptors, are tested for their ability to produce dependence. This may be characterized in the appropriate species, as in humans, by physiological and possibly behavioural changes on withdrawal of the agent.

In addition to the safety pharmacology studies conducted before the first administration of a new active substance to man, an evaluation of effects on other systems, and on potentiation or inhibition of other active agents, is made in later phases of development. Tests include effect on the gastrointestinal system, pro- and anti-convulsant activity, analgesic activity, presumed alteration of drug-metabolizing enzyme capacity (barbiturate sleeping time) and various others. Insofar as these studies detect inappropriate pharmacological properties of the agent, they legitimately comprise an aspect of the overall assessment of adverse-event potential.

Many other investigations are possible, and are pursued according to circumstances of drug chemistry and pharmacology, indication, route of delivery, nature of formulation and a host of additional factors. As in any area of toxicological endeavour, rational selection and valid design of studies remain the goals, rather than prescriptive testing.

3. RISK ASSESSMENT

Risk is the probability of an adverse outcome, i.e. it is quantitative, if in practice often refined only to the extent of being 'high', 'medium' or 'low'. *Hazard* properly should refer to the intrinsic nature of a finding, status or situation that may be subject to measurements or observations on which such an estimate of probability can be based. In the present context, *risk assessment* encompasses a systematic analysis of qualitative and quantitative information about the non-clinical toxicity of a new active substance, and a calculation of the likelihood of its occurrence and severity in humans, including a measure of the degree of uncertainty attending the result. *Risk management* addresses the steps taken to control the impact of the result, and may take a form ranging from regulatory refusal to approve the drug, to warning information in labelling, to routine post-marketing surveillance. Labelling is also one means of *risk communication*, i.e. of transferring the information to the relevant audience in an understandable form.

Risk and risk assessment in chemical toxicity are complex subjects that have been approached in sometimes fundamentally different ways, and any more than very short consideration of them is beyond the scope of this chapter. Although animal models currently remain the best predictors of adverse effects in humans, there are numerous difficulties with quantitative (or qualitative) conclusions about the one based on findings in the other. Carcinogenicity risk analysis is the area that has received probably the most attention. Some of the limitations of carcinogenicity study design in rodents have been pointed out in section 2.2.4 above. If acceptable human cancer risk is placed at around 1 in 10^5 to 1 in 10^6, the problem of extrapolation from a several percent incidence of tumours in rodents given high dose(s) lying on a non-linear response curve in the presence of chronic tissue damage, may be appreciated. An unrealistic percentage of compounds tested are 'positive' in rodent carcinogenicity assays, but the difficulties of calculation tend to produce a conservative

interpretation of human risk if sound mechanistic data are not present to argue otherwise.

Attempts have been made to apply 'safety factor'-based risk analysis to carcinogenicity and other toxicities. In such calculations a divisor (frequently 10) is assigned to inter-individual variation in susceptibility, another to uncertainty of trans-species uncertainty, another to length of study, and so on. The approach is flawed, but pragmatic. It perhaps recognizes honestly that in many situations there is insufficient high-grade information to conduct a satisfactory assessment founded on knowledge of molecular mechanism, and quantitative exposure, biochemistry, physiology and genetic data in animals and humans.

However, for new drugs the best possible estimate of risk to humans must be crafted from in vivo and in vitro non-clinical data. Risk assessment can be improved enormously by elucidation of comparative ADME, dose–response characteristics and threshold versus non-threshold events, biomarker measurement, use of multiple endpoints and understanding of probable pharmacological, physiological or toxicological mechanism of effect. Sufficient clinical and non-clinical data to support such a knowledge-based risk assessment should have been collected by the time of filing an application with a regulatory agency, and will provide the material for both the sponsor's and the agency's critical evaluation of safety.

4. FUTURE CHALLENGES AND NEW TECHNOLOGIES

Commercial pressures, disease demographics, the regulatory environment, the economics of drug supply and patient expectations have changed markedly in recent years, and are continuing to change. In addition to developing safe drugs faster to meet patient needs and maximize patent life in the face of spiralling costs of research and development, fierce competition, price-setting and increased scrutiny by governments, the industry faces other challenges (see Box 2.6).

To meet these challenges the science of toxicology is undergoing a revolution, with an

---

Box 2.6   Future challenges

- The need to characterize higher numbers of chemical leads, due to the use of combinatorial chemistries and high-throughput screening, with lower probability of toxicity and higher probability of success in the clinic, i.e. prediction of toxic liabilities
- Development of in vitro models for reduction of animal use and higher throughput testing, coupled with an earlier understanding of toxicity as it relates to risk to patients in clinical trials, and identification of effective biomarkers of adverse effects
- Increased expectation on the part of regulatory authorities for:
  - improved understanding of mechanisms of toxicity seen in animals and incorporation into the risk-benefit evaluation for humans
  - increased capability for the analysis, integration and management of data from multiple and heterogeneous sources
  - pressure for earlier development of drugs for use in populations perceived as at special risk, such as children or women of child-bearing potential, and addressing 'idiosyncratic' toxicities.
  - improved communication and discussion of risk with regulatory agencies

---

influx of new technologies and ideas.[2] Among many others, these include developments in information technology, genetics (genomics and transgenics), proteomics, metabonomics and imaging. As they mature, these methods should improve predictive toxicology, strengthen risk assessment for humans and reduce animal use.

4.1 Bio-informatics: in silico systems

Recent advances in combinatorial chemistry and high-throughput screening technologies have led to a massive explosion in the numbers of potential drug candidates being produced at the earliest stages of drug discovery. Consequently there is a greater need to acquire alternative methods for the prediction of toxicity in order to be able to cut these numbers rationally to manageable proportions. Computer-based or in silico 'expert systems' for predicting toxicity have been developed to screen new active substances for potential chemical activity before any biological testing. These systems fit broadly into two categories, although there is an overlap between them. The first comprises mathematical models, in which correlations are sought between chemical structure and biological activity; and the second includes predictive models, which rely on existing knowledge in the form of rules describing historical data.

Mathematical approaches address quantitative structure–activity relationships (QSAR). The assumption supporting use of QSARs for prediction of toxicity is that 'biological activity may be described as a function of chemical constitution'. This was first proposed by Crum-Brown and Frazer in 1868,[3] and latterly has been driven by the work of Corwin Hansch (for historical review see Rekker, 1992; Further reading). In the main, one of the most successful applications of QSAR has been genotoxicity, primarily for well-defined congeneric series of chemical structures. Attempts have been made to form non-congeneric models, but the multiplicity, and often uncertainty, of biological endpoints makes this approach far more complex.[4,5]

Rules-based expert systems rely on existing knowledge about chemical structures and their associated toxicological potential, rather than forming empirical relationships. It is fair to state that no system routinely outperforms another. Localized QSAR models for highly conserved congeneric series provide the optimum concordance values, although rules-based systems are applicable to a wider range of chemical entities. The most commonly used systems are summarized below.

DEREK (Deductive Estimation of Risk from Existing Knowledge; LHASA UK Ltd) (http://www.chem.leeds.ac.uk/LUK/derek/de

rek.htm) is a knowledge-based system for the qualitative prediction of a range of toxic endpoints (principally mutagenicity, carcinogenicity and skin sensitization). The system has a rules base consisting of molecular substructures (toxophores) which have been associated with a toxic outcome. A novel structure is presented to the system, and any toxophores are returned with corresponding descriptive text for the user to review.

COMPACT (Computer-Optimized Molecular Parametric Analysis of Chemical Toxicity; Lewis et al, University of Surrey, UK) (http://www.surrey.ac.uk/sbs/research/MTG/index.html) may be used to predict the capability of a compound to act as a substrate for cytochrome P450. Structural characteristics are used to determine the ability of a molecule to fit into the enzyme-binding site and electronic characteristics are used to determine the likelihood of oxidative metabolism. Expert knowledge is then required in order to assess the toxicological significance of such metabolism.

OncoLogic (LogiChem Inc.) (http://www.logichem.com) is a PC-based program for the prediction of carcinogenicity based on human expert knowledge. Predictions are made using a hierarchical decision tree, with four subsystems available for the prediction of fibres, metals or metal-containing compounds, polymers and organic chemicals. The organics module is the most extensive, with in excess of 40 000 discrete rules derived from > 10 000 compounds. The system requires the user to specify the chemical class of the query molecule. It then follows a series of pre-defined rules to produce a mechanism-based evaluation of carcinogenic potential.

TOPKAT (Toxicity Prediction by Computer-Assisted Technology; Health Designs Inc.) (http://www.tripos.com/software/topkat.html) consists of a series of modules for the prediction of a range of acute and chronic toxicity endpoints. Predictions are obtained by either a multiple linear regression approach for continuous measures, or a two-group linear discriminate regression for classification models, e.g. mutagenicity. Topological descriptors are used to define a toxic measure associated with spe-cific chemical substructures. A similarity search is performed to determine whether the test compound is within the optimal prediction space, thus allowing a confidence measure to be applied to the prediction.

ToxSys (SciVision) (http://www.scivision.com/ToxSys.html) comprises a compendium of known toxic effects (RTECS) with batch toxicity prediction and molecular structure/substructure similarity searching that allows a neural network approach for prediction.

HazardExpert (CompuDrug) (http://www.compudrug.com/hazard.html) permits predictions to be made for a series of pre-defined toxicity endpoints. Each endpoint is predicted as one of four levels of toxicity. Predictions are based on the presence of toxicophores within the query structure, compared against those located within the internal toxic-fragments knowledge base. Modulatory substructures and physicochemical parameters such as $\log P$ and pKa are determined, and the user specifies route of exposure and species information to allow a consideration of bioavailability and bioaccumulation in the overall prediction.

M-CASE (Multiple Computer Automated Structure Evaluation; MultiCASE Inc.) (http://www.multicase.com/index.html) analyses the structural fragments of the compounds in a 'training' database to identify biophores, i.e. those fragments responsible for the toxicological endpoint (such as carcinogenicity and mutagenicity) for which data are contained in the database. It compiles a dictionary containing the contribution of each biophore to the particular toxicological outcome. The bioactivity of any compound not in the training database is predicted from the sum of the contributions of the biophores that it contains.

All these systems have their strengths and weaknesses; for example, in rules-based systems the most important attributes are the quality and quantity of the knowledge databases supporting the predictive algorithms. Unfortunately, these are frequently biased toward certain chemical classes and to compounds with positive toxicological outcomes, such that non-toxic compounds are often under-represented. Therefore, when new chemical structures with unknown toxicological potential are analysed, the systems are liable to provide inaccurate predictions. However, the predictive accuracy of these databases is improving as they become more comprehensively populated.

4.2 Genomics, proteomics and metabonomics

4.2.1 Genomics and proteomics

The large-scale sequencing of the genomes of a number of species, particularly those routinely used in biomedical research, will have a major impact on the toxicological sciences. The development of novel tools and methods for the analysis of altered gene and protein expression is beginning to provide new insights into mechanisms by unravelling the molecular basis for toxicity.[2] These techniques have been termed genomics or transcriptomics (mRNA expression analysis) and proteomics (protein expression analysis), respectively, and their use in predictive toxicology has two main applications.

(a) *Provision of new insights into mechanisms of toxicity*

It is envisaged that the application of genomics and proteomics in safety assessment will lead to a much greater understanding, and a holistic view, of the mechanisms of toxicity and therefore improve mechanism-based risk assessment for humans. Furthermore, by establishing relationships between toxicity and the expression of novel genes or proteins, new biomarkers of predictive toxicity may be identified which are more sensitive and representative of specific toxicities compared with traditional endpoints (e.g. histopathology and clinical chemistry), particularly at low doses.[6]

(b) *Provision of characteristic fingerprints of drug-related effects*

Patterns of mRNA, i.e. differential gene expression, or protein expression may yield fingerprints of drug-related effects over a range of exposures – some denoting toxicity (interaction with a toxicophore) and others a pharmacological effect (interaction with a therapeutic target or pharmacophore). It is envisaged that gene/protein expression fingerprinting may provide novel screens for ranking new active substances by therapeutic potential and toxicological liability and thereby support the selection of lead compounds (or backup molecules) from discovery programmes with lower probability of toxicity and higher probability of success in the clinic.

Genomics technologies have been reviewed by Farr and Dunn[7] and Lockhart and Winzeler[8] and at present are based on either:

(a) closed architecture systems, e.g. DNA microarrays, in which both the sequence and number of genes to be screened are known, or

(b) open architecture systems, which do not rely on prior knowledge of the transcriptome (the sum of the genes expressed in any given cell). Examples of these methods include serial analysis of gene expression (SAGE) or total gene expression analysis (TOGA). Although the open architecture systems have the theoretical advantage of screening the complete range of expressed genes within a cell or tissue, coverage remains incomplete, and the analysis time is usually much longer compared with closed architecture systems.

Compared with the genome, the proteome is a far more dynamic system. Proteins are subject to, among other things, post-translational modification such as phosphorylation, glycosylation and sulphation or cleavage. These alterations determine protein activity, stability, localization and turnover, and therefore may change under various conditions of disease and stress. Traditionally, proteomic profiling has involved two stages. First, the proteins in a biological sample are separated by two-dimensional polyacrylamide gel electrophoresis (2D-PAGE). Differentially expressed or modified proteins associated with treatment may be resolved as absent or as new spots on the gel following separation by isoelectric focusing in the first dimension and molecular weight separation in the second, orthogonal dimension. The identity of proteins associated with the changed spots (typically revealed by Coomassie blue, silver or fluorescence staining) may be determined from historical data, or by analysis of the excised spot by either peptide cleavage and sequencing or matrix-assisted laser desorption/ionization (MALDI) mass spectrometry, which results in time-of-flight distribution of the peptides comprising the sample. The identity of individual proteins is then determined by comparison of the mass spectrum with databases containing known profiles. One of the main criticisms of this approach has been the low throughput. More recently, new technologies which dispense with 2D-PAGE have emerged, and these include protein chips (coated with antibodies to specific proteins or peptides) or platforms such as Ciphergen's SELDI ProteinChip® system, which involves the capture of proteins onto proprietary chemical surfaces subsequently subjected to MALDI mass spectrometry. These advances should increase throughput and make the technology more amenable to routine screening and mechanistic studies (for review see ref. 9).

4.2.2 Metabonomics
Metabonomics is a relatively new science that aims to define the status and changes of the endogenous metabolite profile in biofluids or tissues of animals, or in in vitro systems, in response to pathophysiological stimuli or genetic modification.[10] As a component of the study of 'functional genomics', metabonomics allows the impact of altered gene expression on metabolism to be evaluated. The most commonly applied methodology is ^{1}H nuclear magnetic resonance (NMR) spectroscopy, which yields a spectrum describing all relatively low-weight metabolites in urine, plasma or other biological fluids. Multivariate statistical approaches detect metabolite patterns that are diagnostic of site and mechanism of toxicity (or efficacy) after administration of drugs or other chemicals, and indicate biomarkers of effect applicable to animals or, potentially, humans.

Urine is a particularly useful matrix for reflecting metabolic change, as its composition is not under homeostatic control, and it allows non-invasive longitudinal studies of onset, progression and recovery of metabolic change to be monitored easily. Because there is no need for pre-selection of parameters to be measured, metabonomics is applicable to screening for toxicity early in development, and can be used to identify markers in clinical trials as well as non-clinical toxicity studies. Spectra of tissues can be generated on extracts, or can be obtained directly by a technique known as magic angle spinning, which removes the peak broadening that is otherwise characteristic of semi-solid matrices.

4.2.3 Integrated methodologies
It is hoped that the elucidation of pharmacological and toxicological events at the molecular level may improve understanding of mechanism and allow better extrapolation across species. The results of genomic, proteomic and metabonomic technologies all provide key data that are intrinsically amenable to integration. However, the picture is complicated by the temporal relationship of events, in that the processes involved move sequentially, the products have markedly different half-lives, and there are numerous interdependent feedback controls. Moreover, the animal or cell exposed to a second or subsequent dose of an agent will not be the same biochemically or physiologically as when it was exposed to the first. Success is dependent not only on the development of robust experimental technologies, but on advances in bio-informatics to provide comprehensive and sophisticated analysis of the vast quantities of data generated by these approaches. Only then can correlations between toxicity endpoints and transcription, translation, post-translational modification, protein function and metabolite pool balance allow the definition of mechanisms relevant to tissue injury.

These technologies have only relatively recently started to be applied in drug development toxicology. Public availability of the fundamental database is limited, experts who can bridge the gap between the '-omics' and the world of drug development and regulation are few, and neither broad nor specific consensus on the application and interpretation of these data has been reached in international governmental and scientific arenas. As such, there is a pressing need for a coordinated evaluation of the various methods and platforms currently available or in development, in order to deliver their full potential. For a more comprehensive review the reader is referred to ECETOC Document 42 (Carpanini, 2000; Further reading).

4.3 Genetically modified (GM) animals

The main applications of GM animals to non-clinical safety assessment at present lie in the areas of evaluation of drug metabolism and interactions of agents with drug-metabolizing enzymes, general toxicity, mutagenesis, carcinogenesis and teratogenesis. Various appropriate gene knockout and transgenic rodent models have been produced and characterized, including GM animals with transgenic reporter genes.

4.3.1 Drug metabolism
The CYP genes encode the cytochrome P450 enzymes, which are responsible for the initial (Phase I) metabolic steps of oxidative biotransformation of many drugs (see Chapter 4). There are marked species differences, especially between rodents and humans, in the catalytic activity and regulation of these genes. The generation of P450 'humanized' GM mice is in progress, using gene and promoter elements of native human P450s.[11] If successful, such GM animals may obviate the need for higher order mammals (e.g. dogs and primates) to investigate species differences in drug metabolism, and possibly toxicity. In addition, GM mice and associated cell lines lacking expression of the genes encoding various CYP genes (e.g. CYP1A2, CYP2E1 and CYP1B1) have been developed. These cytochrome P450-null mice have marked sensitivities to some acute chemical toxicities and to chemical carcinogenesis.[12] As a result, they provide pointers to the specific contribution of individual enzymes to the activation and/or detoxification of chemical toxins and carcinogens.

4.3.2 General toxicology
GM mouse lines containing a variety of reporter constructs are being developed with genes known to be activated or regulated by particular toxic stresses or their promoter elements. One example is the Tg-HO-1-Luc model, in which a luciferase gene reporter is attached to a 10-kb promoter for the gene encoding murine haem oxygenase-1.[13,14] Emission of light from sites of HO-1 expression can be detected and measured through the body wall of the animal when co-expressed luciferase metabolizes exogenous luciferin. The effects of dose and/or treatment duration on the expression of the reporter construct may be assessed by using various reference compounds of known mechanism of toxicity, in this case involving oxidative tissue damage. This type of GM model promises reductions in animal use, in that the same individual can be monitored non-invasively through onset, progression and regression of effect. In addition, animals with several incorporated promoter-reporter constructs may be useful in drug candidate toxicity screening.

4.3.3 Mutagenesis, carcinogenesis and reproductive toxicology
Several GM rodent (mouse and rat) models have been developed that contain specific prokaryotic 'reporter' genes (e.g. *lac*Z or *sup*F) integrated into their genomes.[15–20] The reporter transgenes can readily be recovered from target tissues by way of various shuttle vector technologies or gene capture, and analysed for mutations by suitable bacterial assays. These GM animals provide an opportunity to assess both spontaneous and chemically induced mutations in virtually any tissue or organ, and provide a relatively simple means to analyse mutations at the molecular level. This can supply mechanistic information about mutagenesis; for example, in cases where a chemical agent causes only a marginal increase in mutation frequency, a unique mutation spectrum may determine whether the agent is a mutagen.

Investigations using repeat doses may provide data with immediate relevance to carcinogenicity. Moreover, appropriate GM models may yield improvements over current methods for the assessment of heritable damage in germ cells, which is currently determined by mouse specific-locus and dominant lethal tests.

The duration of lifetime rodent carcinogenesis studies, the number of animals required, and doubts about the assay's reliability have been subjects of debate and concern in the scientific community, and have led to a search for suitable, shorter-term alternatives. Several mouse models have been developed that have been genetically manipulated to reduce tumour latency for the assessment of carcinogenesis.[21,22] These include tumour suppressor gene knockouts (e.g. p53 +/− hemizygous and XPA null mice) and transgenic animals (e.g. TgHras2, Tg.AC and OncoMouse), which contain additional copies of specific oncogenes (ras and myc). However, whereas these models may reduce the duration of testing to approximately 26 weeks, the issues of biological significance and predictiveness are far from entirely resolved, and are the focus of continuing research. Also, as there are more historical data on carcinogenic mechanisms in rats and more compounds are positive in 'rat only' than in 'mouse only' studies, the development of new murine models raises additional concerns. Despite this, regulatory pressure to use such models is increasing, and results are beginning to influence interpretative thinking. One pharmaceutical (the laxative phenolphthalein) was declared a carcinogen by the US FDA on the strength of results of a classical 2-year carcinogenicity study supported by a short-term study using the p53 +/− hemizygous mouse.

In recent years, it has been recognized that many of the molecular control mechanisms of embryogenesis are conserved during evolution. The relevance of these observations for reproductive toxicology and the application of genetic approaches using mouse mutants as a tool for functional genome analysis is becoming more apparent. GM animals are beginning to be used to screen for teratogenicity; for example, 129/Sv-TgR(ROSA26) mice have been modified with the ROSA26 retroviral insertion, and express lacZ in all tissues of the developing embryo, whereas Syx4 transgenic mice show a strong expression of the lacZ gene in round spermatids and subsequent stages of spermatogenesis.[23,24]

4.4 Imaging

Several imaging modalities familiar in clinical practice are now being applied to the study of toxicity in animals. Probably the most familiar are X-ray transmission and magnetic resonance spectroscopy (MRS) or imaging (MRI). Nuclear magnetic resonance (NMR) relies on the absorption and emission of energy by magnetic nuclei (biologically relevant ones include ^{1}H, ^{13}C, ^{23}Na, ^{31}P and ^{39}K) in applied magnetic fields. MRS in particular, despite its low sensitivity, offers unique insights into pharmacokinetics (the changing concentration of the drug at its site of action), which can be monitored, and metabolism (both activation and detoxification) can be detected in real time. MRI can show anatomical structure, or provide information about fluid flow and diffusion (functional imaging). Contrast media allow depiction of blood vasculature or other vessels as three-dimensional images.[25]

Injection of animals or humans with a biological molecule carrying a positron-emitting isotope (^{11}C, ^{13}N, ^{15}O, ^{18}F) allows highly sensitive positron emission tomography (PET) to be used to locate sites for which the molecule has an affinity. By measuring the annihilation radiation (gamma rays) produced when an emitted positron collides with an electron (usually < 1 mm from the site of emission), PET imaging can be used to quantitate in vivo biochemical and physiological processes. This includes the measurement of the pharmacokinetics of labelled drugs and the assessment of the effects of drugs on metabolism. Because only very low amounts of the radiolabelled drug have to be administered, far below toxicity levels, human studies can be performed and may provide cost-effective predictive toxicology data and information on the metabolism and mode of action of drugs.[26] The technique is particularly useful for studying receptor occupancy and regional metabolism, although the short half-lives of the isotopes require careful consideration. For example, ^{18}F, which may be used to label a fluorine-containing drug candidate in receptor studies, has a half-life of 1.8 hours; that of ^{11}C is only 20 minutes. Single-photon emission computed tomography (SPECT) is also used, but is of lower resolution and sensitivity than PET.

Echocardiography has been applied to the study of effects of new active substances on heart shape and size in dogs and primates. Doppler echocardiography has also been used successfully to monitor stenosis or regurgitation of blood through the heart valves of these larger species, which may be useful either in detecting toxicity, or in excluding animals with pre-existing defects from studies. The techniques use ultrasound reflection to build an image of heart muscle, and direction and speed of blood flow.

Other magnetic, electrical, acoustic or optical imaging methods may be used occasionally, but those described above are the most frequently employed.

5. CONCLUSIONS

The concept of studying non-clinical toxicology in support of the safety of potential new drugs in humans has long been established. The development of regulatory guidelines reflecting the legal obligation to demonstrate safety, efficacy and quality has generally led to little imagination in the way non-clinical safety is approached, while maintaining frustrating differences in regional requirements. The International Conference on Harmonisation (ICH) process has addressed one aspect of this, while something of a revolution in new technologies and new attitudes has encouraged a mechanism- and knowledge-based study of toxicity. Significant post-marketing safety issues affecting drugs in recent years have highlighted the need for appraisal of evaluation of risk.

The non-clinical toxicologist lives in a changing world, with obligations for technological understanding, commercial and ethical awareness, and effective communication with multiple collaborators beyond that of even the recent past. Intelligent use of the 'old' approaches coupled with the use of novel technologies promises better characterization of hazard, and a more accurate estimate of the risk to patient populations. However, the limitations of all methods have to be taken into account, and ultimately humans are the key experimental species for new drugs. This imposes an increased need for non-clinical scientists and clinicians to work together to understand the implications for safety of the new technologies. Data from non-clinical studies should be an improved guide to safe administration of new drugs to humans, and results in patients should support the rational conduct of the next round of laboratory work. The new and powerful approaches becoming available are capable of strengthening this relationship immeasurably, provided that communication and trust continue to be developed among toxicologists, the medical profession, regulators, and – equally importantly – the patient.

REFERENCES

Further reading

D'Arcy PF. Pharmaceutical toxicity. In: Ballantyne B, Marrs TC, Syversen T, eds. *General and Applied Toxicology*, Vol 3. Oxford: Macmillan Reference, 1999.

Kirkland DJ, ed. *Basic Mutagenicity Tests – UKEMS Recommended Procedures*. Cambridge: Cambridge University Press, 1990.

Carpanini F. *Genomics, Transcript Profiling, Proteomics and Metabonomics (GTPM): An Introduction*. ECETOC Document no. 42. Brussels: ECETOC, 2000.

Rekker RF. The history of drug research: from Overton to Hansch. *Quant Struct Act Relat* 1992; **11**: 195–9.

Web-sites

■ http://www.ecetoc.org/entry.htm
ECETOC (European Centre for Ecotoxicology and Toxicology of Chemicals) is a scientific, non-profit making, non-commercial association,

financed by 50 of the leading companies with interests in the manufacture and use of chemicals. A stand-alone organization, it was established to provide a scientific forum through which the extensive specialist expertise in the European chemical industry could be harnessed to research, review, assess and publish studies on the ecotoxicology and toxicology of chemicals.

■ http://www.fda.gov/default.htm
Food and Drug Administration home page.

■ http://www.mca.gov.uk/
The executive agency of the Department of Health, safeguarding public health by ensuring that all medicines on the UK market meet appropriate standards of safety, quality and efficacy.

■ http://www.frame.org.uk
Fund for the replacement of animals in medical experiments.

■ http://www.homeoffice.gov.uk/leg.htm# research
Home Office regulations for animal experiments.

■ http://www.ifpma.org/ich1.html
The International Conference on Harmonisation of Technical Requirements for Registration of Pharmaceuticals for Human Use (ICH) is a unique project that brings together the regulatory authorities of Europe, Japan and the USA and experts from the pharmaceutical industry in the three regions to discuss scientific and technical aspects of product registration.

■ http://www.nlm.nih.gov/pubs/cbm/ thalidomide.html
Potential risks and benefits of thalidomide.

■ http://www.logichem.com
LogiChem Inc. is owned and operated by a group of biochemical and computer science professionals and specializes in providing information about the health hazards of chemicals through the use of sophisticated software. Their flagship product is OncoLogic®, which assesses the potential of chemicals to cause cancer.

■ http://www.compudrug.com
Details of software programs for pK_a, $logP$, $logD$ predictions, metabolism and toxicity, HPLC development: pKalc, PrologP, PrologD, MetabolExpert, HazardExpert, Eluex.

■ http://www.multicase.com
Multicase Inc. develops and licenses computer programs designed to help the user make a decision about the potential pharmacological activity, toxicity and metabolic transformations of chemicals.

■ http://webnet1.oecd.org/EN/home/0,,EN-home-519-14-no-no-no,FF.html
Organisation of Economic Co-operation and Development. This program works on the development and coordination of environment health and safety activities internationally.

■ http://www.scivision.com
Biomedical/discovery software.

■ http://www.tripos.com/
Tripos combines information technology and science to simplify and speed discovery of new chemicals that are important to the life sciences industry, including pharmaceutical, biotechnology and agrochemical companies. The company accelerates molecular research through an integrated platform of discovery services, including discovery software, software consulting services, chemical compound libraries, and discovery research services.

Scientific papers

1. Russell WMS, Burch RL. *The Principles of Humane Experimental Technique*. London: Methuen & Co., 1959.
2. Smith LL. Key challenges for toxicologists in the 21st century. *TIPs* 2001; **22**: 281–5.
3. Crum-Brown A, Frazer T. On connection between chemical constitution and physiological action. *Trans R Soc Edin* 1868–1869; **25**: 151–203.
4. Benigni R, Giuliani A. QSAR studies in genetic toxicology: congeneric and non-congeneric chemicals. *Arch Toxicol Suppl* 1992; **15**: 228–37.
5. Benigni R, Richard AM. QSAR's of mutagens and carcinogens: two case studies illustrating problems in the construction of models for non-congeneric chemicals. *Mut Res* 1996; **371**: 29–46.

6. Rininger JA, DiPippo VA, Gould-Rothberg BE. Differential gene expression technologies for identifying surrogate markers of drug efficacy and toxicity. *Drug Discov Today* 5: 560–8.

7. Farr S, and Dunn RT. Concise review: gene expression applied to toxicology. *Toxicol Sci* 1999; **50**: 1–9.

8. Lockhart DJ, Winzeler EA. Genomics, gene expression and DNA arrays. *Nature* 2000; **405**: 827–36.

9. Pandey A, Mann M. Proteomics to study genes and genomes. *Nature* 2000; **405**: 837–46.

10. Nicholson JK, Lindon JC, Holmes E. 'Metabonomics': understanding the metabolic responses of living systems to pathophysiological stimuli via multivariate statistical analysis of biological NMR spectroscopic data. *Xenobiotica* 1999; **11**: 1181–9.

11. Gonzalez FJ, Corchero J, Granvil C, Pimprale S, Ellizondo G. P450 humanised mice. *Tox Lett* 2000; **132**(Suppl 1/116): 7.

12. Kimura S, Gonzalez FJ. Applications of genetically manipulated mice in pharmacogenetics and pharmacogenomics. *Pharmacology* 2000; **61**: 147–53.

13. Zhang W, Contag PR, Madan A, Stevenson DK, Contag CH. Bioluminescence for biological sensing in living animals. In: Eke, Delpy, eds. *Oxygen Transport to Tissue* XXI. New York: Kluwer Academic/Plenum Publishers, 1999: 775–84.

14. Weng YH, Tatarov A, Bartos BP, Contag CH, Dennery PA. HO-1 expression in type II pneumocytes after transpulmonary gene delivery. *Am J Physiol Lung Cell Mol Physiol* 2000; **278**: L1273.

15. Gossen JA, de Leeuw WJ, Tan CH et al. Efficient rescue of integrated shuttle vectors from transgenic mice: a model for studying mutations in vivo. *Proc Natl Acad Sci USA* 1989; **86**: 7971–5.

16. Kohler SW, Provost GS, Fieck A et al. Analysis of spontaneous and induced mutations in transgenic mice using a lambda ZAP/lacI shuttle vector. *Environ Mol Mutagen* 1991; **18**: 316–21.

17. Dycaico MJ, Provost GS, Kretz PL, Ransom SL, Moores JC, Short JM. The use of shuttle vectors for mutation analysis in transgenic mice and rats. *Mutat Res* 1994; **307**: 461–78.

18. Boerrigter ME, Dolle ME, Martus HJ, Gossen JA, Vijg J. Plasmid-based transgenic mouse model for studying in vivo mutations. *Nature* 1995; **377**: 657–9.

19. Nohmi T, Katoh M, Suzuki H et al. A new transgenic mouse mutagenesis test system using Spi- and 6-thioguanine selections. *Environ Mol Mutagen* 1996; **28**: 465–70.

20. Leach EG, Narayanan L, Havre PA, Gunther EJ, Yeasky TM, Glazer PM. Tissue specificity of spontaneous point mutations in lambda supF transgenic mice. *Environ Mol Mutagen* 1996; **28**: 459–64.

21. Gulezian D, Jacobson-Ram D, McCullough CB et al. Use of transgenic animals for carcinogenicity testing: considerations and implications for risk assessment. *Toxicol Pathol* 2000; **28**: 482–99.

22. Murakami H, Sanderson ND, Nagy P, Marino PA, Merlino G, Thorgeirsson SS. Transgenic mouse model for synergistic effects of nuclear oncogenes and growth factors in tumorigenesis: interaction of c-myc and transforming growth factor alpha in hepatic oncogenesis. *Cancer Res* 1993; **53**: 1719–23.

23. Friedrich G, Soriano P. Promoter traps in embryonic stem cells: a genetic screen to identify and mutate developmental genes in mice. *Genes Dev* 1991; **5**: 1513–23.

24. Brinster RL, Avarbock MR. Germline transmission of donor haplotype following spermatogonial transplantation. *Proc Natl Acad Sci USA* 1994; **91**: 11303–7.

25. Griffiths JR, Glickson JD. Monitoring pharmacokinetics of anticancer drugs: non-invasive investigation using magnetic resonance spectroscopy. *Adv Drug Deliv Rev* 2000; **41**: 75–89.

26. Paans AM, Vaalburg W. Positron emission tomography in drug development and drug evaluation. *Curr Pharm Des* 2000; **6**: 1583–91.

3

The regulator's view: regulatory requirements for marketing authorizations for new medicinal products in the European Union

---

Rashmi R Shah, Sarah K Branch, Christopher Steele

SUMMARY

The primary purpose of all rules governing medicinal products in the European Union (EU) is to safeguard public health. It is important that this objective is achieved by means that do not hinder the development of the pharmaceutical industry or trade in medicinal products within the EU. The primary focus of this chapter will be the regulatory requirements for the registration of typical new active substances (NAS) of chemical origin, often referred to as new chemical entities (NCEs) or new molecular entities (NMEs). The requirements for biotechnology products are not discussed since each of the biotechnology products is unique and requirements are on a case-by-case basis with a relatively greater emphasis on quality issues. A detailed discussion on any particular aspect of regulatory requirements is beyond the scope of this chapter, but included within the text are references to various documents and web-sites to which those interested can refer for detailed information.

The reader is referred to the postscript at the end of this chapter for access to the codified Directive on EU legislation.

1. HISTORICAL ASPECTS OF REGULATORY CONTROLS

1.1 Need for regulatory controls

A medicinal product is defined as any substance or combination of substances presented for treating or preventing disease in human beings or animals or which may be administered in human beings or animals with a view to making a medical diagnosis or to restoring, correcting or modifying physiological functions in human beings or animals. Substance is further defined as any matter which may be of human, animal, vegetable or chemical origin.

It is an unfortunate fact that the progressive introduction of major regulatory controls on and evaluations of medicinal products before they are placed on the market has been stimulated by major public health disasters. In Britain, following the introduction in 1847 of chloroform as an anaesthetic, there was considerable concern about its cardiac safety (well over 100 fatalities by 1864) and there were calls for setting up of a committee to enquire 'into the uses and the physiological, therapeutical and toxicological effects of chloroform'.

Although rudimentary legislation existed in the USA (the Federal Pure Food and Drugs Act of 1906) and in some European countries (for example, the Therapeutic Substances Act of 1925 in Britain and the Royal Decree of 1934 in Sweden), two disasters – the Elixir Sulfanilamide in the USA in 1937 and the thalidomide disaster in Western Europe in 1960 – were to galvanize the introduction of more stringent legislative controls.

1.2 Elixir Sulfanilamide disaster

The Elixir Sulfanilamide disaster in 1937 in the USA, shortly after the introduction of the first sulfa antimicrobial drug (sulfanilamide), occurred when diethylene glycol was used as a diluent in the formulation of a liquid preparation of sulfanilamide known as Elixir Sulfanilamide. One hundred and seven patients, mostly children, died following its therapeutic use. The drug regulations prevalent at that time did not require pre-marketing toxicity testing. In reaction to this calamity, the US Congress passed the 1938 Federal Food, Drug and Cosmetics Act which required proof of safety before release of a new drug.

1.3 Thalidomide disaster

Thalidomide, first introduced in Germany in October 1957 (as a remedy for an anticipated epidemic of Asian flu) and in the UK in April 1958, was heavily promoted as a safe alternative to the barbiturates. There were early reports of a peripheral neuropathy associated with its use. The drug was promoted for use in pregnancy and during lactation for its sedative properties. Following early anecdotal reports of its ability to control nausea and vomiting in the first trimester, it was also quickly and widely promoted for use in early pregnancy. In late 1959, there was the first report of the occurrence of a previously unknown malformation (termed phocomelia because of its resemblance to seal's flippers) in many babies born in north-western Germany. This malformation was characterized by defective and poor growth of the long bones of the limbs that had normal or rudimentary hands or feet. Subsequently, a large number of additional cases were reported in babies born to mothers who had taken this drug during the first trimester of pregnancy. The teratogenic effect was soon recognized to be caused by thalidomide and was reported from every country where thalidomide was on the market. The 'epidemic' of phocomelia and other malformations among the babies reached such a proportion that the drug was withdrawn from the market in Germany in November 1961 and in the UK in December 1961.

The USA was essentially spared the thalidomide tragedy because of the FDA's (Food and Drug Administration) concerns over the neurotoxicity of thalidomide. Following the thalidomide tragedy in Western Europe, a subsequent New Drug Amendment (the Kefauver-Harris Amendment) in 1962 called for the FDA to monitor all stages of drug development. As a result, even investigational drugs then required comprehensive animal testing before extensive human trials could be started. Under the Kefauver-Harris Amendment, proof of efficacy and safety was mandatory and the time constraints on the FDA for disposition of applications for new drugs were removed.

1.4 Consequences for regulatory controls

The consequences that followed the clinical use of thalidomide were to provide the impetus to the introduction, for the first time in most non-US countries (including those in Western

Europe), of regulatory control for drugs to be marketed for clinical use. The resulting tragedy stimulated worldwide, not only an ever-increasing set of regulatory requirements on preclinical (non-clinical) testing of drugs before administration to humans, but also the laws on liability and compensation. In the UK, the result was the Medicines Act, 1968. The original legal basis of applications for marketing authorizations in the EU was set out in Council Directive 65/65/EEC, together with a brief description of the documents and particulars that should accompany such applications in order to establish the quality, safety and efficacy of the product.

Over time, further stringent requirements have evolved in respect of investigations to be carried out during the clinical development of drugs, the data required before they are approved for marketing and subsequently the requirements for safety monitoring during the post-marketing period (pharmacovigilance). Even over the last two or three decades, introductions of some guidelines and requirements can be traced, directly or indirectly, to some tragedies, albeit of perhaps lesser magnitude than Elixir Sulfanilamide or thalidomide. Examples are the need to investigate pharmacokinetics in the elderly after benoxaprofen-induced hepatotoxicity, the guideline on drug interactions after all the concerns about the interaction potential of H_1-antihistamines and most recently, the QT interval prolongation and the risks of torsade de pointes produced by non-cardiovascular drugs.

1.5 Comparison with US FDA requirements

Since regulatory requirements in different regions have evolved over time, it is not surprising that that there is a remarkable degree of uniformity of data required by the major regulatory authorities. This uniformity in requirements is further driven by discussions and agreement at the International Conference on Harmonisation (ICH). The ICH is a tripartite body which is committed to harmonizing the technical requirements for registration of pharmaceuticals in the EU, USA and Japan. The ICH topics include a wide range of safety, quality and efficacy issues. The guidelines adopted within the ICH process are considered as EU Community guidelines once adopted by the EU's Committee for Proprietary Medicinal Products (CPMP) and published. The aim is to avoid unnecessary duplication of experiments and to streamline the process of drug development worldwide.

There are at present, however, some significant differences between the EU and USA regarding the format in which the data should be presented to the regulatory authority. The FDA in the USA usually require original case report forms and they regularly undertake statistical re-analysis of the data. In addition, they also require an Integrated Summary of Efficacy and an Integrated Summary of Safety. In contrast, the EU has a mandatory legal requirement, in accordance with Article 2 of Directive 75/319/EEC, for the three Expert Reports. The prescribing information in the EU is the Summary of Product Characteristics (SPC). It is referred to as the 'label' in the USA, is structured differently and includes the information in great detail.

There are other important procedural differences between the EU and the USA. For example, in contrast to the USA, in the EU there is a mandatory process for 5-yearly renewal of marketing authorizations, requirement to include patient information leaflets, provision of unit of use packaging, user fees for post-marketing regulatory activities and the provision to suspend marketing authorizations while safety concerns are being investigated further.

2. FORMAT FOR APPLICATIONS FOR MARKETING AUTHORIZATIONS IN THE EU

2.1 Legislative framework

A medicinal product may only be placed on the market in the EU when a marketing authorization has been issued by the competent authority of a Member State for its own territory (national authorization) or when an authorization has been granted by the European Commission (EC) for the entire Community (community authorization).

An application for a marketing authorization shall be accompanied, among other items, by specified pharmaceutical, preclinical and clinical particulars and documents (the 'dossier'). Three important summary documents in the dossier are the SPC, a package or patient information leaflet (PIL) and the sales presentation of the product (label). The SPC has a formally prescribed structure (Box 3.1). The SPC is regulated by Directive 75/318/EEC as amended by Directive 83/570/EEC, while the PIL is regulated by Directive 92/27/EEC.

The basic requirements for the contents of the dossier of information accompanying the application are the same whether it is submitted nationally or centrally and are laid out in detail in Directive 75/318/EEC and its subsequent amendments. Provisions are made in Directive 65/65/EEC for the omission of data in certain circumstances where information is already available to the regulatory authorities from other sources, for example, in the case of applications for line extensions to existing products or for generic drugs. Applications which do not include a full dossier of information are referred to as 'abridged applications'. The complex legal basis for the different types of generic or abridged applications for marketing authorizations will not be considered further in this chapter.

Subsequent to Council Directive 65/65/EEC referred to earlier, other directives have extended the legal system for authorizing medicines, introducing new procedures and expanding on existing legislation. Further information may be found in *The rules governing medicinal products in the European Union*, published by the EC. There are 9 volumes. Volumes 1–3 relate to medicinal products for human use while volumes 5–8 relate to veterinary medicinal products. Volume 4 relates to Good Manufacturing Practice and volume 9 relates to Pharmacovigilance (for both human and veterinary use).

For human medicinal products, the relevant legislation is presented in volume 1. Procedures for marketing authorizations are described in volume 2A, the presentation and the content of the dossier are described in volume 2B and various regulatory guidelines in volume 2C of the *Notice to applicants for marketing authorizations for*

Box 3.1 Contents of the Summary of Product Characteristics (SPC)

1. Trade name of the medicinal product
2. Qualitative and quantitative composition (active ingredient)
3. Pharmaceutical form
4. Clinical particulars
   4.1 Therapeutic indications
   4.2 Posology and method of administration
   4.3 Contra-indications
   4.4 Special warnings and special precautions for use
   4.5 Interactions with other medicaments and other forms of interactions
   4.6 (Use during) Pregnancy and lactation
   4.7 Effects on ability to drive and to use machines
   4.8 Undesirable effects (frequency and seriousness)
   4.9 Overdose (symptoms, emergency procedures, antidotes)
5. Pharmacological properties including pharmacokinetics
   5.1 Pharmacodynamic properties
   5.2 Pharmacokinetic properties
   5.3 Preclinical safety data
6. Pharmaceutical particulars
   6.1 List of excipients
   6.2 Incompatibilities
   6.3 Shelf-life (when necessary after reconstitution or opening the container for the first time)
   6.4 Special precautions for storage
   6.5 Nature and contents of container
   6.6 Instructions for use/handling
7. Marketing authorization holder (name and address)
8. Marketing authorization number
9. Date of first authorization
10. Date of (partial) revision of the text

medicinal products for human use in the European Union. Volume 3 of the *Rules governing medicinal products in the European Union* comprises *Quality and Biotechnology (3A), Pharmaco-toxicological (3B) and Clinical (3C) Guidelines* for medicinal products for human use. These three volumes are a compilation of the notes for guidance produced by the CPMP through its Working Parties or its membership of the ICH. None of these guidelines is legally binding and they are intended to be sufficiently flexible as not to impede scientific progress in drug development. However, where an applicant chooses not to follow a guideline, the decision must be explained and justified in the dossier. Justification is not always easy since these guidelines have been prepared by experts, have undergone input from academia and the industry during consultation and have been adopted only thereafter.

These guidance notes are continually being updated and added to, and applicants need to be aware of the current versions when preparing their dossiers. In the EU, the current guidelines already adopted and those draft versions that have been released for consultation are available from the Medicines and Healthcare products Regulatory Agency (MHRA) EuroDirect Publications Service (Room 10-238, Market Towers, 1 Nine Elms Lane, London SW8 5NQ) or the European Medicines Evaluation Agency (EMEA) web-site (http://www.emea.eu.int/index/indexh1.htm).

2.2 Format of the dossier

2.2.1 Current format
Directive 75/318/EEC requires that the dossier shall be presented in four highly structured parts – Parts I, II, III and IV. Volume 2B of the *Rules governing medicinal products* gives a detailed breakdown of the structure of a European regulatory dossier. This format is valid until end of June 2003 when a new format will become mandatory (see section 2.2.2 below).

Part I takes the form of a summary of the information presented in the whole dossier and includes particulars on fees, various declarations and the type of application as well as par-

ticulars of the marketing authorization (IA), proposed SPC (IB1), proposals for packaging, labels and package or patient information leaflets (IB2) and any SPCs already approved in the Member State(s) (IB3). Also included are separate Expert Reports on chemical and pharmaceutical (IC1), toxico-pharmacological (preclinical) (IC2) and clinical documentations (IC3). They are the summaries of the dossier with a critical appraisal of the data presented by an expert on behalf of the applicant. Detailed regulatory guidance, supported by various Directives, is available on the content of each of these documents.

Part II relates to the quality of the product and gives details of its chemical, pharmaceutical and biological testing. In cases where the active ingredient is made by a manufacturer other than the applicant or product manufacturer, some of the information required in Part II may be presented in a separate file, the Drug Master File, to maintain the confidential nature of the synthetic process. Part III describes the toxicological and pharmacological tests conducted with the drug in animals (preclinical tests). Part IV describes the clinical documentation. The detailed regulatory requirements for each of these three parts are discussed below.

2.2.2 Common Technical Document
Following agreement at the ICH meeting in November 2000, the format of the EU dossier described above will change to conform to the new format known as the 'Common Technical Document'. This new format (CTD) will be common to all the three major regions of drug regulation (EU, USA and Japan) and most other major non-ICH authorities have also agreed to accept the dossier in CTD format. Information on the CTD can be accessed from the EC web-site (http://pharmacos.eudra.org/F2/ pharmacos/docs.htm).

The CTD consists of four (2–5) modules, preceded by a module 1 which is region-specific and includes administrative and prescribing information. Module 2 comprises CTD Summaries and Overviews of the quality, non-clinical (preclinical) and clinical data, module 3 contains data on Quality, module 4 consists of the Non-clinical Study Reports and module 5 comprises the Clinical Study Reports. There are guidelines on the details to be included in each module and these are summarized in Box 3.2. Before the CTD can be introduced, certain legislative changes are required in each of the three regions. The non-clinical and clinical overviews and summaries are equivalent to the present Expert Reports described above. It is anticipated that submission of dossier in CTD format will become mandatory by July 2003, although applicants had the option to use this format from July 2001.

The objectives behind the CTD are to reduce the time and resources needed to compile applications, to facilitate electronic submissions, regulatory reviews and communications and to facilitate exchange of information between regulatory authorities. It is not intended to indicate what studies are required – these are essentially the same as before – but to indicate merely an appropriate format for the presentation of the data that have been generated.

2.3 Product literature and clinical prescribing

The literature associated with the product (and considered an integral part of the marketing authorization) consists of the finally approved

---

Box 3.2 Summary of the contents of the modules of the Common Technical Document (CTD)

Module 1 EU-specific requirements
1.1 Module 1 Comprehensive table of contents (modules 1–5)
1.2 Application form
1.3 Product literature
    1.3.1 Summary of product characteristics
    1.3.2 Labelling
    1.3.3 Package leaflet
    1.3.4 Mock-ups and specimen
    1.3.5 SPCs already approved in the Member States
1.4 Information about experts
1.5 Specific requirements for different types of applications
Annex Environmental risk assessment

Module 2 CTD summaries
2.1 CTD Table of contents (Modules 2–5)
2.2 CTD Introduction
2.3 Quality overall summary
2.4 Non-clinical overview
2.5 Clinical overview
2.6 Non-clinical written and tabulated summary
    Pharmacology
    Pharmacokinetics
    Toxicology

2.7 Clinical summary
    Biopharmaceutics and associated analytical methods
    Clinical pharmacology studies
    Clinical efficacy
    Clinical safety
    Synopsis of individual studies

Module 3 Quality
3.1 Module 3 Table of contents
3.2 Body of data
3.3 Key literature references

Module 4 Non-clinical study reports
4.1 Module 4 Table of contents
4.2 Study reports
4.3. Literature references

Module 5 Clinical study reports
5.1 Module 5 Table of contents
5.2 Tabular listing of all clinical studies
5.3 Clinical study reports
5.4 Literature references

SPC, packaging, labels and package or patient information leaflets. Information permitted to be included in these documents should fully reflect the scientific and objective assessment of the data contained in the dossier. The SPC forms the basis for *authorized* clinical prescribing of the medicinal product concerned.

3. CHEMICAL AND PHARMACEUTICAL REQUIREMENTS

The information to be submitted on the quality aspects of a new medicinal product containing a new chemical active ingredient can be broadly divided into two: (a) details of the individual ingredients of the preparation and (b) details of the dosage form itself. The headings under which data should be provided in Part II of the dossier are given in Box 3.3.

3.1 Active ingredient

The information provided on the chemistry of an NAS should include details of the synthesis of the drug, its characterization (including evidence of structure and physicochemical properties), control of its quality and its stability. The quality of the active ingredient is established by testing against a specification which lists a series of tests and the limits that must be complied with before the material is acceptable for use in the manufacture of the medicinal product. The drug substance specification generally will include tests for appearance, identification, impurities (drug-related compounds, inorganic residues and residual solvents) and an assay for content. Other tests may be added for particular drug substances where necessary. An example of such an additional test is measurement of particle size where this is a critical parameter for performance of the medicinal product, e.g. in inhalers or to ensure proper dissolution from a tablet. Different crystal forms of an active ingredient may also have different physicochemical characteristics such as solubility that may affect the behaviour of the finished product and thus require control in the specification. Drug substances that are chiral may also require identification and control of unwanted

> **Box 3.3   Chemical, pharmaceutical and biological testing of medicinal products**
>
> IIA   Qualitative and quantitative particulars of the constituents
>   1. Composition of the medicinal product
>   2. Brief description of container
>   3. Clinical trial formulae
>   4. Development pharmaceutics
>
> IIB   Description of the method of preparation
>   1. Manufacturing formula
>   2. Manufacturing process
>   3. Validation of the process
>
> IIC   Control of starting materials
>   1. Active substance
>   2. Excipients
>   3. Immediate packaging material
>
> IID   Control tests on intermediate products
>
> IIE   Control tests on the finished product
>   1. Specifications and routine tests
>   2. Scientific data
>
> IIF   Stability tests
>   1. Stability tests on the active substance
>   2. Stability tests on the finished product
>
> IIQ   Other information
>   1. Bioanalytical methods
>   2. Synthesis of radiolabelled material

stereoisomers. The applicant must be able to demonstrate that drug substance of a suitable quality can be manufactured by the proposed synthetic route in a reproducible manner. The data given in the dossier must justify the limits in the proposed specification and this is frequently a subject of negotiation between the regulatory authority and the applicant. The applicant must also show that the drug substance continues to meet the specification following storage for a stated length of time under controlled conditions.

3.2 Excipients or inactive ingredients and containers

Information is also required for other ingredients used to prepare the dosage form. Generally, these materials comply with well-recognized pharmacopoeial standards but where a new excipient is used, the same information must be provided as for a new 'active' substance, including details of toxicological testing. Details of the packaging intended for the medicinal product must be provided and its suitability for pharmaceutical or food use demonstrated.

3.3 Finished product

The information needed for the finished product includes a description of the development of the formulation and its composition, its manufacture, control of its quality and its stability. The rationale for the pharmaceutical development of the medicinal product should be explained. The applicant needs to demonstrate an understanding of the physicochemical behaviour of the active ingredient in the formulation, show that the excipients chosen are suitable for their purpose and that the finished product will perform as expected (e.g. tablets will disintegrate or dissolve in a timely fashion, transdermal patches will release the active ingredient in a controlled manner, inhalers will deposit particles of a suitable size). Scale-up of the manufacturing process should also be described and an understanding of the critical process parameters should be displayed.

Often during the development of a product, the composition changes as the clinical programme advances. If this is the case, then it is important that at each stage the performance of the new formulation is compared to the old one, unless the changes are trivial, to demonstrate that they are bioequivalent. This comparison ensures that the data from earlier clinical trials remain valid for the final product.

3.4 Consistency of quality and shelf-life

The applicant must show that the medicinal product is manufactured consistently and is of suitable quality. The quality is controlled by testing against a pre-set specification, as for the drug substance, before the product is released onto the market. The finished product specification generally will include tests for appearance, identification and assay of the active ingredient and impurities. Other tests are included which are specific to the dosage form, thus, a disintegration or dissolution test will be needed for tablets and capsules, sterility and endotoxin tests for parenteral products and a viscosity test for topical creams, ointments or gels. The specification that applies during the shelf-life of the product may allow for some degradation of the active ingredient, with associated increase in impurities, or change in physical parameters within reasonable limits. The declared shelf-life is based on the data collected from stability studies conducted by storing the product in the intended commercial packaging under defined conditions of temperature and humidity. If the product is a preparation intended for use over a period of time by the patient, e.g. an oral liquid, then additional tests mimicking 'in use' conditions may be required to establish the stability and shelf-life after opening. Parenteral products intended for reconstitution or dilution before administration must be investigated for their compatibility with the intended solvents or diluents. Their physicochemical stability when reconstituted/diluted and any incompatibilities with likely additives must also be established.

3.5 Control of impurities

Control of impurities in both the drug substance and the finished product is of particular importance. Impurities may take the form of heavy metals, residual solvents or substances related to the active ingredient that can arise either from its synthesis or from its degradation. Related substances require identification only if they occur in the drug substance above a certain specified level. In addition, above specified thresholds depending on the maximum daily dose of the drug, the proposed limits for impurities must be qualified by adequate testing in preclinical and/or clinical studies. Thus, if a substance containing a certain level of an impurity has been used in clinical studies, then this level of impurity is considered qualified for use in the medicinal product. To assist assessment of qualification, a full list of all the batches of drug substance and finished product used in toxicological and clinical studies must be provided together with details of their analysis according to their specifications.

Great importance is attached to the analytical techniques used to control the drug substance and medicinal product and to measure the levels of drug and metabolites in the preclinical and clinical studies. All these methods must be adequately validated to demonstrate that they are suitable for their intended purpose.

3.6 Information in product literature

While details of the manufacturing process for the drug substance or the medicinal product are considered commercially confidential, certain information related to the chemical and pharmaceutical aspects of the product is stated in its associated literature. The name of the product, the quantitative content of the active ingredient, the pharmaceutical form (selected from an approved list) and description of the product are stated in the first three sections of the SPC. Inactive ingredients are listed in section 6.1 although quantitative details are not given. Certain excipients, known to cause problems in some patients (e.g. wheat starch), must be stated on the package label and must be accompanied by warnings in the patient information leaflet. The shelf-life of the product, based on the stability studies referred to above, is declared in section 6.3 of the SPC with any special conditions for storage being stated in section 6.4. The nature of the container and its contents (i.e. pack sizes) are given in section 6.5. Provision is also made for declaring any known incompatibilities with likely co-administered drugs (section 6.2) and, under instructions for use/handling (section 6.6), recommendations can be given for reconstituting products with particular solvents or diluents.

4. PRECLINICAL REQUIREMENTS

The preclinical section of an NAS application will typically consist of data qualifying and quantifying the pharmacodynamic, pharmacokinetic and toxicity profile of the new drug. As already described in the Introduction, the nature of these studies is to a large extent governed by guidelines issued by regulatory authorities. However, the studies can be 'tailored' to a specific product and the whole process should be governed by what is *scientifically* appropriate. Most authorities are sufficiently flexible to accept this and will not insist on a 'box ticking' exercise. In addition, the guidelines are being continuously updated with the advances in toxicology. A recent example of this is the inclusion of tests for immunotoxicity incorporated into the guideline for repeated-dose toxicity tests.

4.1 Pharmacodynamic studies

These studies to demonstrate preclinical efficacy will usually include in vitro, ex vivo and in vivo experiments to demonstrate that the NAS has suitable activity. Each therapeutic area has animal models specific to it. So, for example, for the development of a new medicine for the treatment of type II diabetes, strains of mice such as ob/ob or rats such as the Zucker fatty rat (which are themselves diabetic) will be used. It is a disappointing fact that as these experiments proceed from simple in vitro systems to the complexity of a whole animal the efficacy of the compound diminishes. This process reaches its peak when the application is assessed by the advisory committees (in the UK, the Committee on Safety of Medicines) and may be rejected, at least for some of the proposed indications, for lack of clinical efficacy.

4.2 Safety pharmacology studies

The full list of safety pharmacology studies for an NAS application is shown in Table 3.1. Other organ systems may be required to be investigated where there is cause for concern. For some applications a more restricted package is

Table 3.1   Safety pharmacology studies

Studies	Parameters
Core battery of tests	
Central nervous system	Motor activity, behavioural changes, coordination, sensory/motor reflexes, body temperature
Cardiovascular system	BP, heart rate, ECG and possibly methods for detecting repolarization and conductance abnormalities
Respiratory system	Respiratory rate, and other measures such as tidal volume or haemoglobin oxygen saturation
Follow-up studies	
Central nervous system	Behavioural pharmacology, learning and memory, ligand-specific binding, neurochemistry, visual and auditory examinations, etc.
Cardiovascular system	Cardiac output, ventricular contractility, vascular resistance etc.
Respiratory system	Airway resistance, compliance, pulmonary arterial pressure, blood gases, blood pH, etc.
Supplementary studies	
Renal/urinary system	Urinary volume, specific gravity, osmolality, pH, fluid/electrolyte balance, proteins, cytology and clinical biochemistry of blood (blood urea nitrogen, creatinine, plasma proteins)
Gastrointestinal system	Gastric secretion, gastrointestinal injury potential, bile secretion, transit time in vivo, ileal contraction in vitro, gastric pH measurement
Autonomic nervous system	Binding to relevant receptors, functional responses to agonists or antagonists, direct stimulation of autonomic nerves and measurement of cardiovascular responses (baroreflex testing, heart rate variability)

undertaken but will usually include an assessment of the effects on cardiovascular, respiratory and central neurological functions. Safety pharmacology studies may not be needed for locally applied agents (e.g. dermal or ocular) where the pharmacology of the test substance is well characterized and systemic exposure or distribution to other organs or tissues is demonstrated to be low.

4.3 Pharmacokinetic studies

Pharmacokinetic studies on absorption, distribution, metabolism and excretion must demonstrate that the animal species used in toxicity studies (typically rats, mice, rabbits and another non-rodent such as the dog, marmoset or Cynomolgus monkey) are relevant to humans in terms of exposure to the parent compound and metabolites. Comparison of exposure must be in terms of plasma Cmax and/or area under the curve (AUC). For oral dosing it has long been unacceptable to make comparisons in terms of mg/kg. If exposure is substantially different in humans, then appropriate alternative animal models may be included in the preclinical studies. Alternatively, for example, it may be the case that metabolites are produced in humans that have not been detected in animal species. In this instance, chemists could be asked to synthesize these and pivotal toxicity studies may be repeated by dosing with these metabolites directly. This may seem a time-consuming process and would probably cost several million pounds but in terms of the overall development time and cost it is in effect of relatively little consequence.

Interaction with cytochrome P450 enzymes is possibly the most critical aspect of the pharmacokinetic studies. It must be established in preclinical studies which cytochrome P450 enzyme (if any) is responsible for metabolism of the parent compound, which (if any) it inhibits and which (if any) it induces. This is generally determined with in vitro human microsomal preparations or a cell line of any origin genetically modified to express human cytochrome P450 isozymes. The importance of this aspect of drug development will increase as the study of pharmacogenomics enables drug companies to tailor drugs to subpopulations with specific cytochrome P450 activity.

4.4 Toxicity studies

The toxicity studies usually take a minimum of 5 years to complete. They consist of the following usually conducted in a rodent (rat) and non-rodent (dog, primate) species.

4.4.1 Acute toxicity
These are single-dose studies that provide valuable information on the potential clinical consequences of overdosage. The focus is more on clinical signs than on identifying target organs. They are also used to determine doses for subsequent repeated-doses studies.

4.4.2 Repeated-doses toxicity
In these studies the purpose is to identify target organs and to establish (hopefully) safety margins with respect to clinical exposure. Since many of the parameters are monitored during volunteer studies or during clinical trials the preclinical data are usually superseded by clinical findings by the time of the marketing authorization application. The maximum dosing period is 1 year and recovery groups are often included to determine whether adverse effects are reversible.

4.4.3 Reproductive toxicity
The point covering preclinical data being superseded does not apply to the reprotoxicity studies (nor to genotoxicity/oncogenicity) since, with the possible exception of a few unexpected pregnancies, no data are available in humans. Fertility and early embryonic development, teratogenicity and pre- and post-natal studies are conducted in rats. The teratogenicity study, now called the embryofetal study, is also repeated in a non-rodent, more often than not the rabbit.

The pre-ICH3 nomenclature of Segment I, II and III studies to describe the reprotoxicity studies is unfortunately no longer used. However, such studies are still submitted and are acceptable to all regulatory authorities.

4.4.4 Genotoxicity
A full genotoxicity package comprises in vitro tests of mutagenicity in bacteria (Ames test) and mammalian cells as well as a test for clastogenicity for which human lymphocytes are commonly used. An in vivo micronucleus test in rats or mice usually completes the package, although it is becoming more frequent to receive an Unscheduled DNA Synthesis assay, particularly when one of the other genotoxicity tests is positive. Suitable positive controls are included in all genotoxicity tests.

4.4.5 Oncogenicity
Lifetime studies to detect oncogenic potential are conducted in rats and mice, usually using dietary administration. These are critical studies and to have to repeat them would cost money and time and delay the receipt of a marketing authorization. For this reason applicants take great care to get the doses right such that at the high dose (at least) there are signs of toxicity but sufficient animals have survived to the end of the study. While drug companies will discuss this with the FDA before initiating the studies, this is not routine in the EU. However, companies may request guidance from any one or more national authority on this or any other issue relevant to the development of an NAS during such a meeting. A more formal alternative is to seek the Scientific Advice from the CPMP.

The tumour profiles of different strains of rats and mice are well known. In addition, the induction of some tumours, usually by some epigenetic mechanism, has been well established. This enables positive results from oncogenicity studies to be put into context and not be considered a risk in clinical use. Frequently encountered explanations are: exaggerated pharmacological activity (i.e. a class effect), reversibility, safety margin, 'stress', known mechanism, acceptable clinical data, infection, spontaneous occurrence in control animals (i.e. sensitivity of test species) and epiphenomenona. These can all be valid provided that they are supported by the data (which may be bibliographic or from investigative studies).

There is an increasing number of alternative tests models for oncogenicity including transgenic and 'knockout' animals. Although these have advantages, particularly in terms of time taken to complete the study, they have yet to be as fully validated as the standard rat and mouse studies, and interpretation of the results (whether positive or negative) can be problematical.

Unless the toxicity profile is well understood, as for example with effects on the rat thyroid, investigative studies will be necessary to explain any adverse effect seen in toxicity studies. The nature of these will be determined on a case-by-case basis. This also applies to the impurities and degradation products.

4.4.6 Other studies

Other toxicity studies will include an assessment of irritancy and tolerance as well as an Environmental Risk Assessment. The latter is often based on calculations alone but if experiments are submitted they tend to consist of toxicity to micro-organisms (algae), fish (trout) and plants (algae). Consideration of potential contamination of both water and soil is required.

The duration of toxicity testing in animal species for any given period of treatment in humans varies between countries and is shown in Table 3.2.

An important consideration, perhaps the most important consideration for applicant and regulator alike, is the interpretation of positive results. There will be plenty of these since one of the objectives of the toxicity studies is to dose at toxic levels. A toxicity study with no signs of toxicity – albeit only something insignificant such as a slight reduction in body weight gain or minor histopathological changes at the site of injection – is almost certainly an invalid study and will have to be repeated. An exception might be a particularly non-toxic substance that has been administered at abnormally high unphysiological doses such as 2000 mg/kg. At

Table 3.2   Duration of repeated-dose toxicity studies to support Phase III clinical trials in the EU

Duration of clinical trials	Minimum duration of repeated-dose toxicity studies	
	Rodents	Non-rodents
Up to 2 weeks	1 month	1 month
Up to 1 month	3 months	3 months
Up to 3 months	6 months	3 months
>3 months	6 months	Chronic*

*This table also reflects the marketing recommendations in the three ICH regions except that a chronic non-rodent study is recommended for clinical use for longer than 1 month.

the other end of the dose scale, a study that does not have a 'no observed effect level' is similarly probably invalid and will have to be repeated.

Unlike the other preclinical studies, the conduct of the toxicity studies should be compliant with Good Laboratory Practice. In practice, however, the development of a new drug is such a long and difficult process that non-GLP compliant studies conducted before the initiation of GLP are still being submitted. Often these are accompanied by a statement by an independent assessor that the studies were conducted in the spirit of GLP. Provided that there are not too many like this and that they do not comprise the most critical studies in terms of adverse results then this can be acceptable.

4.5 Information in product literature

Although it is often the case that one or two pregnant women end up taking an NAS (despite stringent efforts to avoid this occurring) such data that are obtained are of little use. The information from the reprotoxicity studies alone therefore forms the basis of what is written in section 4.6 of the SPC giving advice on use in pregnancy and lactation. More often than not the use of the NAS is contra-indicated in these conditions.

Clinical trials will not have been conducted for a sufficiently long period to be able to make an assessment of the carcinogenic potential in humans. So, as for section 4.6, section 5.3 of the SPC is a description of preclinical data, in this instance the genotoxicity/oncogenicity studies and information from general toxicity studies on potential target organs. However, in the latter case, clinical data will have superseded preclinical findings.

5. CLINICAL REQUIREMENTS

The clinical requirements and the data provided in the dossier are divided into Part IVA which is the detailed clinical pharmacology of the medicinal product and Part IVB which describes in detail the clinical experience. In addition, there is of course Part IC3 which is the Clinical Expert Report. Details of the requirements are set out in the Commission Directives 75/318/EEC as modified by 91/507/EEC.

In addition, there is a wide range of guidelines and 'points to consider' documents produced by the Efficacy Working Party of the CPMP. These include, for example, pharmacokinetic studies in man, drug interactions, studies in the elderly, dose-ranging studies, investigations of drugs in specific therapeutic areas, biostatistics and the extent of safety database required. These guidelines and documents provide comprehensive guidance on conduct of clinical trials, choice of endpoints and comparators and duration of studies in the therapeutic areas concerned. In areas of uncertainty or controversy or areas that are highly innovative, there is a mechanism in place for obtaining Scientific Advice from CPMP well in advance of commencing the clinical development or the pivotal clinical trials programme. The requirements and the procedures for seeking Scientific Advice are highly structured. Although not binding on either side, this Advice from CPMP provides a consensus view of all the Member States of the EU.

Studies should be conducted in accordance with the Good Clinical Practice (GCP) guidelines. The Clinical Expert is asked to confirm that all studies are undertaken in accordance with GCP guideline and comment on those that are not and give a clear statement as to why they are not. Any deficiencies in these studies should be clearly identified and commented upon.

Data are required on the characteristics of the population and the dose ranges studied. Documentation should include clinical and laboratory results as a function of dose and/or concentration as relevant to the efficacy and the safety of the drug. Each study in the clinical dossier, whether clinical pharmacology or clinical experience, should be presented in a structured manner to include a summary, study objectives, detailed study design (including doses selected, duration, planned number of patients, assessment times and statistical methods), results, conclusion and bibliography if necessary. The results should include information on patients screened, patients enrolled and their disposition, the characteristics (with respect to demography, disease under investigation, co-morbidity and co-medications) of the population randomized, data on each of the pre-specified efficacy endpoints with appropriate statistical analyses, clinical safety and laboratory changes. Any amendments to the protocol should be clearly identified with a comment on the reason for and the effect of each amendment.

5.1 Phasic development of drugs

Traditionally, the clinical development of a drug is divided into four phases. Phase I studies are usually in healthy volunteers, aimed at characterizing the clinical pharmacology and tolerance of a drug. Phase II studies are early or pilot efficacy studies in patients, aimed at confirming an effect in the disease of interest – the so-called 'proof of principle' studies – and at defining the optimal dose. Phase I and II studies form the core clinical pharmacology package. Phase III studies are the pivotal studies, against placebo and/or active comparators, that constitute the core dataset forming the basis of indications and safety. Phase IV studies are post-approval studies aimed at confirming the efficacy and safety during uncontrolled clinical use of the drug. Additional indications (or a new target population) may be claimed after an initial approval by conducting appropriate studies in the proposed new indication (or new target population) as an extension to the original clinical development programme.

5.2 Use in children

Unless a drug is exclusively for use in children, it is usual to find that the clinical documentation focuses on adults. There is now a greater emphasis on investigations of a drug in children. Of course, the time for commencing investigations in children is dependent on the preclinical profile of the drug and the likelihood of its use in children. Even if children are not included in the initial clinical documentation within the dossier, it is imperative that if a drug is likely to be used in children the applicant should present at the outset a well thought out paediatric clinical development programme.

5.3 Clinical pharmacology

Clinical pharmacology data should provide characterization of the pharmacodynamics and the pharmacokinetics of the drug. It is not only the primary pharmacology (responsible for the therapeutic effect of the drug) but also its secondary pharmacology (responsible for unwanted effects) that needs to be investigated. Considerable information will have been gained during preclinical in vitro and in vivo investigations. Compounds are tested in high-throughput systems for activity at a wide range of receptors and enzymes. There are of course no guidelines on activities that need to be characterized but one is guided by chemical structure and effects of other previous drugs in the same pharmacological or therapeutic class. An example would be the investigation of an H_1-antihistamine not only as an antagonist of the effect of histamine but also its effects on cardiac electrophysiology, mental alertness and muscarinic receptors.

Pharmacokinetics of the drug require full characterization, with all the aspects that embody the term pharmacokinetics in its broadest sense, together with the effect of age, gender, renal or hepatic dysfunction and food. Genetic factors are assuming greater importance and information should be provided on the ethnic structure of the trial population. Arising from pharmacokinetic studies, there should be a detailed and well-designed programme of drug interaction studies. This is still an area that is poorly addressed. It is not only the interactions with drugs that are the substrates of the same drug-metabolizing enzyme as the new drug under investigation that matter. These studies should carefully consider the in vitro data obtained (and included in Part III of the dossier) to elucidate the potential of the new drug to inhibit various drug-metabolizing enzymes. In addition, it is important to consider the drugs most likely to be used by the target population. Renal drug interactions are now becoming an equally important cause for concern as the metabolic interactions. Depending on the therapeutic margin of the drug, the possibility of clinically significant renal drug interactions should be investigated if the renal clearance of the drug is about 30% or more of the total body clearance.

5.4 Dose–response and dose selection studies

The next important requirement is the demonstration in early pilot studies that the drug does work in patients of interest (proof of concept studies) and a discussion of the rationale for selection of dose for the pivotal efficacy studies. This is often another area that is poorly addressed in many clinical dossiers. A well-designed programme of dose-finding studies makes evaluation so much easier. The parameters of interest are the minimal effective dose and maximum dose beyond which safety is a concern, additional benefits do not accrue or the risk-benefit ratio is adversely affected. It is important that the dose schedule is scientifically supported by the pharmacokinetics and pharmacodynamics of the drug and its metabolite(s). Equally critical are the considerations of the time to steady-state and whether the pharmacodynamic effects lag behind changes in plasma concentrations. An ideal dose-ranging studies programme should provide definitive information on the risk-benefit of a range of doses and dose regimens. Well-supported data on subtherapeutic doses become important if it ever becomes necessary, for reasons of unforeseen risks, to lower the doses during the post-marketing period.

5.5 Pivotal clinical trials on efficacy

The Phase III clinical trials form the core of efficacy studies and a large part of the clinical documentation. Typically, the studies include a number of placebo-controlled studies as well as active-controlled studies. Although there are no rules on the number of studies, it is usual to see two or three placebo-controlled studies, three or four active-controlled studies or any combination thereof. It is recognized that the use of placebo in some indications may not be feasible or ethical. Placebo-controlled studies provide an absolute measure of efficacy while active-controlled studies provide a measure of efficacy relative to the widely used alternatives. A good statistical input before the protocols are finalized obviates questions on the power and statistical robustness of the Phase III programme. Needless to say, if the Phase III programme cannot withstand regulatory scrutiny, the entire application is jeopardized.

Efficacy analysis should include subset analysis if it is likely that the overall benefit observed is driven by efficacy in a subset. Furthermore, the indication needs to be carefully crafted to ensure that it fully reflects not only the population and the disease studied but also any pre-specified subgroups most likely to benefit.

Data on long-term efficacy are also required if the medicinal product is likely to be used long-term. In this context, long-term use may be defined as chronic or repeated intermittent use for longer than 6 months. This evidence usually comes from double-blind controlled studies of at least 6 months' duration and/or open-label studies of least 12 months' duration.

Typically, the trial population exposed to the drug is of the order of 2500 patients but this very much depends on the disease under investigation and the range of its clinical presentation. Does the drug show efficacy in patients who are unresponsive to previous therapy? Is the drug intended to be administered as a monotherapy or as an add-on therapy? Is it intended to be a first-line or second-line therapy? It is important to consider whether the treatment is prophylactic, curative or symptomatic. Clinical trials may only include, for example, patients with mild chronic cardiac failure who are already receiving ACE inhibitors or patients with asthma who do not respond to low dose inhaled steroids or patients with nocturnal asthma. Under these circumstances, claims of indications in broad terms such as 'cardiac failure' or 'asthma' cannot be sustained.

5.6 Safety database

The safety database should be presented overall and by subpopulation exposed in terms of dose, duration, age, gender and special populations such as those with hepatic dysfunction or renal impairment. For drugs intended for long-term administration, it is required that at least 300 patients should have been exposed to the drug for at least 6 months and at least 100 patients for a minimum of 12 months.

Safety should be documented across all studies in terms of all adverse events, serious adverse events, adverse events leading to discontinuation of treatment and deaths. Studies should also document withdrawals due to failure of efficacy. Adverse events should be characterized in terms of severity, reversibility and their relationship to dose and duration of therapy and demographic parameters.

The data should be presented in terms of adverse events irrespective of causality and those considered by investigators to be related to study medications. The outcome of patients with serious adverse events and events leading to discontinuation of study medications should be carefully documented. Full narratives of patients who died should be available including, where possible, data from autopsy.

Changes in laboratory parameters constitute an important safety component. It is required that studies should monitor a broad range of laboratory parameters.

For patients who develop serious laboratory changes, it avoids questions if the data are presented for each patient in a chronological order beginning with baseline values and subsequently after administration of the drug and if appropriate, after its discontinuation. To facilitate interpretation, information on associated changes should also be presented. Typical examples would be information on dizziness or palpitation in a patient developing QT interval prolongation or changes in bilirubin and other hepatic function parameters in a patient developing high values of the liver enzyme, alanine transferase (ALT).

Safety data should also include post-marketing experience from countries (EU and non-EU) where the medicinal product is already approved and is on the market. To put these data in perspective, data should be included on the estimated patient exposure. Every attempt should be made to obtain details of the serious adverse events and those that resulted in deaths.

5.7 Clinical Expert Report

A Clinical Expert Report should be a critical analysis not exceeding 25 pages. It must include (as appendices) tabular formats of the studies and may be supplemented by a written summary of clinical pharmacology, efficacy and safety data. The Expert Report should contain a critical assessment of the methodology, results and conclusions of all studies. Precise references to specific studies or other relevant information contained in the dossier should be cross-referenced by volume(s) and page number(s).

The expert should begin by focusing on clinical practice and give useful information on currently available treatment modalities, including any unmet clinical needs, followed by a commentary on the contribution of the medicinal product in question. This should be followed by a critical discussion on the clinical pharmacology of the drug, assessment of individual studies together with their GCP status, global analysis of efficacy and then the global analysis of safety.

The clinical expert should discuss any post-marketing experience and other relevant information. The conclusion should cover therapeutic justification of the product, its efficacy and safety, dose regimen proposed, a risk-benefit analysis and when relevant, the position of the new drug in current therapeutic strategy. Exceptionally, small supplementary report(s) have been provided by the applicants to clarify specific issues but ideally, these should form part of the one Clinical Expert Report.

Lastly, there should be information on the clinical expert. Although only one clinical expert may assume the responsibility for the report, others may contribute to it (identified by name and contribution). In the CTD format, the Clinical Overview has been designed to replace the EU Expert Report.

5.8 Information in product literature

Clinical assessment of the dossier requires that the efficacy and the safety of the drug are carefully evaluated and the risk-benefit of the drug is considered and compared to existing therapeutic modalities. If the drug is unsafe or its risk-benefit ratio is unacceptable, approval may be denied. The SPC is the critical interface between the prescriber on one hand and the regulator and the marketing authorization holder on the other. If approvable, the SPC, label and package leaflet are carefully scrutinized so that the clinical information allowed or required to be included fully reflect the scientific data and the risks and benefits of the drug with all other prescribing restrictions and recommendations.

6. INTEGRATED REGULATORY ASSESSMENT

A typical dossier for an NAS includes 4–6 volumes of Part I, 6–10 volumes of Part II, 20–40 volumes of Part III and 100–200 volumes of Part IV data. During the regulatory assessment process, there is a documented interactive dialogue between each assessor and the applicant to clarify points that are complex or ambiguous or to enable the applicant to provide additional raw data, statistical appendices and detailed protocols to facilitate the assessment process.

However, none of these four parts of the dossier are stand-alone or independent of others. There are areas within each that are intricately linked to the others. In preparing a comprehensive and integrated regulatory assessment report, it is important that these areas of common interest are appropriately addressed by the assessors.

6.1 Integration of preclinical and pharmaceutical dossier

The drug substance and finished product specification of any product allow for the presence of low levels of impurities, depending on daily dose and duration of treatment. The permitted levels are specified. It is important that the safety of these allowable impurities is con-

firmed. The preclinical dossier requires careful scrutiny to ensure that these impurities were present in the test product administered to animals and in quantities sufficient to provide a confident and reassuring margin of safety during the clinical use.

If this has not been done, then the impurities present in relatively high concentration(s) need to be isolated or synthesized and a limited programme of toxicity studies, probably consisting of acute toxicity and genotoxicity, should be conducted directly with these.

6.2 Integration of preclinical and clinical data

The clinical dossier has to be scrutinized to ensure that the effects observed in preclinical general toxicity studies have been looked for in the clinical studies and, if present, the level of the risk has been established. Typical examples would include the preclinical effect of the drug on drug-metabolizing enzymes or specific target organs for toxicity. Likewise, it is easier to appreciate the significance of an unexpected finding in the clinical studies if there was a corresponding finding in the animal studies.

Often, unusual preclinical findings may require specific studies in man to exclude their clinical significance. For others, such as testicular or thyroid tumours in animals, the mechanism of their induction is sufficiently well understood that usually no additional studies are warranted.

Of course, any metabolite-related toxicity can only be relied upon if the metabolic profile of the drug in man and in the animal species concerned was similar. While some drug-metabolizing isoforms show polymorphism in man, the same may not apply to the animal species used in the preclinical programme. As with impurities, any unusual metabolite, if found at a significant level in man, would have to be tested preclinically in separate studies. This is more likely if the impaired metabolism of a drug in man is likely to activate alternative pathways and generate atypical metabolites. In the case of drugs with chiral centre, the enantioselectivity in pharmacokinetics in man and in animals should be similar if the findings from clinical and preclinical studies are to be correlated.

The most important areas of preclinical and clinical integration are the results of the genotoxicity, oncogenicity and reproductive studies. The findings from the latter studies are central to approving the use of the drug during pregnancy and lactation and in children.

6.3 Integration of pharmaceutical and clinical data

Frequently, the formulation used in clinical trials is not the one that is ultimately marketed. The pharmaceutical dossier is scrutinized for these variations and to ensure that studies have been carried out to prove the bioequivalence of the two. The same applies if more than one dose strength or dosage form are to be marketed, e.g. tablets for adults and liquid preparations for use in children.

Devices used for delivery of the drug (e.g. inhalers) are another area requiring an integrated clinical and pharmaceutical assessment for their performance, ease of use and implications for safety and efficacy.

The content uniformity and the finished product specifications are critical for drugs with a very narrow therapeutic index. In such cases, the specifications may have to be tightened.

7. PROCEDURES

7.1 Clinical trials in the UK

The primary legislation regarding the clinical trials in the UK at present is the Medicines Act 1968, which includes the definition of a clinical trial and of a medicinal product. Clinical studies involving healthy volunteers do not meet this definition of a clinical trial and, as a result, do not come under the remit of the Medicines Act 1968 or the Medicines and Healthcare products Regulatory Agency. Such studies are subject to self-regulation by the pharmaceutical industry. However, effective from 1 May 2004, the legislative basis and the procedures involved in initiating clinical trials in the UK will change following the introduction of the EU directive

(see section 7.2) relating to the implementation of good clinical practice in the conduct of clinical trials on medicinal products for human use.

At present there are four ways of seeking approval for the commencement of clinical trials in the UK. These are by means of a Clinical Trial Certificate (CTC), a Clinical Trial Exemption (CTX), a Doctors and Dentists Exemption (DDX) or as a Clinical Trial on a Marketed Product (CTMP). Each requires provision of a detailed protocol of the proposed trial.

7.1.1 Clinical Trial Certificate

A Clinical Trial Certificate (CTC) is granted for a period of 2 years and may be renewed. Variations to the Certificate are possible. The applicant for a CTC is required to provide full information on the quality and safety of the product to be used in the trial along with any early evidence of efficacy. This information is provided under the same headings as a marketing authorization application and, thus, consists of data on the chemical or biological/biotechnological and the pharmaceutical aspects of the drug substance and drug product (Part II), preclinical data on the pharmacodynamics, pharmacokinetics, safety pharmacology and toxicology of the material (Part III) and any clinical data already generated (Part IV).

The full data package is submitted and is assessed by assessors from each of the three disciplines. Their assessment report is then considered by the Committee on Safety of Medicines and its Subcommittees. If the decision is positive then a Certificate is issued. If the decision is negative, then the applicant has the same appeal rights as those that apply to a marketing authorization application (see section 8.4).

The disadvantage of the CTC approach is that it can be slow. There are no statutory timelines for the process. As a result, most applicants now use the CTX scheme. However, CTC is required for any proposed trials involving xenotransplantation.

7.1.2 Clinical Trial Exemption

This is an exemption from the need to hold a CTC and this scheme has been available since

1981. It was introduced in an attempt to avoid delay to medical research and has the advantage of statutory timelines. Summary data, under the same headings as for a CTC, are submitted and are assessed by assessors from each of the three disciplines on behalf of the Licensing Authority. If the Exemption is granted, it is valid for a period of 3 years. If it is refused then the applicant can submit a revised application, taking account of the reasons for refusal, which are always on safety grounds. This process can be repeated as often as is required until an Exemption can be granted. In the event of a refusal, the applicant also has the option of applying for a CTC. The advantage of the CTX scheme is its speed, since a decision has to be made by the Licensing Authority within 35 days with the possibility of one 28-day extension to this period. The maximum time for determination of a CTX application is therefore 63 days.

7.1.3 Doctors and Dentists Exemption

This is an exemption which is available to doctors or dentists who are undertaking clinical trials initiated by them and not at the request of a pharmaceutical company. Outline information about the trial is required and a decision is made within 21 days. Where the product to be used is unlicensed and is complex, further information may be requested and the 21-day period may be extended.

7.1.4 Clinical Trials on Marketed Products (CTMG)

Where a clinical trial is proposed with a marketed product then the CTMP scheme can be used. This is a streamlined process based on the fact that there are no quality issues with a product that has already been granted a marketing authorization. The applicant submits a copy of the trial protocol, provides information on the investigators and, depending on whether or not the applicant is the marketing authorization holder, information on the procedures for reporting adverse drug reactions. It is only possible to use this approval for UK marketed products. It does not apply to unauthorized products manufactured specifically for trial nor to products that are licensed only in countries other than the UK.

7.2 EU Clinical Trials Directive

With a view to harmonizing the conduct of clinical trials, an EU Directive on clinical trials (2001/20/EC) was finally agreed on 14 December 2000 by the Health Council and was formally adopted in May 2001 with a 3-year transition period for its implementation.

The Directive contains specific provisions regarding the conduct of clinical trials, including multi-centre trials, on human subjects. It sets standards relating to the implementation of Good Clinical Practice and Good Manufacturing Practice with a view to protecting clinical trial subjects. All clinical trials, including bioavailability and bioequivalence studies, shall be designed, conducted and reported in accordance with the principles of good clinical practice. It proposes introduction of procedures in the Community that will provide an environment where new medicines can be developed safely and rapidly. The Directive is very detailed and comprehensive in terms of clarifying ethical and scientific standards.

It defines 'clinical trial' as any investigation in human subjects intended to discover or verify the clinical, pharmacological and/or other pharmacodynamic effects of one or more investigational medicinal product(s), and/or to identify any adverse reactions to one or more investigational medicinal product(s) and/or to study absorption, distribution, metabolism and excretion of one or more investigational medicinal product(s) with the object of ascertaining its (their) safety and/or efficacy. It defines 'subject' as an individual who participates in a clinical trial as either a recipient of the investigational medicinal product or a control. Thus, healthy volunteer studies are included.

The Directive lays down specific obligations for the Member States and proposes drawing up detailed guidance on the application format and documentation to be submitted. The competent authority shall consider a valid request of an application for a clinical trial as rapidly as possible and this period may not exceed

60 days. No further extension to this period shall be permissible except in the case of trials with medicinal products involving gene or cell therapy, for which an extension of a maximum 30 days shall be permitted. For these products, this 90-day period may be extended by a further 90 days under certain circumstances. If the competent authority of the Member State notifies the sponsor of grounds for non-acceptance, the sponsor may, on one occasion only, amend the content of the request to take due account of the grounds given. There are specific measures before commencement and end or early termination of a clinical trial. It is important to note that the Directive allows for 'The Member States may lay down a shorter period than 60 days within their area of responsibility if that is in compliance with current practice' and that 'The competent authority can nevertheless notify the sponsor before the end of this period that it has no grounds for non-acceptance'. The Directive contains detailed articles on conduct of a clinical trial, exchange of information between Member States, EMEA and the Commission, the reasons and procedures for suspension of the trial by a Member State and notification of adverse events including serious adverse reactions.

7.3 Application procedures for marketing authorizations

The marketing authorization holder (MAH) must be established within the European Economic Area (EEA) which consists of the EU plus Norway, Iceland and Liechtenstein.

The applications for national authorizations are submitted to the national competent authority which in the UK is the Licensing Authority (LA), whose functions are discharged by the Medicines and Healthcare products Regulatory Agency (MHRA) of the Department of Health. The LA/MHRA are advised by the Committee on Safety of Medicines (CSM), a multidisciplinary scientific body consisting of clinical, preclinical and pharmaceutical members well known for their expertise in their respective fields. Lay members are also included.

The applications for community authorizations are submitted to the EMEA, based in

Canary Wharf, London. The EMEA is advised by the CPMP, a scientific body which consists of two delegates from each Member State of the EU. These delegates are chosen by reason of their role and experience in the evaluation of medicinal products and they represent their competent authorities and may be accompanied by their experts. In addition to providing objective scientific opinions, these members ensure that there is appropriate coordination between the tasks of EMEA and the work of the competent national authorities, including the consultative bodies. While NASs or innovatory medicinal products *may* use this 'centralized' procedure, all medicinal products developed by biotechnological processes *must* go through this 'centralized' procedure and can be the subject of only the community authorizations.

7.4 UK national authorizations

When an application is received, it is validated to ensure that it is submitted in the correct format with all requirements for contents and procedure satisfied and that the appropriate fees have been paid.

The data are then assessed and an integrated assessment report is prepared for discussion at the CSM. It is possible to appoint special member(s) for the day in case of drugs that require unique expertise at the Committee. Following in-depth discussion, the Committee formulates and communicates to the applicant its *provisional* advice. This may be: (a) a refusal to grant a marketing authorization and the reasons for this decision, (b) grant of a marketing authorization (b) or, as is more often the case (c) grant of a marketing authorization subject to any number of amendments to the SPC and other conditions for data to be provided.

In the event of a refusal or a conditional grant, the applicant has a right of appeal. This appeal is supported by additional data or clarification of concerns from data already available. Most or all of the CSM concerns/conditions may (or may not) be resolved and the outcome following the deliberations of the appeal data is the *final* advice which the CSM communicates to the LA/MHRA. If the applicant is still unhappy with refusal or revised conditions, the only option available to the applicant is an appeal to the Medicines Commission. The Commission will consider only the outstanding issue(s) and their decision is final. If the applicant is still not content with the outcome, the only course open is to seek a judicial review in the High Court. The High Court is concerned primarily with ensuring that the due legal processes were adhered to and is not concerned with the science behind the rejection.

Apart from some differences in detail, similar procedures operate for national authorization in almost all EU Member States.

When an applicant has obtained one national authorization (within an EU country), any ongoing assessment of that product in other EU Member States is suspended and the first authorization granted is entered for mutual recognition by all or selected (depending on the wishes of the applicant) Member States.

7.5 Mutual recognition procedure

Information on the mutual recognition procedure can be accessed from the EC web-site (http://pharmacos.eudra.org/F2/pharmacos/docs.htm).

During this procedure, the original competent authority and the applicant act jointly. The applicant submits an application and the updated dossier to each Member State from whom the applicant seeks a marketing authorization. The original competent authority (now called the Reference Member State, RMS) transmits the assessment report (updated if required) to each Member State (now called the Concerned Member States, CMS), together with the SPC approved by it.

From then on, each CMS treats the application almost as a national application with the important differences that (a) they deal with the RMS in respect of any concerns, queries or need for clarification and (b) the procedure is driven by predetermined immutable deadlines (Fig. 3.1).

By day 50, all CMS are required to have communicated their concerns to the RMS. By day 60, the applicant, with the help of the RMS, responds to all CMS, addressing their concerns and enclosing a revised SPC (that requires approval by the RMS). At day 75, outstanding issues of major concerns are discussed at a face-to-face meeting between the RMS, CMS and applicant. The SPC is still revised further if justified. By day 89, any CMS who still has major public health concerns declares their position and reasons for concerns. The procedure is closed on day 90 with a final revision to SPC and the applicant having withdrawn from those CMS (on average, one or two) who still have major public health concerns. Until the day the procedure is closed, the applicant has the right to withdraw the application from these Member States. If the applicant refuses to withdraw the application from a CMS who has major public health concerns, the CMS has no choice but to refer the application to CPMP for arbitration. The applicant too is free to refer the application to arbitration if it considers some major objections to be unreasonable. The arbitration procedure has its own timetable.

It is easy to see why an SPC coming out of this procedure is usually a highly effective document in terms of the therapeutic claims allowed, a dose schedule which is carefully scrutinized and detailed safety information and/or monitoring requirements. In rare instances, the SPC comes out too restricted or unbalanced because of the differences in medical practices and cultures among the Member States.

Once a product goes through the mutual recognition procedure, all its post-approval activities are undertaken by the same RMS and goes through this procedure.

7.6 Community authorizations

Information on the centralized procedure can be accessed from the EC web-site (http://pharmacos.eudra.org/F2/pharmacos/docs.htm).

Conceptually, the procedure for community authorizations resembles a hybrid of the national procedure and the mutual recognition procedure with the differences that (a) the application is submitted to EMEA, (b) the medicinal product undergoes a detailed assessment

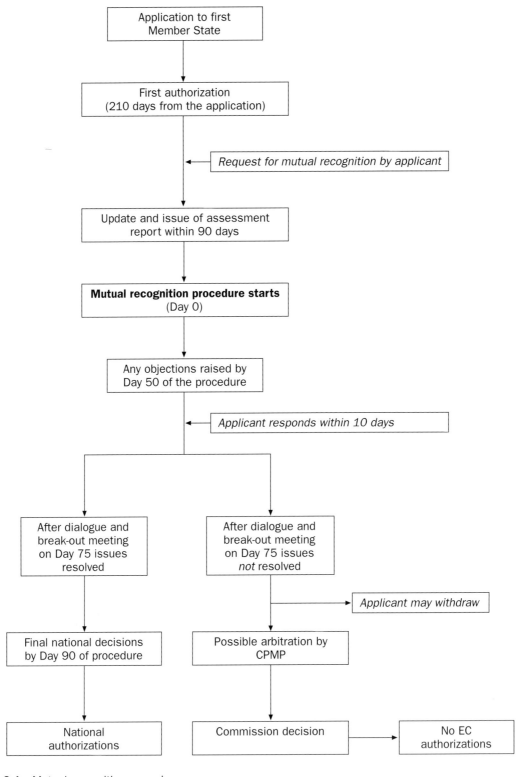

Fig. 3.1 Mutual recognition procedure.

by the CPMP before approval in any Member State of the EU, (c) it provides the applicant with an opportunity for clarifying any issues raised by any of the EU Member States (d) the procedure naturally has an extended time-frame but with predetermined deadlines and (e) the applicant ends up with an approval or a refusal to market the product in all or any Member States of the EU.

The CPMP appoints one of its members to act as Rapporteur for the coordination of the evaluation of an application for a marketing authorization. In such cases, the CPMP will also appoint a second member to act as Co-Rapporteur.

A member of staff of the Human Medicines Evaluation Unit of the EMEA is officially appointed as EMEA project manager and the applicant is notified of the project manager's identity. The project manager remains responsible for providing procedural guidance during the pre-submission phase, coordinating the validation of the application submitted, monitoring compliance with the time-frame and coordinating all the activities (between the applicant, EMEA, CPMP and the Rapporteurs) with regard to the progression and final determination of the application.

On receipt of a valid application by EMEA, the Rapporteur and the Co-Rapporteur both prepare their separate detailed assessment reports which are circulated to the EMEA and other Member States by day 70 of the start of the procedure (Fig. 3.2). By day 100, the Rapporteur, Co-Rapporteur, other CPMP members and EMEA receive comments from members of the CPMP. A draft Consolidated List of Questions is prepared by the Rapporteur and circulated to the members by day 115. A final Consolidated List of Questions is agreed by the CPMP on day 120 and communicated to the applicant and the clock of the procedure is stopped. This Consolidated List includes any major public health concerns, points for clarification and changes to the SPC, raised by all the Member States. The applicant, after seeking clarification from the Rapporteur if necessary, responds to these issues (the maximum time allowed for responding is no longer than

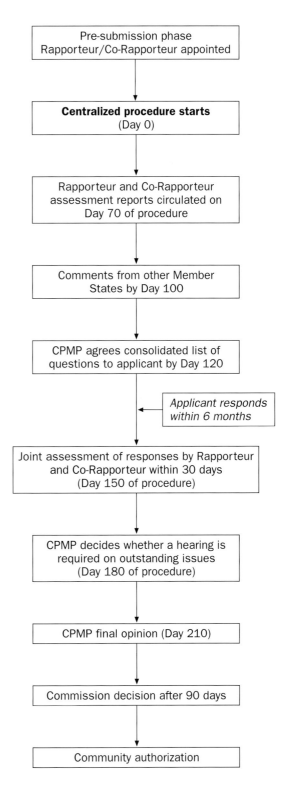

Fig. 3.2 Centralized procedure.

6 months) and the clock is re-started. The Rapporteur and the Co-Rapporteur prepare a joint assessment of responses which is circulated by day 150 to all members of the CPMP. The deadline for comments from CPMP members to be sent to Rapporteur and Co-Rapporteur, EMEA and other CPMP members is day 170. Any issue(s) still outstanding are discussed on day 180 of the procedure at the CPMP. These are communicated to the applicant and may be addressed at a hearing before the CPMP and a decision is made on whether to issue a positive or a negative opinion. The deadline for adopting an opinion is day 210 of the procedure. A positive opinion requires at least 16 positive votes in support; otherwise a negative opinion is issued.

A negative opinion may be the subject of an appeal, a procedure that has its own time-frame. The EMEA immediately informs the applicant when the opinion of the CPMP is that the application does not satisfy the criteria for authorization set out in the Regulation. The following documents are annexed and/or appended to the opinion: (a) the appended CPMP assessment report stating the reasons for its negative conclusions and (b) when appropriate, the divergent positions of committee members with their grounds. The applicant may notify the EMEA/CPMP of their intention to appeal within 15 days of receipt of the opinion (after which if the applicant does not appeal, the applicant is deemed to have agreed with the opinion and it becomes final opinion). The grounds for appeal must be forwarded to the EMEA within 60 days of receipt of the opinion. If the applicant wishes to appear before the CPMP for an oral explanation, this request should also be sent at this stage. The CPMP may decide to appoint a new Rapporteur and Co-Rapporteur, for whom applicants can express their preference, to coordinate the appeal procedure, accompanied if necessary by additional experts. Within 60 days from the receipt of the grounds for appeal, the CPMP will consider whether its opinion is to be revised. If considered necessary, an oral explanation can be held within this 60-day time-frame. Once the CPMP issues a final opinion, it

is forwarded (with the required annexes) within 30 days of its adoption to the Commission, the Member States, Norway and Iceland and the applicant, stating the reasons for its conclusion.

The opinion is issued by the CPMP and is transmitted to the European Commission, which issues a decision that is binding upon all Member States.

Once a product goes through the centralized procedure, all its post-approval activities are undertaken by the same Rapporteur and goes through this procedure.

7.7 Review 2001

Regarding all activities for the regulation of the pharmaceuticals at the EU level, Article 71 of Regulation EEC/2309/93 required that 'Within six years of the entry into force of this Regulation, the Commission shall publish a general report on the experience of the procedures laid down in this Regulation, in Chapter III of Directive 75/319/EEC and in Chapter IV of Directive 81/851/EEC'. The tender was awarded to a consortium of Cameron McKenna and Arthur Anderson. The general objectives of the review were to provide answers to the following questions:

- Have the centralized and decentralized procedures contributed in a qualitative and quantitative sense to the creation of a harmonized Community market in medicinal products?
- Have these procedures provided a high degree of safety of use for patients? Is the quality of the evaluation carried out in the two procedures of a comparable level?
- Have the availability of the new medicinal products and patients' access to such products been improved by the introduction of the new Community system and are they satisfactory at the present time?
- What are the benefits of the two procedures (cost-benefit ratio)? Are they carried out with sufficient transparency?

The full Report from Cameron McKenna 'Evaluation of the Operation of Community

Procedures for the Authorization of Medicinal Products' is a comprehensive and highly constructive document and all interested parties have formulated and discussed a number of strategies aimed at further improving the regulatory requirements and control for marketing authorizations for new medicinal products in the EU. The EC has already proposed a comprehensive set of reforms to the two pivotal pieces of legislation (Council Regulation EEC/2309/93 and Directive 2001/83/EC) (see postscript below)

8. CONCLUSIONS

For all practical purposes, the most important document is the SPC. Its terms are carefully scrutinized by the competent authority in light of the dossier accompanying the application. The approved SPC sets out the agreed position of the medicinal product as distilled during the course of the assessment process. It is the definitive statement between the competent authority and the marketing authorization holder and it is the common basis of communication between the competent authorities of all Member States. As such, the content cannot be changed except with the approval of the originating competent authority. The agreed SPC forms the basis for subsequent marketing of the medicinal product and all information that may/should be made available to health professionals and patients.

Involving as it does the scrutiny of pharmaceutical, preclinical and clinical assessors from each of the Member States, the Euro-SPC of an NAS is a highly effective document, doing full justice to the efficacy of the product and delineating precise indications and dose schedules for its clinical use, while providing all information aimed at or necessary for safeguarding the public.

The marketing authorization holder needs the approval of the competent authority should it wish to vary the terms of the SPC. Such variations require supporting data.

There are, of course, special provisions when a Member State can suspend or revoke an authorization where the product proves to be harmful in the normal conditions of use or where its therapeutic efficacy is found to be lacking or where its qualitative and quantitative composition is not as declared. An authorization may also be suspended or revoked where the particulars in the dossier are incorrect or have not been amended or when the controls on finished product have not been carried out.

During its first reading in October 2002 of the proposed changes to the pharmaceutical legislation, the European Parliament had already approved 144 of the 167 amendments to Regulation EEC/2309/93 and 160 of the 202 amendments to Directive 2001/83/EC. It is anticipated that these changes will result in an even more robust and efficient system of regulatory controls for human medicinal products in the EU.

POSTSCRIPT

Throughout the text, we have referred to various pieces of legislation by their original reference. However, these have been frequently amended. Therefore, for clarity, a whole range of the latest versions of the Directives was codified by assembling them in a single text that is known as Directive 2001/83/EC of 6 November 2001. Therefore, the reader should also refer to Directive 2001/83/EC which codifies the following:

Council Directive 65/65/EEC
Council Directive 75/318/EEC
Council Directive 75/319/EEC
Council Directive 89/342/EEC
Council Directive 89/343/EEC
Council Directive 89/381/EEC
Council Directive 92/25/EEC
Council Directive 92/26/EEC
Council Directive 92/27/EEC
Council Directive 92/28/EEC
Council Directive 92/73/EEC

Directive 2001/83/EC can be accessed at:
http://www.emea.eu.int/htms/human/qrd/qrdlegal.htm

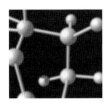

Section 2

Clinical Pharmacology

4

Principles of pharmacokinetics

Andrew G Renwick

Summary • Introduction • The different approaches to pharmacokinetic analysis • Non-compartmental analysis – a combination of physiological insights and data fitting • Conclusions and future directions • Abbreviations • References

SUMMARY

This chapter provides an introduction to the basic principles of pharmacokinetics. It describes both the biology of the processes and how the plasma concentration-time curve data can be analysed to extract appropriate pharmacokinetic parameters. The concepts discussed apply mainly to the fate of low molecular weight, organic molecules and other processes will be involved in the biodisposition of therapeutic macromolecules.

1. INTRODUCTION

The term 'pharmacokinetics' describes the movement of a drug or medicine around the body, and therefore relates to its absorption from the site of administration, its distribution around the body, and its elimination, usually by either metabolism or excretion. The relationship between the external dose of a drug and the therapeutic response can be divided into two aspects (Fig. 4.1); *pharmacokinetics*, which relates to the delivery of the chemical to its site of action, and *pharmacodynamics*, which relates to the interaction between the drug at its site of

action and the final therapeutic outcome or pharmacological response. There are a large number of factors that can influence the relationship between the external dose and that delivered to the site of action. The extent of inter-patient variability in pharmacokinetics is similar to the variability in pharmacodynamics,[1] so that pharmacokinetics are important in determining the magnitude of clinical response in a patient. Factors that can have a significant influence on pharmacokinetics include age (both the very young[2] and the elderly[3]), renal and liver disease,[4] pregnancy,[5,6] gender (to a minor extent in humans[7]), ethnicity[8] and food.[9–11] There are major differences in pharmacokinetics between humans and the animal species normally used in toxicity tests,[12] so that the interpretation of animal studies and their extrapolation to humans requires considerable expertise.[13] The doses used initially in Phase I human studies are normally at least an order of magnitude below doses that do not produce effects in test animals, and the human doses are then escalated until a response is seen. Prediction of the expected pharmacokinetics in humans can increase confidence in dose selection for 'first-into-man' studies.

Determination of the pharmacokinetics of a

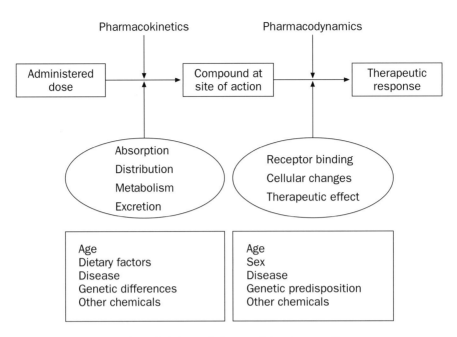

Fig. 4.1 The relationship between the administered dose and the therapeutic response.

drug requires the definition of the concentration time course for the drug in the body (Fig. 4.2), and therefore is based on measurements of the time course for the changes in drug concentration in accessible body fluids, such as blood and urine. The different processes of absorption, distribution and elimination (Fig. 4.3) can

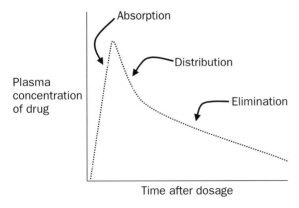

Fig. 4.2 Theoretical plasma drug concentration–time curve after a single oral dose.

be characterized from an analysis of the increases and decreases in the concentrations of the drug present in such body fluids. Early studies on the fate of drugs in the human body simply defined the extent of absorption, metabolism and elimination by measurement of the drug and its metabolites in urine and faeces with occasional, but not systematic, measurements of the concentrations in the general circulation. Such data were not adequate to define the rates or extents of the different processes shown in Fig. 4.3. The subsequent development of pharmacokinetics as a subject was dependent on the development of analytical methods that were able to measure the low concentrations of the drug present in the plasma, and the generation of mathematical models able to describe the increases and decreases in concentrations measured. An additional impetus to the study of pharmacokinetics was the development of automated analytical facilities capable of processing the large number of samples that are developed as a result of the multiple sequential blood sampling, which is a feature of pharmacokinetic studies. The development of an ade-

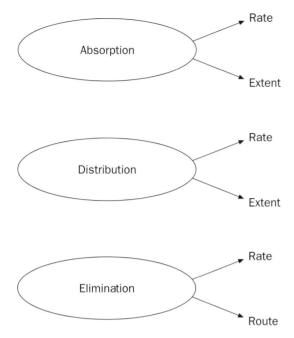

Fig. 4.3 The fundamental processes that determine the nature of the plasma concentration-time for a drug and its pharmacokinetic properties.

partmental analytical method (see below), combined with measurements such as the area under the plasma concentration-time curve (AUC). The output of such models includes the parameters that are the most frequently reported, such as bioavailability, clearance, elimination half-life and the apparent volume of distribution. These parameters are particularly useful because they determine drug dosage regimens, and in addition reflect physiological changes in drug disposition that may be produced by a variety of clinical conditions. Prediction of human pharmacokinetics from animal studies can be undertaken by simply scaling the different pharmacokinetic parameters (Y) in animals according to body weight (W) raised to a power function ($Y = aW^b$) to reflect intermediary metabolism, surface area or can be derived empirically from the available animal data.[13]

quate analytical method is critical to the generation of valid pharmacokinetic data, and a number of aspects have to be taken into consideration (Table 4.1).

2. THE DIFFERENT APPROACHES TO PHARMACOKINETIC ANALYSIS

Historically, three different approaches have been used to analyse the plasma concentration-time curves to define the basic processes described in Fig. 4.3.

2.1 Non-compartmental analysis

In non-compartmental analysis the pharmacokinetics of the drug are described by parameters that reflect the processes given in Fig. 4.3. The parameters are derived by a combination of determining the terminal rate constant from the concentration-time curve by a process equivalent to a simplified version of the multi-com-

2.2 Multi-compartmental analysis

Compartmental analysis involves the fitting of simultaneous exponential equations to the plasma concentration-time curve data, without an a priori determination of the relationship between the rate constant and any physiological or metabolic processes. As illustrated in Fig. 4.4, the entry of the drug into the system is usually

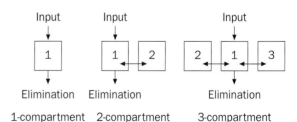

Fig. 4.4 Simple multi-compartmental models. The number of exponential terms required to fit the model to the data determines the number of compartments. The one-compartment model would require two exponentials (to describe input and output), whereas the two-compartment model would require three exponential terms. Most therapeutic drugs require a two- or three-compartment model.

Table 4.1   Aspects of the analytical method used in pharmacokinetic studies

Aspect	Parameter	Comments
Chemical moiety measured	Parent compound	It is usual for the pharmacokinetics of a compound to be defined in relation to the concentrations of parent compound in the biological sample(s). This is of greatest relevance when the parent compound is the active pharmacological agent.
	Active metabolite	The circulating concentrations of an active metabolite are the most relevant measurement in the case of a pro-drug that undergoes extensive first-pass metabolism during absorption. Under these circumstances the pharmacokinetic parameters should be defined as relating to the metabolite not to the parent compound (but this needs to be defined clearly in data reporting).
	Inactive metabolites	The measurement of inactive metabolites is not an important part of pharmacokinetic measurements, and the main criterion is that the analytical method should clearly separate the parent compound from its metabolites. Methods that measure both parent drug and inactive metabolites will not produce valid pharmacokinetic measurements.
	Stereoisomers	Many drugs possess an asymmetric carbon atom and exist as optical isomers. In some cases the therapeutic activity resides with one of the two isomers, and there may be major differences in the metabolism and pharmacokinetics of the two isomers. An analytical method that measures the racemic compound (both optical isomers) may be misleading because the quantitation of drug would be for both active and inactive isomers, and the terminal half-life could in some cases may be determined primarily by the inactive isomer (and therefore irrelevant).
Biological sample	Plasma	The vast majority of pharmacokinetic analyses are based on measurements of the total concentration of drug in plasma (free plus protein-bound). Because the unbound and bound drug concentrations are in essentially instantaneous equilibrium, any process that actively adds drug to or removes drug from the plasma will increase both free and bound drug proportionately. Free concentrations of drug can sometimes provide valuable additional information and this is normally specified in the description of the pharmacokinetic parameter. Measurements based on free drug may be particularly valuable when patients show altered plasma protein-binding (e.g. in pregnancy), so that there is a different relationship between the total concentration and the free concentration able to interact with the target site.

Table 4.1 Continued

Aspect	Parameter	Comments
	Blood	Analysis of drug concentrations in blood is less common than in plasma, primarily because there is the potential for the compound to enter and to be sequestered into erythrocytes, such that the total concentration in blood will not adequately represent changes in the concentration in plasma. (In other words, the blood compartment could contain elements of both rapidly and slowly equilibrating compartments – see later).
	Urine	Measurements of the concentrations of drug and its metabolites in urine can provide valuable information on the role of the kidneys in the elimination of the compound, but do not provide information on the concentrations delivered to the target site. Because the concentration in the urine reflects the concentration in plasma, sequential analysis of urinary samples can be used to describe the rates of absorption and elimination.
Analytical method	Specificity Sensitivity	The analytical method must measure only the compound of interest (see above). The method must be able to define adequately the terminal elimination phase of the plasma concentration-time curve.

described by a simple rate constant, which may be either first-order or zero-order (see below). In most models the drug is assumed to enter a central compartment (the equivalent to blood plus rapidly equilibrating tissues), before distributing into a second compartment (usually representing slowly equilibrating, poorly perfused tissues). Elimination is normally from the central compartment and is usually assumed to be a first-order reaction (see later). A strength of compartmental analysis is that it allows the plasma concentration-time curve data to be extrapolated, so that the concentration present at any time after dosing can be calculated from the model fitted to the experimental data. A disadvantage of compartmental analysis is that it is not readily related numerically to physiological or metabolic processes that occur within the body. In addition, it is not easy to predict the influence of diseases on drug disposition with this approach.

2.3 Physiologically based pharmacokinetic models (PBPK models)

PBPK models, as illustrated in Fig. 4.5, use a series of equations to describe each of the processes involved in the absorption, distribution and elimination of the compound. The absorption rate is based on the physicochemical properties of the compound and the site of administration; distribution is described by a series of equations relating to the blood flow (Q) to the major body organs, and the partition coefficient for the uptake of the chemical by the tissue (usually measured from in vitro studies); elimination is described by appropriate rate constants, which can include Michaelis-Menten constants. The development of such a model requires a detailed understanding of the biological fate of a chemical in the body, for example, the sites of tissue distribution and the enzymes involved in its elimination. Thus a large amount of chemical-specific information is necessary to develop an appropriate physiologically based model before comparing the output of the model with the actual measured plasma concentration-time curve. In consequence, PBPK modelling has not been applied to any

great extent to the clinical pharmacokinetics of therapeutic drugs, primarily because there is inadequate definition of many of the physiological and metabolic variables that would be an inherent part of any model that would be useful for clinical conditions. PBPK modelling has been used most in relation to the analysis of data deriving from animal toxicity studies and their extrapolation to potential human exposures. Because of the complexity of the numerous tissue compartments with their blood flow and partition coefficients, it is usual to combine or pool tissues that share similar perfusion rates and partition coefficients, as illustrated in Fig. 4.5. Human pharmacokinetics can be predicted based on the incorporation of in vitro data on enzyme activity and partition coefficients and in vivo physiological data into a PBPK model.[14] Studies on drug metabolism and predicted pharmacokinetics are increasingly important at an early stage of drug design and develop-

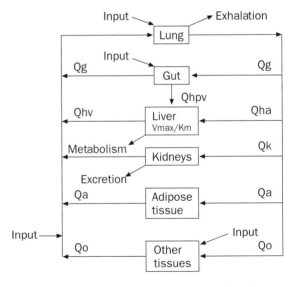

Fig. 4.5 Physiologically based pharmacokinetic models. The model requires general information on organ volume and blood flows plus drug-specific data on tissue affinity, partitioning and rates of metabolism. The model can be refined in relation to the delivery of the compound to specific sites of action, providing that the blood flow and partition coefficients for that site are known.

ment,[15] and there have been important recent developments in high-throughput screening for these aspects.[16]

3. NON-COMPARTMENTAL ANALYSIS – A COMBINATION OF PHYSIOLOGICAL INSIGHTS AND DATA FITTING

The following text describes the processes in Fig. 4.3 in relation to their underlying biology, and the derivation of appropriate pharmacokinetic parameters using primarily non-compartmental methods. The plasma concentration-time curve presented in Fig. 4.2 is represented as a series of sequential processes; however, in reality as soon as any of the dose has been absorbed it will be undergoing both distribution to tissues and elimination. In consequence, the processes in Fig. 4.2 are occurring concurrently, as indicated in Fig. 4.6, and in order to be able to analyse absorption or distribution it is necessary to separate the contribution of the elimination process from the absorption process. Because the rate of elimination is (usually) slower than either absorption or distribution, these processes will be essentially complete long before elimination, and therefore later time points are determined by the elimination rate constant only. In consequence, the following text starts with a description of the elimination of drugs from the general circulation and subsequently considers

the distribution of drugs to tissues and then their absorption from the site of administration into the general circulation. The text describes both the biology of the processes and how the plasma concentration-time curve data can be analysed to extract appropriate pharmacokinetic parameters. The descriptive text relates primarily to the fate of low molecular weight, organic molecules, and readers should be aware that other processes will be involved in the biodisposition of therapeutic macromolecules.

3.1 The elimination of drugs and elimination rate constants

3.1.1 The biological processes involved in the elimination of drugs
The processes involved in the elimination of drugs from the general circulation depend on the physicochemical properties of the molecule (Table 4.2).

3.1.1.1 Elimination via the airways
The principal determinant of the extent of elimination of volatile compounds via the airways is the partition coefficient between plasma and alveolar air in comparison with the partitioning of the chemical into adipose tissue, and its elimination via other processes such as metabolism. The blood:gas partition coefficient ranges from <1 for nitrous oxide to 10–14 for methoxyflurane (Table 4.3). In general, compounds with a high blood:gas partition coefficient also show high oil:gas partitioning and such anaesthetics are retained in the body to a greater extent, and there is a decrease in the percentage eliminated in the expired air accompanied by an increase in the extent of metabolism. In the case of halothane its retention is associated with hepatic metabolism, which can occasionally result in toxicity.

3.1.1.2 Metabolism
The elimination of low molecular weight, lipid-soluble compounds involves metabolism by pathways that have evolved for the removal of unwanted foreign chemicals that enter the body from the diet and the environment. Drug

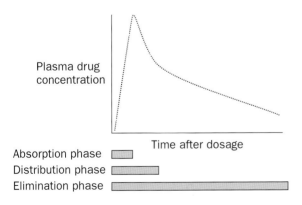

Fig. 4.6 Theoretical plasma drug concentration–time curve after a single oral dose.

Table 4.2 Biological processes involved in the elimination of drugs

Physicochemical characteristics	Principal route of elimination
Low molecular weight volatile compounds	Volatile compounds are administered via inhalation and they are eliminated, at least in part, in the expired air at the end of the treatment period. Volatile drugs tend to be lipid-soluble molecules and may also undergo metabolism.
Low molecular weight lipid-soluble drugs	Lipid-soluble compounds are not rapidly eliminated from the body and will tend to accumulate in adipose tissue. Elimination of such molecules is dependent on their conversion in the body, via metabolism, into water-soluble excretory products. The products of metabolism are usually eliminated from the body either in the urine or in the bile.
Low molecular weight water-soluble compounds	Water-soluble drugs are usually eliminated unchanged in urine.
High molecular weight organic compounds	Large molecules (> 500 Da) are eliminated largely in the bile.
Macromolecules	Macromolecules may be eliminated from the body by a combination of hydrolysis within the circulation, and uptake and degradation by the liver and other processes involved in the removal of foreign proteins.

Table 4.3 The relationship between physicochemical properties of general anaesthetics and the extent of their elimination by exhalation

Anaesthetic	Blood:gas partition coefficient	Oil:gas partition coefficient	Percentage eliminated in exhaled air
Nitrous oxide	0.47	1.4	100
Sevoflurane	0.65	50	95
Isoflurane	1.4	91	95
Enflurane	1.9	99	80
Halothane	2.3	224	60–80
Methoxyflurane	10–14	825–970	20

Data abstracted from the 'Clinical pharmacology' web-site (http://www.cp.gsm.com/fromcpo.asp).

metabolism characteristically involves two phases, an initial phase I reaction, usually oxidation, reduction or hydrolysis, following by a phase II reaction in which a normal cell constituent is covalently bound to the drug molecule, thereby increasing its water solubility and/or masking active functional groups.

By far the most important enzyme system involved in the oxidation of drugs is the microsomal cytochrome P450 family (Table 4.4). The cytochrome P450s are a family of membrane-bound enzymes[17] present in the smooth endoplasmic reticulum, which have an affinity for drug substrates and molecular oxygen (because they are haemoproteins). They catalyze the oxidation of drugs, usually at specific parts of the drug molecule, and may produce a number of different metabolites. The enzymes may be induced by certain other drugs and by some environmental chemicals, and may be inhibited by different drugs[18,19] (see Table 4.5). The basal expression of enzyme activity is determined genetically (see Chapter 5). Some of the forms of cytochrome P450, for example CYP2D6 and CYP2C19, show genetic polymorphism, such that some individuals will have an impaired ability to oxidize substrates for these particular isoenzymes.[20] CYP3A4 is the most abundant form of cytochrome P450 in both the liver and the intestine and shows wide inter-individual variability.[21]

In addition to cytochrome P450-mediated reactions, there are a variety of other phase I enzymes that can metabolize drugs, including esterases, proteases, reductases, flavine mono-oxygenases, and enzymes involved in the metabolism of specific structural groups, e.g. monoamine oxidase and alcohol dehydrogenase.

The Phase II or conjugation reactions involve the addition of an endogenous functional group, such as glucuronic acid, sulphate, acetyl, methyl-, or amino-acid group to the drug structure. The different processes are summarized in Table 4.6. The synthesis of a chemical bond between the drug and the endogenous compound requires the introduction of energy in the form of a high energy compound; in most cases it is the endogenous substrate that is activated. However, for amino-acid conjugation the drug forms a high energy drug–CoA complex which then interacts with the amino-acid to form, for example, a glycine conjugate. Glucuronidation is probably the most important Phase II enzyme; it is located in the

---

Table 4.4   The P450 gene superfamily

Component	Comments
Cytochromes P450	1.4 billion years; 1% change per $2–4 \times 10^6$ years
Families 1–4	Hepatic microsomal enzymes
Families 17, 19, 21, 22	Steroid biosynthesis
CYP1A	Induced by benzo [a] pyrene; substrate – aromatics
CYP2A	Induced by benzo [a] pyrene; substrate – testosterone
CYP2B	Induced by phenobarbitone – many substrates
CYP2C	Constitutive – many substrates
CYP2D	Debrisoquine hydroxylation (CYP2D6)
CYP2E	Ethanol-induced
CYP3A	Many substrates – cyclosporine/nifedipine
CYP4	Clofibrate-induced (in rodents)

Table 4.5 Interactions affecting cytochrome P450

P450	Substrate	Inducer	Inhibitor
CYP1A2	Caffeine Phenacetin Theophylline	Polycyclics Omeprazole	Fluoroquinolones Fluvoxamine
CYP2A6	Coumarin		
CYP2C9	Ethoxycoumarin Phenytoin S-Warfarin	Rifampicin Phenobarbitone	Amiodarone Ketoconazole Sulphenazole
CYP2C19	S-Mephenytoin Omeprazole	Rifampicin Phenobarbitone	Omeprazole Fluoxetine
CYP2D6	Debrisoquine Dextromethorphan		Quinidine
CYP2E1	Ethanol Paracetamol	Ethanol Acetone	Disulfiram
CYP3A4	Terfenadine Nifedipine Erythromycin	Rifampicin Carbamazepine Dexamethazone	Erythromycin Ketoconazole

Table 4.6 The main drug conjugation reactions

Reaction	Activated species	Functional group	Product
Glucuronidation	UDP-Glucuronic acid	$-OH$, $-COOH$ $-NH_2$	Drug$-C_6H_9O_6$
Sulphation	PAPS	$-OH$, $-NH_2$	Drug$-O-SO_3^-$ Drug$-NH-SO_3^-$
Acetylation	Acetyl–CoA	$-NH_2$, $NHNH_2$	Drug$-NH-COCH_3$
Methylation	S-Adenosyl methionine	$-OH$, $-NH_2$	Drug$-O-CH_3$ Drug$-NH-CH_3$
Amino-acid conjugation	Drug–CoA complex	$-COOH$	Drug$-CO-NH-AA$

endoplasmic reticulum and conjugates many of the metabolites formed by cytochrome P450. It is present in the liver and intestines and can be induced by certain pretreatments.[22,23]

3.1.1.3 Renal excretion

The renal excretion of water-soluble drugs and their metabolites may involve three processes: glomerular filtration and renal tubular secretion,[24,25] which serve to transfer the drug from the blood to the renal tubule contents, and passive reabsorption, which is a pH-dependent process transferring drug from the renal tubule back into plasma. This last process depends on the lipid solubility of the molecule and is the reason why lipid-soluble molecules are not excreted in the urine. In recent years there has been increased interest in the functioning of drug transporters, such as P-glycoprotein, in the kidney, intestine and other organs,[26,27] and as a mechanism of resistance in cancer cells.[28,29] Such transporters can be important sites for drug interactions.[30]

3.1.1.4 Biliary excretion

Drugs and drug conjugates that have a molecular weight greater than about 500 Da are eliminated in bile, rather than urine. Drug conjugates that are excreted in bile may undergo hydrolysis by the bacterial flora of the lower bowel, and the drug may be reabsorbed into the circulation, a process known as enterohepatic circulation.[31] Enterohepatic recirculation in humans is characterized by the presence of secondary peaks in the plasma concentration-time curve after about 6–12 hours. These arise because the drug conjugate is released into the intestine episodically as the gall bladder contracts, and this results in a bolus of drug conjugate undergoing hydrolysis and reabsorption. Enterohepatic recycling has the effect of reducing the drug clearance, by increasing the area under the plasma concentration-time curve (see below).

3.1.2 Clearance and processes involved in removing the drug from the body

Each of the processes given above can be described in terms of a blood flow to the organ performing the elimination process combined with an ability of that organ of elimination to extract and eliminate the drug molecule. Elimination of the drug can be achieved by either removal of that molecule from the body in exhaled air, urine or bile, or conversion of the drug molecule into a metabolite that is no longer measured by the analytical method (see Table 4.1). Most biochemical and physiological processes are first-order reactions at low concentrations (see Fig. 4.7) and therefore the rate of elimination from the body by any process is proportional to the plasma concentration. This proportionality (for first-order process – see Fig. 4.7) can be expressed as an equation:

$$\text{Clearance} = \frac{\text{rate of elimination by that process}}{\text{plasma concentration}}$$

The concept of clearance[32,33] is most easily illustrated by the clearance of drugs by the kidneys, because renal clearance (CL_R) can be calculated directly from measurements of the concentration of the drug in urine, the urine flow and the plasma concentration, as illustrated in Fig. 4.8. Theoretically, the clearance by hepatic metabolism could be measured as:

$$\frac{\text{Rate of hepatic metabolism}}{\text{Plasma concentration}}$$

However, in reality the rate of hepatic metabolism cannot be measured readily, and metabolic clearance in vivo has to be estimated as the difference between plasma clearance and renal clearance. Hepatic metabolic clearance can be estimated from in vitro data on enzyme activity, combined with physiological scaling for liver weight and blood flow.[34,35]

Plasma clearance is the most valuable and relevant clearance parameter because it represents the sum of all the different clearance processes. Plasma clearance is calculated as indicated in Fig. 4.9. Plasma clearance reflects the abilities of all the organs of elimination to remove the drug from the body, and the total dose that is used in the calculation of clearance must be 100% available to the organs of elimination, and therefore has to be given intravenously. Because plasma clearance represents the sum of all clearance processes it is one of the main pharmacokinetic parameters that

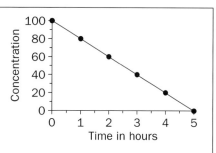

(a) Zero-order reactions

The rate is constant and independent of concentration

$$-\frac{dC}{dt} = k$$

(b) First-order reactions

The rate is proportional to concentration

$$-\frac{dC}{dt} = k \times conc.$$

$$\frac{dC}{dt} = -k \times C_t \qquad \begin{aligned} C_t &= \text{concentration} \\ &\quad \text{at time} = t \\ k &= \text{rate constant} \\ t &= \text{time} \end{aligned}$$

or

$$C_t = C_0 \times e^{-kt} \qquad \begin{aligned} C_0 &= \text{concentration at time zero} \\ e &= \text{exponential} \end{aligned}$$

Taking natural logarithms

$$\ln C_t = \ln C_0 - kt$$

A plot of C_t against t on a log scale will be a straight line

Intercept = C_0
Slope = $-k$

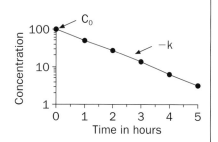

Fig. 4.7 Zero- and first-order reactions. (a) Zero-order reactions proceed at a fixed and constant rate and are seen at high doses when an enzymic reaction is saturated. (b) First-order reactions are a characteristic of passive diffusion and of most metabolic and physiological processes at low (non-saturating) substrate concentrations.

$$CL_R = \frac{Cu \times Fu}{C} \qquad \begin{aligned} Cu &= \text{concentration in urine} \\ Fu &= \text{urine flow} \\ C &= \text{plasma concentration} \end{aligned}$$

For weak acids and bases, the ratio Cu/C is dependent on urine pH; therefore CL_R can be altered by changes in urine pH

CL_R = can also be calculated as:

$$CL_R = \frac{\text{Amount excreted in urine as unchanged parent drug}}{\text{AUC}}$$

provided that the urinary excretion and the AUC (see later) relate to the same time interval

Fig. 4.8 Calculation of renal clearance (CL_R) from plasma and urine data.

$$CL = \frac{\text{rate of elimination from the body}}{\text{plasma concentration}}$$

CL is calculated as $\dfrac{\text{dose}_{\text{intravenous}}}{\text{AUC}_{0-\text{infinity}}}$

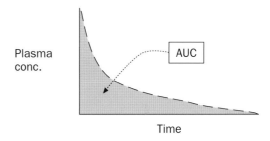

- is independent of concentration or dose

- is a specific value for each drug

- depends on how good the body is at eliminating that drug

- is the volume of plasma cleared of drug per minute (or per hour)

- is the parameter that best reflects the relationship between the blood and the organs of elimination

- for many drugs equals the sum of metabolic clearance and renal clearance

$$CL_{\text{plasma}} = CL_{\text{metabolic}} + CL_{\text{renal}} + CL_{\text{etc.}}$$

- approaches liver blood flow for very rapidly metabolized drugs (1500 ml/min)

- approaches renal blood flow for drugs secreted by the renal tubule (650 ml/min)

- approaches glomerular filtration rate for drugs eliminated by filtration (120–130 ml/min)

Fig. 4.9 Plasma clearance (CL), its calculation and characteristics.

determines the slope of the terminal plasma concentration-time curve, which in turn determines dose interval and prescribing practice.

3.1.2.1 Elimination half-life

The half-life of a drug is the most frequently reported pharmacokinetic parameter, and is perhaps the term most easily understood. The term 'half-life' refers to the time taken for the plasma concentration to decrease by 50% during the terminal log-linear decrease in the plasma concentration-time curve. It is related to the rate constant for the exponential decrease by:

$$t\tfrac{1}{2} = \frac{0.693}{\lambda_z}$$

where λ_z refers to the slope of the terminal phase. The usual convention is to describe the terminal slope for a one-compartment model as k and for a two-compartment model as β (the initial slope is termed α). For three or more compartments it is usual to describe the rates as $\lambda_1, \lambda_2, \lambda_3$, etc. to λ_z, where λ_1 is the fastest rate, λ_2 the next fastest rate, etc. The data for many drugs can be fitted by a simple two-compart-

ment model (see Fig. 4.4), for which the two exponential rate constants after an intravenous bolus dose are described as α and β (see later).

The terminal half-life is inversely proportional to the clearance of the drug because the greater the ability of the organs of elimination to remove the drug (the clearance) from the circulation, the shorter will be the time taken for plasma concentrations to decrease by 50% (the half-life). However, clearance processes can act only on the concentrations and amounts of drug that remain in the circulation after distribution, i.e. the proportion of the total body load that is present in the general circulation. If a drug shows extensive distribution to slowly equilibrating compartments such as the adipose tissue (Fig. 4.5) or compartments 2 or 3 in a multi-compartment model (Fig. 4.4), then mobilization of the drug from these compartments will become an important factor influencing the overall rate of elimination from the body and therefore the half-life (Fig. 4.10). The parameter that describes the extent of reversible distribution from plasma into tissues is the apparent volume of distribution.

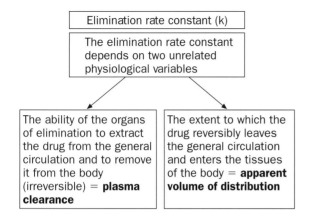

Fig. 4.10 Factors determining the elimination half-life of a drug.

3.2 Distribution of drugs

Drug distribution relates to the *reversible* movement of drug from the systemic circulation into the body tissues. Uptake into an organ that results in elimination is part of the clearance process, because the drug is not available to re-enter the circulation if the blood levels were to decrease.

3.2.1 Biological processes involved in drug distribution

The rate of drug distribution (Fig. 4.3) is determined by the rate for uptake from the general circulation into those tissues that have a high affinity for the drug. For water-soluble drugs the rate of diffusion across the cell membrane into well-perfused tissues may be rate limiting. For lipid-soluble drugs the primary determinant of the rate of distribution is the rate of blood flow to those body tissues that have a high affinity for the drug, for example, adipose tissue. The rate of entry and removal from adipose tissue is largely determined by the perfusion rate of the tissue, rather than the diffusion rate of the drug into and out of the cells. Body tissues may be subdivided into well-perfused tissues such as the lungs, kidneys, liver, heart and brain, which all have perfusion rates >0.5 ml/g tissue per minute, and poorly perfused tissues such as fat, resting muscle, skin

and bone, which have perfusion rates of 0.02–0.03 ml/g tissue per minute. The rate of distribution depends on the relative uptake by well-perfused and poorly perfused tissues, and this would influence the initial slope following an intravenous bolus dose (see Fig. 4.11).

The extent of distribution of a drug between plasma and body tissues depends on the relative affinity of the drug for plasma and tissue. Factors that can influence partitioning into tissues include plasma protein binding,[36] tissue protein binding, dissolution in plasma lipids and dissolution in tissue and cell lipids. Compounds with more extensive tissue uptake will show a more extensive decrease in plasma concentrations during the distribution phase and lower plasma concentrations before equilibration and during the elimination phase (Fig. 4.11). Plasma protein binding may be altered by liver disease[37] and renal disease[38] via changes in serum albumin, while inflammatory diseases can influence the concentrations of α_1-acid glycoprotein, which binds basic drugs.[39]

3.2.2 The rate of distribution

When a drug concentration-time curve fits a single compartment model (Fig. 4.4) there is essentially instantaneous distribution between the blood and all body tissues, so that a discrete distribution phase is not detected (Fig. 4.12). However, for the majority of drugs distribution into slowly perfused tissues results in a discrete distribution phase, so that a concentration-time curve (plotted on a logarithmic scale) shows two exponential rates comprising a rapid distribution phase (described as the rate constant α) and a slower elimination phase (described as the rate constant β) (Fig. 4.13). During the terminal phase of the concentration-time curve for a two-compartment model, the rate of distribution is not contributing to the concentration-time curve (because the term $Ae^{-\alpha t}$ is essentially zero when t is a high value), and the slope is dependent purely on the elimination rate ($Be^{-\beta t}$). Between dosage and the establishment of the terminal phase, the slope is determined by both rate constants α and β (Fig. 4.14). The distribution rate constant (α) can be determined by the difference between the measured plasma

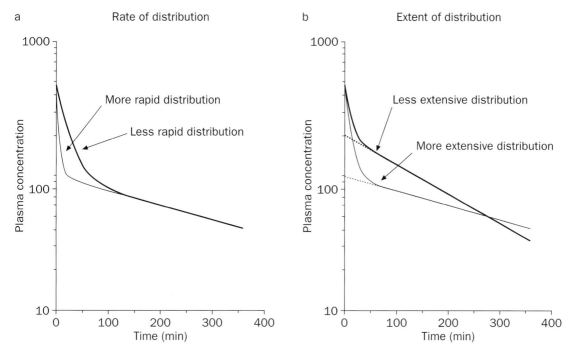

Fig. 4.11 The influence of the rate of distribution (a) and the extent of distribution (b) on the plasma concentration-time curve after an intravenous bolus dose. (Note: in (b) the drug with more extensive distribution shows a slower elimination half-life.)

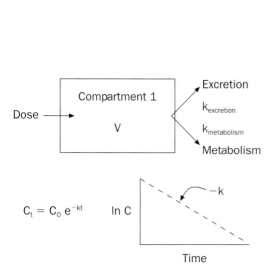

Fig. 4.12 The one-compartment model. The drug dose equilibrates very rapidly with all body tissues so that a discrete distribution phase is not detected.

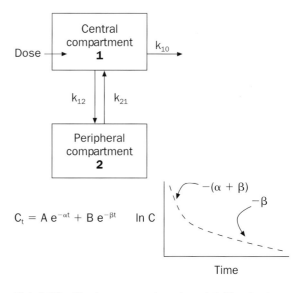

Fig. 4.13 The two-compartment model. The drug takes a finite time to reach equilibrium with some body tissues, and these represent a second compartment. This results in a bi-exponential decrease in the plasma concentration-time curve.

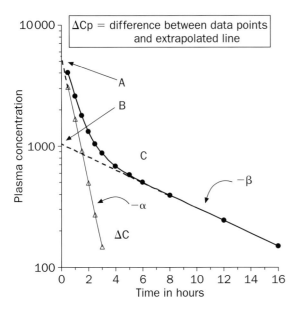

Fig. 4.14 Determination of the rate constant α and β by the method of residuals.

concentrations and the concentrations determined by back extrapolation of the terminal phase through to time = zero (see Fig. 4.14). The extrapolated line represents the elimination of the drug that would occur if distribution to the tissues had been instantaneous. The position of the intercept of the extrapolated line is dependent on the extent of distribution from blood into tissues (Fig. 4.11) and the lower the plasma concentration of the intercept the greater will be the distribution into tissues.

3.2.3 The extent of distribution – the apparent volume of distribution

The apparent volume of distribution is conceptually a difficult term, because it is the volume of plasma in which the body load of the drug *appears* to be distributed. It can be regarded as a 'dilution factor' because it represents the ratio between the total amount of drug in the body and the plasma concentration (C), i.e.:

$$V = \frac{Ab}{C}$$

where V is the apparent volume of distribution and Ab is the amount of drug in the body. The value of V is a characteristic of the drug and is independent of concentration, because it represents the equilibrium between the tissues and blood plasma and at equilibrium an increase in plasma concentration must be accompanied by an equal increase in all tissue concentrations. The value of V can range from about 0.1 litre per kg up to > 50 litres per kg.

In reality, the only time that the amount of drug in the body is known is immediately following an intravenous bolus dose, but at that time the drug will not have distributed to the tissues, and any measurement of plasma concentration would simply reflect the total plasma volume (before drug distribution). In consequence, the concentration needed for such a calculation is the concentration that would be obtained if all the drug instantly distributed to the body tissues. Such a value is given by the intercept B shown in Fig. 4.14, and this is one method of calculating the apparent volume of distribution.

The greater the apparent volume of distribution, the slower will be the overall rate of elimination (Fig. 4.11), and the longer the half-life (because the clearance processes have a larger apparent volume of plasma to turn over). Thus, the overall rate of elimination and the half-life can be regarded as depending on two key pharmacokinetic parameters (Fig. 4.10). Firstly, the plasma clearance (the greater the clearance the shorter the half-life) and secondly, the apparent volume of distribution (the greater the value the longer the half-life).

$$t_{\frac{1}{2}} = \frac{0.693 \times V}{CL}$$

This equation essentially reduces the mathematics of pharmacokinetics to a 'bucket and tap' model in which the tap represents the clearance, turning over a certain volume of plasma per minute, and the bucket represents the apparent volume of distribution (see Fig. 4.15).

In practice the apparent volume of distribution is not usually calculated by the dose divided by the back-extrapolated initial plasma concentration after distribution, but is based on the equation given in Fig. 4.15 which relates clearance, volume of distribution and the elimi-

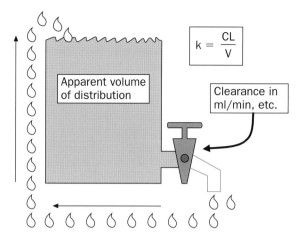

$$k = \frac{CL}{V}$$

Apparent volume of distribution

Clearance in ml/min, etc.

Fig. 4.15 The 'bucket and tap' model of pharmacokinetics. (Note: the plasma has to be recycled back into the bucket because the apparent volume of distribution is independent of concentration; the tap can be regarded as equivalent to the liver or kidneys.)

nation rate constant. Thus, V is usually calculated as:

$$V = \frac{CL}{k} \qquad \text{or} \qquad V = \frac{CL}{\beta}$$

It is apparent from this equation that the analytical method (Table 4.1) must be of sufficient sensitivity to define adequately the terminal slope k or β. An alternative approach, which provides a more robust measure of the apparent volume of distribution, is given under statistical moment analysis (see below).

3.3 The absorption of drugs and absorption rate constants

3.3.1 Biological properties

The rate of absorption of a drug into the general circulation depends on both the physicochemical properties of the drug and the site of administration (Table 4.7). Although the estimation of absorption is independent of the site of administration, there are very great metabolic and physiological differences affecting absorption from the intestine[9,10,11] compared with the dermal route[40–42] or inhalation.[43–45] The rate of absorption from the intestine may also be determined by the formulation of the drug;[11] sustained-release formulations give a rate of absorption that is slower than the rate of elimination (see below). The extent of absorption (which is measured as the bioavailability, see below and Box 4.1) is determined by both the physicochemical properties of the compound in relation to its transfer from the site of administration, and also its potential for degradation or metabolism between the site of administration and the general circulation (first-pass metabo-

Table 4.7   The characteristics of drug absorption from different routes of administration

Route	Characteristics and bioavailability (F)
Oral	Delay; lipid-soluble = fast; water-soluble = slow; F = variable
Intravenous	Instantaneous; F = 1
Subcutaneous	Lipid-soluble = slow; water-soluble = fast; F = 1
Intramuscular	Lipid-soluble = slow; water-soluble = fast; F = 1
Inhalation	Lipid-soluble = fast; high F
Trans-dermal	Very slow; low F
Nasal	Rapid; lipid-soluble; high F cf oral
Other	Mainly for local effects

(Note: F is the bioavailability – see Box 4.1.)

lism). In pharmacokinetic terms, first-pass metabolism is part of the absorption process and is not a part of clearance. However, because the liver is important in both first-pass metabolism and elimination, interactions that alter hepatic metabolism may alter both bioavailability after oral dosage and systemic clearance. The oral bioavailability of a drug may also be reduced by efflux pumps in the gut wall.[46]

3.3.2 Absorption rate constant

The absorption rate constant (ka) may be determined from the plasma concentration-time curve by back extrapolation of the terminal elimination phase to time = zero, when the absorption rate constant is given by the slope of the difference between the actual plasma concentration data and the extrapolated line (ΔC – Fig. 4.16). However, this method of analysis is most appropriate for simple one-compartment models, or cases where the rate of distribution exceeds the rate of absorption, such that a discrete distribution phase is not detected after oral dosing. Misleading data would be obtained by this simple approach if a distinct distribution phase were apparent after oral dosage, or if the rate of absorption were less than the rate of elimination. In the latter case the terminal slope would be determined by the absorption rate

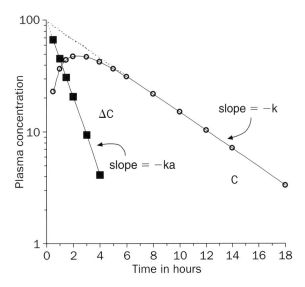

Fig. 4.16 Calculation of the absorption rate constant (ka) by the method of residuals for a compound absorbed by a first-order process. With flip-flop kinetics the dissolution rate is limiting (slowest) and this determines the rate of decrease after the peak: the increase to peak is determined by the faster (elimination) rate. (Note: see statistical moment analysis for an alternative, model-independent method of estimation.)

constant and not the elimination rate constant. This phenomenon, known as 'flip-flop' kinetics, applies most to data for sustained-release formulations (Fig. 4.17).

Calculation of the absorption rate constant requires the determination of an adequate number of measurements of concentration during the initial increase phase, as well as sufficient during the elimination phase to define the terminal slope. For some formulations the absorption phase does not represent either a first-order or zero-order process, and therefore it is difficult to fit a standard compartmental model to oral data. Under these circumstances, a useful estimate of the rate of absorption is the mean absorption time (MAT), which is calculated by statistical moment analysis (see later).

3.3.3 Extent of absorption

The extent of absorption, or bioavailability, is the fraction of the administered dose entering

---

Box 4.1 Bioavailability: definition and factors affecting oral bioavailability

Bioavailability = Fraction of dose passing from the site of administration into the general circulation **as the parent compound** (intravenous = 1.0)

Common reasons for low oral bioavailability

1. Decomposition in the gut lumen
2. First-pass metabolism in the gut wall
3. First-pass metabolism in liver
4. Not absorbed from the gut lumen
5. Tablet does not completely dissolve

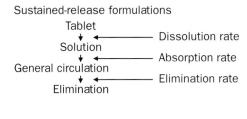

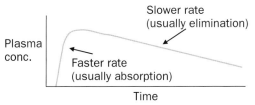

Fig. 4.17 Flip-flop kinetics – the pharmacokinetic basis of sustained-release formulations. Flip-flop kinetics are also found whenever the rate of absorption is lower than the rate of elimination and is most commonly observed for topical drug application.

the systemic circulation as the parent compound (see Table 4.7). Calculation of the bioavailability for a route of administration requires comparison of the blood concentrations after dosing by that route with those found after an intravenous dose (where the bioavailability is by definition 1.0 or 100%). Because the plasma concentration-time curve will have a different shape depending on the route of administration, the bioavailability is calculated by comparisons of the area under the concentration-time curve or AUC (Fig. 4.18). As indicated in Fig. 4.18, calculation of drug bioavailability by comparison of the AUCs after oral and intravenous dosage is dependent on an assumption that the clearance from the circulation is the same on both occasions. In consequence, the bioavailability of a drug is usually determined by a cross-over design, in which each individual is studied after oral and intravenous dosage and the data are analysed by a paired statistical analysis. 'Relative bioavailability' is sometimes reported for comparison between two different oral formulations, in which case the AUC is measured after each oral formulation and not referred to a systemic dose. To avoid confusion the true bioavailability, based on a comparison of oral and intravenous data, is often called the

'absolute bioavailability'. The term bioavailability is one of the most misused pharmacokinetic terms, and it means only what is given above. It is *not* the amount delivered to the site of action (although for a systemic effect the amount at the site of action will be affected by the bioavailability). For pro-drugs the blood concentrations of the parent drug, or absolute bioavailability, are of limited importance, and the AUC of the active metabolite is sometimes referred to as the 'bioavailability', but it is not the true pharmacokinetic bioavailability of the drug.

3.4 Repeated dosage and chronic administration

At the start of an intravenous infusion, the plasma concentrations are zero and at this time the rate of elimination, which equals [plasma

Extent of absorption – bioavailability – F

F – is the fraction of an oral dose which reaches the systemic circulation as the parent compound

F – is calculated as the ratio of the AUC_{oral} to the AUC_{iv} (F = 1 for an iv dose)

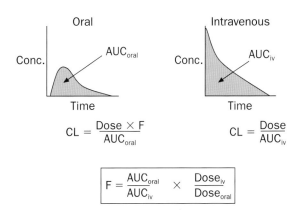

Fig. 4.18 Calculation of the bioavailability of a drug from oral and intravenous data. (Note: the method is applicable to all non-vascular routes. Criteria for application of this method are that the AUC values are extrapolated to infinity, and that the plasma clearance is the same for each route; for example, there is not saturation of systemic clearance with the intravenous bolus dose. The intravenous dose can be given as a bolus, or as an infusion – see Fig. 4.19.)

clearance × plasma concentration] is zero. As the infusion is started, the plasma concentrations will increase, and at any time after the start of the infusion the rate of elimination from the body equals [plasma clearance × plasma concentration at that time]. Plasma concentrations will continue to increase until an equilibrium will be reached in which the product of [plasma clearance × plasma concentration] produces a rate of elimination that exactly balances the rate of the infusion. This concentration will then be maintained unless there is a change in either the rate of infusion or the plasma clearance, i.e. an equilibrium or steady-state is reached (Fig. 4.19) where:

$$\frac{\text{Rate of}}{\text{infusion (R)}} = \frac{\text{rate of elimination}}{(\text{CL} \times C_{ss})}$$

where C_{ss} is the plasma concentration at steady-state. If the infusion is stopped, the plasma concentrations will decrease at a rate dependent on the overall rate of elimination and the elimination half-life. The time taken to reach the steady-state equilibrium concentration (see Fig. 4.19) represents the inverse of the elimination phase because 50%, 75%, 87.5%, etc. of the final steady-state is reached after an infusion for 1, 2, 3, etc. times the elimination half-life. Plasma clearance can be calculated from infusion data using the AUC for the total infusion plus elimination period as:

$$\text{CL} = \frac{\text{total infused dose}}{\text{total AUC}}$$

Most repeated-dose and chronic treatment regimens involve oral administration, and in this case the plasma concentration-time curve resembles that shown in Fig. 4.19 except that there is an increase immediately after dosage and a decrease between the peak concentration and the subsequent dose (Fig. 4.20). Again, an average steady-state concentration is reached, at which point the rate of input into the circulation:

$$\frac{\text{dose} \times \text{bioavailability}}{\text{dose interval}}$$

is exactly balanced by the rate of drug elimination [clearance × average steady-state drug concentration]. As indicated in Fig. 4.20 the AUC for a dose interval at steady-state is determined by the dose, bioavailability and clearance, and therefore is equivalent to the AUC for a single dose extrapolated to infinity. This relationship is true only if chronic administration does not change either the systemic clearance or the bioavailability. Comparison of the AUC for a dose interval at steady-state with the AUC for

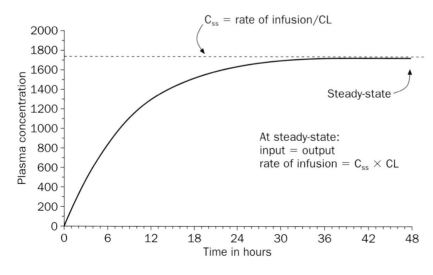

Fig. 4.19 The accumulation of a drug during a constant intravenous infusion (the elimination half-life of the drug is 6 hours).

Average plasma concentration at steady-state (C_{ss}) depends on:
  dose
  bioavailability
  clearance

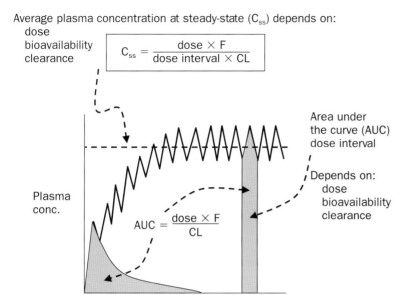

$$C_{ss} = \frac{\text{dose} \times F}{\text{dose interval} \times CL}$$

$$AUC = \frac{\text{dose} \times F}{CL}$$

Plasma
conc.

Area under
the curve (AUC)
dose interval

Depends on:
  dose
  bioavailability
  clearance

Time

Fig. 4.20 The accumulation of drug during repeated oral dosage. The AUC for a single dose extrapolated to infinity (shown for the first dose of treatment) is equal to the AUC for a dose interval at steady-state (provided that F and CL remain constant).

a single dose indicates the extent of any enzyme induction or inhibition arising from chronic treatment with the drug.

The time taken to reach steady-state depends on the elimination half-life, and it takes approximately four or five times the elimination half-life to reach approximately 94–97% of the final steady-state condition. An increase in either the rate of intravenous infusion or oral dosage will simply increase the steady-state concentration, but after the same time interval. In order to avoid the delay between starting therapy and achieving therapeutic steady-state drug concentrations, a single large dose can be given as a first dose (a loading dose) which will have the effect of producing the desired body load and plasma concentration, and this can then be maintained by lower doses. This is illustrated in Fig. 4.21.

3.5 Zero-order kinetics

All the pharmacokinetic analyses described above have assumed that the interaction between the drug and proteins (such as enzymes, transporters, etc.) are first-order with respect to substrate; in other words that the

For drugs with long half-lives, the delay in the time to steady-state concentrations may be unacceptable. The delay can be avoided by giving a large first dose (loading dose) which has the effect of 'topping-up' the apparent volume of distribution

$$\text{Loading dose} = C_{ss} \times V$$

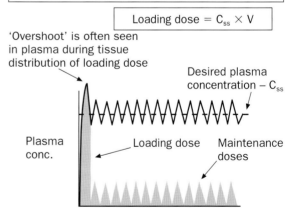

'Overshoot' is often seen in plasma during tissue distribution of loading dose

Desired plasma concentration – C_{ss}

Plasma conc.

Loading dose   Maintenance doses

Fig. 4.21 The loading dose: a method of avoiding the slow build up to steady-state during chronic treatment (see Fig. 4.19).

drug dosage does not result in saturation of the enzyme or transporter system. In the absence of saturation, the basic pharmacokinetic parameters such as bioavailability, clearance and apparent volume of distribution are constant, characteristic of the drug, and are independent of either dose or plasma concentration.

However, for some drugs in clinical practice and for many drugs during preclinical, high-dose animal toxicity testing, there is the possibility that the concentration presented to the enzyme or transporter will saturate that process so that the rate of elimination proceeds at the maximum rate (Vmax). The possible consequences of saturation of interactions between drug and enzymes, etc. are summarized in Table 4.8.

The principal parameter that is affected when the dose of drug results in zero-order kinetics is the AUC and consequently the clearance, which is calculated as dose/AUC. With zero-order kinetics the clearance decreases with increase in dose, and therefore the AUC increases disproportionately with increasing dose. The terminal elimination half-life does not change with increasing dose because this is always measured in the terminal phase of the plasma concentration-time curve, and therefore corresponds to low plasma concentrations that do not result in saturation of the enzyme (Fig. 4.22).

3.6 Statistical moment analysis

The non-compartmental analyses outlined above can provide information on most of the important pharmacokinetic parameters. However, in many cases oral data cannot be fitted readily to the models, and determination of the absorption rate, and the influence of formulation, are difficult to quantitate. The AUC is a robust measurement provided that the concentration-time course is followed for sufficient time so that extrapolation from the last measured time point to infinity represents only a small percentage of the total AUC measured by the trapezoidal rule (see Fig. 4.23). However, the AUC does not have a time-base and represents the overall exposure, so it cannot be used to derive rates of absorption or elimination. A

related method that can provide a time-base for determination of the duration of exposure to the drug is statistical moment analysis (see Gibaldi & Perrier, 1982; Further reading) in which the concentration at each time point is multiplied by the time of sampling, and this product (concentration × time) is plotted against time (see Fig. 4.23). The area under this curve is the area under the first moment curve (AUMC) and has units of (concentration × time^2). Dividing the AUMC (concentration × time^2) by the AUC (concentration × time) gives a parameter with units of time. This parameter is called the mean residence time (MRT) and it represents the duration of exposure for the total time course, and includes absorption, distribution and elimination phases. (Like the AUC, the AUMC can be measured by the trapezoidal rule up to the last time point and then has to be extrapolated to infinity as indicated in Fig. 4.23).

The major advantage of measuring the

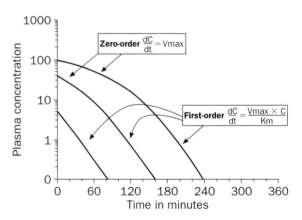

Fig. 4.22 Plasma concentration-time curves for three intravenous bolus doses of a drug illustrating saturation of elimination. The compound fits a simple one-compartment model with a Km for the clearance process equivalent to a plasma concentration of 20 units. The doses resulted in initial plasma concentrations of 5, 40 and 100 units. (Note: assuming a constant value for V the doses would be in the same ratios; the AUC increases disproportionately to the doses, but the terminal slope and half-life (at concentrations below 5) are not affected by the dose.)

Table 4.8   The sites and consequence of saturation of drug–protein interactions

Site	Process saturated	Possible consequences of saturation of drug-protein interaction
Absorption	Active transport (uptake)	Reduced uptake; a decrease in AUC after oral but not intravenous dosage: reduced bioavailability.
	Active transport (elimination) (e.g. P-glycoprotein)	Increased uptake; an increase in AUC after oral but not intravenous dosage; increased bioavailability.
	First-pass metabolism	Increased plasma concentrations; an increase in AUC after oral but not intravenous dosage; increased bioavailability.
Distribution	Plasma protein-binding	Increased unbound drug concentration in plasma which can lead to an increased entry into tissues or an increased apparent volume of distribution; increased glomerular filtration and increased hepatic clearance.
	Tissue protein-binding	Increased unbound concentrations in tissue leading to increased concentrations in all other compartments including the plasma, resulting in a decreased apparent volume of distribution.
Metabolism	Enzyme reactions	Decreased clearance leading to an increase in AUC at high doses. The AUC/dose ratio increases with increasing dose; the AUC for the metabolite may decrease with increase in dose, if alternative pathways are available. Affects both oral and intravenous administration.
Excretion	Renal tubular secretion	Decreased renal clearance resulting in an increased AUC at high doses for both oral and intravenous administration. Non-renal routes of administration may become more important.
	Biliary excretion	Decreased biliary elimination may result in a reduced enterohepatic circulation and increased elimination via the renal route; the ratio of the AUC:dose will increase for both oral and intravenous doses.

AUMC and MRT is that it allows two further calculations which produce valuable pharmacokinetic parameters. The apparent volume of distribution at steady-state (V_{ss}) is calculated as:

$$V_{ss} = CL \times MRT = \frac{\text{dose} \times AUMC}{AUC^2}$$

This measure of the apparent volume of distribution is a more reliable estimate than that given by the dose divided by the initial intercept C_0 or B, or $\dfrac{CL}{k}$ or $\dfrac{CL}{\beta}$ because it represents both central and peripheral compartments. It is particularly valuable when only a small propor-

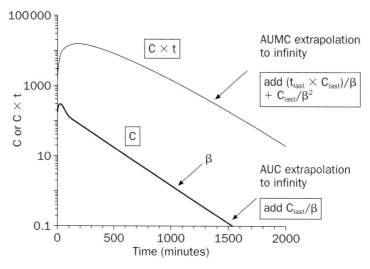

Fig. 4.23 The plasma concentration-time curve (C) and the first moment of the plasma concentration-time curve (C × t) for the oral administration of a drug that fits a two-compartment model. The area under each curve for the period of observations is determined by the trapezoidal rule, in which the areas for each time interval are summed. The area for each time interval equals the duration of the time interval multiplied by the average concentration – for the first time interval this is given by $[(t_2 - t_1) \times (C_1 + C_2)/2]$. Extrapolation to infinity is based on the last observed measurement and the terminal slope (β), but different calculations are necessary for C and C × t.

tion of the body load of the drug enters the slowly equilibrating compartments, and the majority of the drug is associated with rapidly equilibrating tissues. Under these circumstances half-lives and apparent volumes of distribution based on the terminal, and quantitatively minor component of the overall concentration-time curve will be misleading in relation to the exposure of more rapidly equilibrating tissue (which may represent the site of drug action).

The use of statistical moment analysis also allows calculation of an absorption parameter without fitting either first- or zero-order components to the absorption phase. The mean absorption time (MAT) can be calculated as the difference between the MRT after oral dosing and the MRT after intravenous dosing, i.e.:

$$MAT = MRT_{oral} - MRT_{iv}$$

Comparisons of MAT and MRT_{iv} (or MRT_{oral} and MRT_{iv}) will give an indication of the extent to which the absorption rate is governing the overall plasma concentration-time curve and body exposure to the drug. Comparisons of the MRT after oral dosage of different formulations can provide useful insights into the extent to which the formulation is increasing the duration of exposure and therefore acting as a sustained-release formulation.

4. CONCLUSIONS AND FUTURE DIRECTIONS

In this chapter the basic principles of pharmacokinetics have been outlined such that the non-specialist can appreciate the method of determination of the major pharmacokinetic parameters reported in most published papers. There are now a number of software packages available. WinNonlin is a PC-based program suitable for non-compartmental and compartmental methods, which incorporates statistical moment analysis, but not PBPK modelling. Pharmacokinetics is a complex and evolving field and a number of developments are likely to be of increasing importance in the future.[47]

4.1 PBPK modelling

PBPK modelling has been outlined and is illustrated in Fig. 4.5. Historically it has been used primarily for comparison of the kinetics in different test species and for extrapolating from test species to humans. Most research with PBPK models has been carried out on non-pharmaceutical compounds, particularly industrial solvents. However, this approach has great potential for analysing the possible influences of physiological factors such as age, and diseases of the liver or kidneys on the overall biodisposition of the compound in humans. This can be achieved without the need for direct experimentation, provided that the influence of the disease process has been studied in relation to the enzymes and processes that govern the fate of that compound, and which are part of the PBPK model.

4.2 Population analysis

The text given above describes the analysis of data from specifically designed pharmacokinetic studies in which the concentration-time course for the drug is followed in each individual. Phase II and Phase III clinical trials frequently involve the collection of single blood samples from different individuals; for example, in order to monitor compliance. Population-based approaches[48–51] allow such single-point data for different subjects to be combined and analysed to indicate the overall pharmacokinetics of the compound, providing that the time interval between the previous dose and the blood sample is well documented. The pooling of such individual data can also be useful for the identification of subgroups within the overall patient population which show abnormal pharmacokinetic characteristics. For example, the individual time points for patients with renal disease could be analysed separately and compared with the overall population average data, to determine whether this represents an 'at risk' group.

4.3 Pharmacokinetic-pharmacodynamic (PKPD) modelling

PKPD modelling allows the analysis of each of the major steps between dosage and therapeutic response indicated in Fig. 4.1. Such modelling requires both concentration-time course data and response-time course data. It involves the initial fitting of a model to the concentration-time curve data, following which an effect model is added to analyse the pharmacodynamics of the drug in relation to the circulating plasma concentrations. Such dynamic data can be particularly valuable because they provide an indication of concentration-response relationship in vivo in humans and can be used to define inter-patient variability in target organ or receptor sensitivity and response.[52–54] Such models are most readily fitted to acute effects following a single dose but may also be developed using a population-based analysis.[55–58]

ABBREVIATIONS

α The rate constant (with units of time^{-1}) for the distribution phase for a 2-compartment model; it is a composite term that is not simply the rate of transfer from compartment 1 into compartment 2 (see Renwick, 2001; Further reading).

AUC   Area under the concentration-time curve (with units of concentration $\times$ time); usually relates to the plasma or serum drug concentration-time curve; measured by the trapezoidal rule with extrapolation to infinity.

AUMC   Area under the first moment of the concentration-time curve (with units of concentration $\times$ time^2); used to calculate MRT, V_{ss} and MAT.

β The elimination rate constant (with units of time^{-1}) for a 2-compartment model; it is a composite term and is not simply the rate of removal (by metabolism or excretion) from compartment 1 (see Renwick, 2001; Further reading).

CL	Plasma clearance (with units of volume × time^{-1}); volume of plasma cleared of drug per unit time (by all processes combined); it is a characteristic of the drug and is independent of dose (at low doses); major determinant of elimination half-life and steady-state concentrations during repeat dosage.
CL$_R$	Renal clearance (with units of volume × time^{-1}); volume of plasma cleared of drug by the kidneys in unit time; a useful parameter because $(CL - CL_R)$ usually reflects metabolic clearance.
F	Bioavailability; the fraction of the administered dose that reaches the systemic circulation unchanged; sometimes given as a percentage instead of a fraction.
k	A first-order rate constant (with units of time^{-1}); the nature of the process to which it refers is usually indicated by a subscript: k_a = absorption rate constant, k_{el} = elimination rate constant.
MAT	Mean absorption time (with units of time); a useful parameter that reflects the duration of the absorption phase but does not require fitting to a particular model; calculated as $(MRT_{oral} - MRT_{iv})$.
MRT	Mean residence time (with units of time); reflects the overall duration of exposure and not simply the terminal (post-distribution) phase; calculated by statistical moment analysis.
t$\frac{1}{2}$	Half-life (with units of time); can be described for any rate constant and calculated as 0.693/rate constant; usually taken to mean the elimination half-life, in which case it is calculated as $0.693/\beta$ or $0.693/k$ or $0.693/\lambda_z$ (see text).
V	Apparent volume of distribution (with units of volume); the volume of plasma in which the body load of drug appears to have been distributed; it is a characteristic of the drug and is independent of dose (at low doses); an important parameter that

relates dose to plasma concentration, and is a determinant of the elimination half-life. There are various methods of calculating V which have different abbreviations (V_β, V_{ss}) and give slightly different values.

REFERENCES

Web-sites

■ http://www.cp.gsm.com/fromcpo.asp
Drug information web-site.

■ http://bnf.vhn.net/
Electronic British National Formulary.

■ http://emc.vhn.net/
Electronic compendium of drugs.

■ http://www.vet.purdue.edu/depts/bms/courses/
Lecture course on pharmacokinetics.

■ http://www.summitpk.com
Pharmacokinetics and metabolism software.

Further reading

Ioannides C, ed. *Cytochrome P450. Metabolic and Toxicological Aspects*. Boca Raton, FL: CRC Press, 1996.

Gibaldi M, Perrier D. *Pharmacokinetics*, 2nd edn. New York: Marcel Dekker, 1982.

Krishnan K, Andersen ME. Physiologically based pharmacokinetic modeling in toxicology. In: Hayes AW, ed. *Principles and Methods of Toxicology*, 4th edn. Philadelphia: Taylor & Francis, 2001: 193–242.

Renwick AG. Toxicokinetics: pharmacokinetics in toxicology. In: Hayes AW, ed. *Principles and Methods of Toxicology*, 4th edn. Philadelphia: Taylor & Francis, 2001: 137–92.

Scientific papers

1. Renwick AG, Lazarus NR. Human variability and noncancer risk assessment – an analysis of the default uncertainty factor. *Regul Toxicol Pharmacol* 1998; **27:** 3–20
2. Loebstein R, Koren G. Clinical pharmacology and therapeutic drug monitoring in neonates and children. *Pediatr Rev* 1998; **19:** 423–8.
3. Hammerlein A, Derendorf A, Lowenthal DT.

Pharmacokinetic and pharmacodynamic changes in the elderly. Clinical implications. *Clin Pharmacokinet* 1998; **35**: 49–64.

4. Morgan DJ, McLean AJ. Clinical pharmacokinetic and pharmacodynamic considerations in patients with liver disease. An update. *Clin Pharmacokinet* 1995; **29**: 370–91.

5. Loebstein R, Lalkin A, Koren G. Pharmacokinetic changes during pregnancy and their clinical relevance. *Clin Pharmacokinet* 1997; **33**: 328–43.

6. Perucca E. Drug metabolism in pregnancy, infancy and childhood. *Pharmacol Ther* 1987; **34**: 129–43.

7. Tanaka E. Gender-related differences in pharmacokinetics and their clinical significance. *J Clin Pharm Ther* 1999; **24**: 339–46.

8. Johnson JA. Predictability of the effects of race or ethnicity on pharmacokinetics of drugs. *Int J Clin Pharmacol Ther* 2000; **28**: 53–60.

9. Welling PG. Effects of food on drug absorption. *Annu Rev Nutr* 1996; **16**: 383–415.

10. Singh BN. Effects of food on clinical pharmacokinetics. *Clin Pharmacokinet* 1993; **37**: 213–55.

11. Fleisher D, Li C, Zhou Y, Pao LH, Karim A. Drug, meal and formulation interactions influencing drug absorption after oral administration. Clinical implications. *Clin Pharmacokinet* 1999; **36**: 233–54.

12. Lin JH. Species similarities and differences in pharmacokinetics. *Drug Metab Dispos* 1995; **23**: 1008–21.

13. Mahmood I, Balian JD. The pharmacokinetic principles behind scaling from preclinical results to phase 1 protocols. *Clin Pharmacokinet* 1999; **36**: 1–11.

14. Iwatsubo T, Hirota N, Ooie T, Suzuki H, Sugiyama Y. Prediction of in vivo drug disposition from in vitro data based on physiological pharmacokinetics. *Biopharm Drug Dispos* 1996; **17**: 273–310.

15. Smith DA, Jones BC, Walker DK. Design of drugs involving the concepts and theories of drug metabolism and pharmacokinetics. *Med Res Rev* 1996; **16**: 243–66.

16. White RE. High-throughput screening in drug metabolism and pharmacokinetic support of drug discovery. *Annu Rev Pharmacol Toxicol* 2000; **40**: 133–57.

17. Cupp MJ, Tracy TS. Cytochrome P450: new nomenclature and clinical implications. *Am Fam Physician* 1998; **57**: 107–16.

18. Lin JH, Lu AYH. Inhibition and induction of cytochrome P450 and the clinical implications. *Clin Pharmacokinet* 1998; **35**: 361–90.

19. Michalets EL. Update: clinically significant cytochrome P-450 drug interactions. *Pharmacotherapy* 1998; **18**: 84–112.

20. Daly AK, Cholerton S, Gregory W, Idle JR. Metabolic polymorphisms. *Pharmacol Therap* 1993; **57**: 129–60.

21. de Wildt SN, Kearns GL, Leeder JS, van den Anker JN. Cytochrome P450 3A. Ontogeny and drug disposition. *Clin Pharmacokinet* 1999; **37**: 485–505.

22. de Wildt SN, Kearns GL, Leeder JS, van den Anker JN. Glucuronidation in humans. Pharmacogenetics and developmental aspects. *Clin Pharmacokinet* 1999; **36**: 439–53.

23. Tukey RH, Strassburg CP. Human UDP-glucuronosyltransferases: metabolism, expression and disease. *Annu Rev Pharmacol Toxicol* 2000; **40**: 581–616.

24. Bendayan R. Renal drug transport: a review. *Pharmacotherapy* 1996; **16**: 971–85.

25. Dresser MJ, Leabman MK, Giacomini KM. Transporters involved in the elimination of drugs in the kidney: organic anion transporters and organic cation transporters. *J Pharm Sci* 2001; **90**: 397–421.

26. Zhang L, Brett CM, Giacomini KM. Role of organic cation transporters in drug absorption and elimination. *Annu Rev Pharmacol Toxicol* 1998; **38**: 431–60.

27. Leveque D, Jehl F. P-glycoprotein and pharmacokinetics. *Anticancer Res* 1995; **15**: 331–6.

28. Krishna R, Mayer LD. Multidrug resistance (MDR) in cancer. Mechanisms, reversal using modulators of MDR and the role of MDR modulators in influencing the pharmacokinetics of anticancer drugs. *Eur J Pharm Sci* 2000; **11**: 265–83.

29. Aszalos A, Ross DD. Biochemical and clinical aspects of efflux pump related resistance to anticancer drugs. *Anticancer Res* 1998; **18**: 2937–44.

30. Bonate PL, Reith K, Weir S. Drug interactions at the renal level. Implications for drug development. *Clin Pharmacokinet* 1998; **34**: 375–404.

31. Smith RL. *The Excretory Function of Bile. The Elimination of Drugs and Toxic Substances in Bile.* London: Chapman & Hall, 1973.

32. Wilkinson GR. Clearance approaches in pharmacology. *Pharmacol Rev* 1987; **39**: 1–47.

33. Rowland M, Benet LZ, Graham GG. Clearance concepts in pharmacokinetics. *J Pharmacokinet Biopharm* 1973; **1**: 123–36.

34. Worboys PD, Bradbury A, Houston JB. Kinetics of drug metabolism in rat liver slices. II.

Comparison of clearance by liver slices and freshly isolated hepatocytes. *Drug Metab Dispos* 1996; **24**: 676–81.

35. Ito K, Iwatsubo T, Kanamitsu S, Nakajima Y, Sugiyama Y. Quantitative prediction of in vivo drug clearance and drug interactions from in vitro data on metabolism, together with binding and transport. *Annu Rev Pharmacol Toxicol* 1998; **38**: 461–99.

36. Lindup WE. Drug-albumin binding. *Biochem Soc Trans* 1975; **3**: 635–40.

37. Rodighiero V. Effects of liver disease on pharmacokinetics. An update. *Clin Pharmacokinet* 1999; **37**: 399–431.

38. Ibrahim S, Honig P, Huang SM et al. Clinical pharmacology studies in patients with renal impairment: past experience and regulatory perspectives. *J Clin Pharmacol* 2000; **40**: 31–8.

39. Piafsky KM, Borga O, Odar-Cederlof I, Johansson C, Sjoqvist F. Increased plasma protein binding of propranolol and chlorpromazine mediated by disease-induced elevations of plasma α_1 acid glycoprotein. *N Engl J Med* 1978; **299**: 1435–9.

40. Harvell JD, Maibach HI. Percutaneous absorption and inflammation in aged skin: a review. *J Am Acad Dermatol* 1994; **31**: 1015–21.

41. Schaefer H. Penetration and percutaneous absorption of topical retinoids. A review. *Skin Pharmacol* 1993; **6**: 117–23.

42. Roberts MS. Targeted drug delivery to the skin and deeper tissues: role of physiology, solute structure and disease. *Clin Exp Pharmacol Physiol* 1997; **24**: 874–9.

43. Witek TJ. The fate of inhaled drugs: the pharmacokinetics and pharmacodynamics of drugs administered by aerosol. *Respir Care* 2000; **45**: 826–30.

44. Berridge MS, Lee Z, Heald DL. Regional distribution and kinetics of inhaled pharmaceuticals. *Curr Pharm Des* 2000; **6**: 1631–51.

45. Cochrane MG, Bala MV, Downs KE, Mauskopf J, Ben-Joseph RH. Inhaled corticosteroids for asthma therapy: patient compliance, devices, and inhalation technique. *Chest* 2000; **117**: 542–50.

46. Suzuki H, Sugiyama Y. Role of metabolic enzymes and efflux transporters in the absorption of drugs from the small intestine. *Eur J Pharm Sci* 2000; **12**: 3–12.

47. Peck CC, Barr WH, Benet LZ et al. Opportunities for integration of pharmacokinetics, pharmacodynamics, and toxicokinetics in rational drug development. *Clin Pharmacol Ther* 1992; **51**: 465–73.

48. Vozeh S, Steimer JL, Rowland M et al. The use of population pharmacokinetics in drug development. *Clin Pharmacokinet* 1996; **30**: 81–93.

49. Racine-Poon A, Wakefield J. Statistical methods for population pharmacokinetic modelling. *Stat Methods Med Res* 1998; **7**: 63–84.

50. Aarons L. Software for population pharmacokinetics and pharmacodynamics. *Clin Pharmacokinet* 1999; **36**: 255–64.

51. Rousseau A, Marquet P, Debord J, Sabot C, Lachatre G. Adaptive control methods for the dose individualisation of anticancer agents. *Clin Pharmacokinet* 2000; **38**: 315–53.

52. Van-Peer A, Snoeck E, Huang ML, Heykants J. Pharmacokinetic-pharmacodynamic relationships in phase I/phase II of drug development. *Eur J Drug Metab Pharmacokinet* 1993; **18**: 49–59.

53. Shaw LM, Bonner HS, Fields L, Lieberman R. The use of concentration measurements of parent drug and metabolites during clinical trials. *Ther Drug Monit* 1993; **15**: 483–7.

54. Girard P, Nony P, Boissel JP. The place of simultaneous pharmacokinetic pharmacodynamic modelling in new drug development: trends and perspectives. *Fundam Clin Pharmacol* 1990; **4** (Suppl. 2): 103S–15S.

55. Mandema JW, Verotta D, Sheiner LB. Building population pharmacokinetic-pharmacodynamic models. I. Models for covariate effects. *J Pharmacokinet Biopharm* 1992; **20**: 511–28.

56. Sheiner LB, Ludden TM. Population pharmacokinetics/dynamics. *Annu Rev Pharmacol Toxicol* 1992; **32**: 185–209.

57. Yuh L, Beal S, Davidian M et al. Population pharmacokinetic/pharmacodynamic methodology and applications: a bibliography. *Biometrics* 1994; **50**: 566–75

58. Olson SC, Bockbrader H, Boyd RA et al. Impact of population pharmacokinetic-pharmacodynamic analyses on the drug development process: experience at Parke-Davis. *Clin Pharmacokinet* 2000; **38**: 449–59.

5

The use of pharmacogenetics to maximize therapeutic benefit

Christian Meisel, Matthias Schwab

SUMMARY

Individual variability in drug response and drug toxicity can to a considerable extent be ascribed to inter-individual differences in the genetic make-up of drug-metabolizing enzymes, drug transporters and – increasingly recognized during recent years – drug targets. About 40% of currently used drugs are metabolized by cytochrome P450 (CYP) 2C9, CYP2C19 or CYP2D6, enzymes that are important in Phase I drug metabolism and are expressed polymorphically. Similarly, enzymes such as thiopurine S-methyltransferase (TPMT), important in Phase II drug metabolism, and the MDR1 gene product P-glycoprotein (P-gp), important in drug transport across compartments, exhibit polymorphism. There are many examples of drugs in which polymorphic expression of metabolizing enzymes (e.g. CYP2D6, TPMT) are responsible for therapeutic failure, exaggerated drug response or serious toxicity after taking a standard dose. There is an increasing expectation that polymorphisms in drug targets such as receptors may also have an important influence on responsiveness to drug therapy and may ultimately lead to rational drug selection criteria. Taken together, pharmacogenetics offers the prospect of safer and more efficient drug therapy tailored to individual patients. The ability to identify, prospectively, individuals at risk of adverse drug events before drug treatment is not only an advantage for the patient but is also economically efficient, reducing the need for hospitalization and its associated cost. However, prospective studies in a broad population of patients are necessary to prove the benefit of genotype-based dose recommendations and pharmacogenetic-based drug selection for individual patients.

1. INTRODUCTION

The response of individual patients to the same drug given in the same dose varies considerably for many substances. Many patients will experience the desired drug effect, some may suffer from well-known adverse drug reactions, others may experience no effects, and very rarely a patient will die from severe side-effects. It is currently very difficult for physicians to prescribe the optimal drug in the optimal dose for each patient, since prediction of a patient's response to any one specific drug is rarely possible.

From a clinical point of view, excessive numbers of patients suffer from adverse drug reactions. In the USA, such reactions are estimated to be from the fourth to sixth leading cause of deaths in hospital patients.[1] In addition, the cost burden is tremendous. A large percentage of health budgets are spent on inefficient drug therapy. The application of pharmacogenetic knowledge offers the opportunity for individually tailored, safe and efficient drug treatment.

After an introductory brief historical overview, this chapter discusses relevant determinants of individual drug response, including the influence of genetic polymorphism on drug metabolism, drug transport and drug targets (Fig. 5.1). The current status of the clinical application of pharmacogenetics will be outlined, including a brief outlook at its impact on the future of drug therapy.

2. HISTORICAL BACKGROUND

Pharmacogenetics is actually not a novel field in clinical pharmacology. Indeed, the term 'pharmacogenetics' was coined by the German geneticist Friedrich Vogel no fewer than 40 years ago.[2] Important inherited differences in

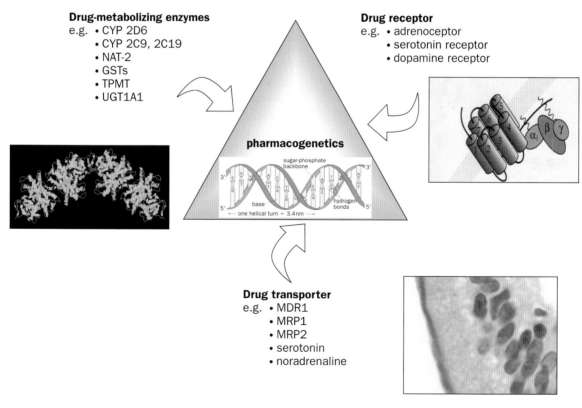

Drug-metabolizing enzymes
e.g. • CYP 2D6
• CYP 2C9, 2C19
• NAT-2
• GSTs
• TPMT
• UGT1A1

Drug receptor
e.g. • adrenoceptor
• serotonin receptor
• dopamine receptor

pharmacogenetics

sugar-phosphate backbone

base

hydrogen bonds

one helical turn = 3.4 nm

Drug transporter
e.g. • MDR1
• MRP1
• MRP2
• serotonin
• noradrenaline

Fig. 5.1 Current research areas in pharmacogenetics. Pharmacogenetics currently comprises the study of polymorphic drug-metabolizing enzymes and drug transporters (pharmacokinetics) and drug targets such as drug receptors (pharmacodynamics).

drug response first emerged during the 1950s. The astute observation of prolonged postoperative muscle relaxation after administration of suxamethonium was attributed to an atypical variant of plasma cholinesterase (butyrylcholinesterase).[3] During this period it was shown that the haemolysis observed in a significant fraction of patients treated with antimalarial drugs such as primaquine or chloroquine co-segregated with an anomaly of erythrocyte glucose 6-phosphate dehydrogenase activity – which was also shown to be under genetic control. Studies likewise disclosed that the pharmacokinetics and side-effects of isoniazid (such as peripheral neuropathy) are influenced by inherited variants of arylamine N-acetyltransferase (NAT2).[4,5]

The field of pharmacogenetics experienced an enormous increase in attention in 1977 when two independent research groups in London and Bonn observed markedly increased side-effects in some volunteers given the antihypertensive drug debrisoquine[6] and the antiarrhythmic agent sparteine.[7] Both drugs are catalyzed by the cytochrome P450 2D6 (CYP2D6) isozyme and it was shown that side-effects resulted from reduced oxidative metabolism, which in turn was shown to be under monogenic control. Phenotyping larger numbers of individuals – by administration of probe drugs such as debrisoquine and sparteine and measurement of the ratio of parent to metabolite in the urine – disclosed that 5–10% of the white population exhibit the poor metabolizer ('PM') phenotype.[8] The genetic basis of the CYP2D6 (debrisoquine/sparteine) polymorphism,[9] and the application of the first reliable genotyping methods,[10] were established about ten years later. The introduction of routine genotyping methods including the development of high-throughput techniques and the availability of sequence data from the human genome project has led to an exponential increase in research in this field during the last few years. Thus, it has been proposed that by the year 2010, personalized medicines based on pharmacogenetics should be part of routine clinical practice.[11]

3. INDIVIDUAL VARIATION IN DRUG RESPONSE

To understand why individual patients respond differently to drugs, it is helpful to envisage the progress of a particular drug from its administration to its observed effect (Fig. 5.2). The effect of a drug will depend firstly on its systemic concentration and its concentration at the drug target. Drug concentration at its target will in many cases represent a mere function of the systemic concentration. Active transport processes, however, may influence local target concentrations; for example, the blood–brain barrier is an important determinant of drug concentration in the cerebrospinal fluid.[12]

The systemic concentration of a drug depends on several pharmacokinetic factors, commonly referred to by the acronym ADME (drug absorption, distribution, metabolism and elimination). It has long been known that a wide variety of individual patient factors may influence the pharmacokinetics of a drug and must therefore be taken into account when determining dosage for a given patient. Box 5.1 shows some of these traditional determinants. In addition, it has come increasingly clear that hereditary variances in drug-metabolizing enzymes and drug transporters can exert considerable influence on drug concentrations and accordingly will be discussed extensively below.

The second crucial determinant of an observed drug effect is the response of the drug

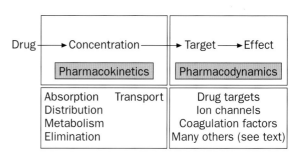

Fig. 5.2 Understanding individual variance in drug response (see text).

Box 5.1   Selected traditional factors influencing the pharmacokinetics of drugs

- Age
- Sex
- Weight
- Body fat
- Alcohol consumption
- Concomitant drugs
- Nutritional status
- Liver function
- Renal function
- Cardiovascular function
- Environmental pollutants

---

target to a given drug concentration. Hereditary variants have been discovered and characterized in receptors, drug transporters, ion channels, lipoproteins, coagulation factors and many other factors involved in immune response, cell development, cell cycle control and other functions, that significantly influence the manifestation and course of diseases. Many of these polymorphic structures are at the same time targets of specific drugs and can thus potentially influence the effect that a specific drug concentration will exert at the drug target. Knowledge in this field is still accumulating rapidly and this area will be discussed in the light of current examples.

3.1 Drug-metabolizing enzymes

3.1.1 Phases and enzymes of xenobiotic metabolism

A large number of enzymes play a role in xenobiotic metabolism – in which drug metabolism is included. In brief, drug metabolism takes place in two phases. In Phase I metabolism, the xenobiotic is subject to oxidation, reduction or hydrolysis, leading to modifications in the functional chemical groups of the drug. Phase II of xenobiotic metabolism comprises conjugation reactions with small endogenous molecules,

resulting in increased solubility in water and facilitating elimination of the drug. The reactions involved in xenobiotic metabolism lead in most cases to inactivation of the drug. However, there are also examples, of inactive pro-drugs that are metabolized to the functionally active drug by drug-metabolizing enzymes (bioactivation). During the last ten years, polymorphisms have been described in genes coding for most drug-metabolizing enzymes. Table 5.1 shows a list of drug-metabolizing enzymes in Phase I and Phase II metabolism with functionally relevant polymorphisms and lists examples of drugs that may be affected.[13,14]

3.1.2 The cytochrome P450 enzyme system

Of this group of enzymes, the cytochrome P450 (CYP) enzyme system has undergone the most extensive study. The cytochrome P450s are a group of haem-containing mono-oxygenases that are divided into families and subfamilies based on their sequence homology (see www.drnelson.utmem.edu/CytochromeP450.html). More than 1200 CYP sequences are now known. In humans, 17 families of CYP genes and 42 subfamilies with 55 CYP genes and 20 pseudogenes are currently recognized. Of this group, CYP families 1–3 are involved primarily in xenobiotic metabolism, whereas the other CYP families are involved mainly in the biosynthesis of endogenous compounds. CYP family 2, the largest family in humans, comprises about one-third of human CYPs. Of these, CYP2C9, CYP2C19 and CYP2D6 are involved in the metabolism of >40% of drugs currently in use and they have been characterized most extensively. This share will probably increase with the discovery and characterization of further polymorphisms in genes of the CYP2 family (e.g. *CYP2B6* and *CYP2C8*).

The most highly expressed subfamily is CYP3A, which includes the isoforms CYP3A4, CYP3A5, CYP3A7 and CYP3A43.[15] These isoforms account for as much as 30% of total P450 content in the liver and are involved in the metabolism of at least 50% of all drugs. Hepatic expression of CYP3A4 varies by >50% between individuals but the causes of the variability in constitutive CYP3A expression are unknown.

Table 5.1 Selected polymorphic drug-metabolizing enzymes and drugs affected by polymorphic metabolism

Phase I	Relevant for	Phase II	Relevant for
CYP2A6	Nicotine, halothane	Arylamine N-acetyltransferase 2 (NAT2)	Isoniazid, hydralazine, sulfonamides, procainamide, dapsone
CYP2C9, CYP2C19, CYP2D6	See Table 5.2	UDP-glucuronosyl transferase 1A1	Irinotecan
Flavine-dependent mono-oxygenase 3	Perazine, sulindac, albendazole	Glutathione S-transferases (GST) (GST M1, T1, P1, Z1)	Hypericin phototoxicity (?) Epirubicin (GST P1)
Alcohol dehydrogenase	Ethanol	Catechol O-methyltransferase	Oestrogens, L-dopa, α-methyldopa
Butyrylcholinesterase	Succinylcholine	Thiopurine S-methyltransferase	Azathioprine, 6-mercaptopurine
Dihydropyrimidine dehydrogenase	5-Fluorouracil	Sulfotransferases (SULT 1A1, SULT 1A2)	Steroids, oestrogens, acetaminophen

For details see refs 13 and 14; (a more comprehensive listing, related to the latter article, is available at http://www.sciencemag.org/feature/data/1044449.shl).

One analysis suggests that depending on the drug studied, 60–90% of person-to-person variability in CYP3A function is caused by genetic factors. As of now, the few reported mutations in the coding or promotor region of *CYP3A4* have not been shown to have a profound effect on the expression level or the function of the enzyme.[15]

3.1.2.1 CYP2D6

One of the best-studied isozymes of the CYP family is CYP2D6, which is involved in the metabolism of many clinically important drugs: e.g. beta-blockers, antiarrhythmics, antipsychotics and antidepressants, as well as a variety of other substances (see Table 5.2). The *CYP2D* gene locus in humans is comprised of three highly homologous genes – two pseudogenes and the *CYP2D6* gene – the latter consisting of nine exons and eight introns.[16] The *CYP2D6* gene is highly polymorphic, and systematic analysis in a large number of individuals with the so-called extensive metabolizer (EM) or

Table 5.2	Cytochrome P450 enzyme-specific drug metabolism
Enzymes	**Substrates**
CYP2C9	Antihypertensives: losartan, irbesartan, torasemide Antidepressants: fluoxetine, amitriptyline Antiepileptics: phenytoin Antidiabetics: tolbutamide, glimepiride, rosiglitazone NSAIDs: ibuprofen, naproxen, piroxicam, indomethacin, celecoxib Anticoagulant: S-warfarin
CYP2C19	Neuropsychiatric agents: amitriptyline, imipramine, citalopram, moclobemide, diazepam phenobarbital, hexobarbital, mephenytoin Antimalarial: proguanil Betablockers: propranolol Proton pump inhibitors: omeprazole, lansoprazole, pantoprazole Anticoagulant: R-warfarin HIV protease inhibitor: nelfinavir
CYP2D6	Antiarrhythmics: ajmaline, n-propylajmaline, flecainide, mexiletine, propafenone, sparteine Antidepressants: amitriptyline, clomipramine, desipramine, imipramine, trimipramine, nortriptyline, maprotiline, fluoxetine, fluvoxamine, paroxetine, trazodon, venlafaxine Antiemetics: ondansetron, tropisetron Antihypertensives: debrisoquine, urapidil, alprenolol, carvedilol, metoprolol, propranolol, timolol Neuroleptics: haloperidol, perphenazine, perazine, risperidone, thioridazine, zuclopenthixol, chlorpromazin Opioids: codeine, dihydrocodeine, dextromethorphan, oxycodon, ethylmorphine, tramadol Others: perhexiline, amphetamine, metamphetamine, MDMA 'ecstasy', dexfenfluramine, tamoxifen, lidocaine

poor metabolizer (PM) phenotypes has so far led to the discovery of >70 different alleles (www.imm.ki.se/CYPAlleles/). At least 15 of these encode non-functional gene products. Homozygous carriers of two non-functional alleles as well as compound heterozygous carriers display severely decreased or diminished enzyme activity, resulting in the PM phenotype. Moreover, 2–3% of the German population carry a duplicated/multiplied *CYP2D6* gene and display ultra-high enzyme activity – resulting in ultra-rapid metabolism (UM) of CYP2D6 drug substrates. These differences in enzyme activity can have dramatic con-

sequences on plasma concentrations, as shown >30 years ago for the tricyclic antidepressant nortriptyline.[17] A >30-fold difference in nortriptyline steady-state plasma concentrations was observed between poor and ultra-rapid metabolizers if nortriptyline was prescribed in a standard daily dose of 100–150 mg .[18,19]

Among Caucasians, about 7–10% of individuals can be identified as PM, about 10–15% of persons are intermediate metabolizers (IM) and at the opposite end of the spectrum up to 10% of individuals have a UM phenotype. The remainder are classified as 'extensive' or 'rapid'

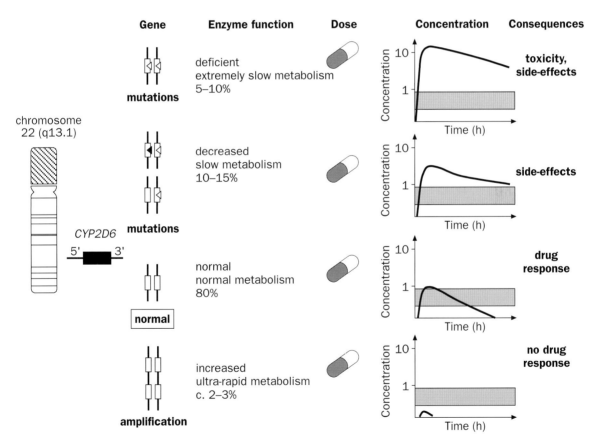

Fig. 5.3 The genetic polymorphism of CYP2D6 (debrisoquine/sparteine polymorphism) and its clinical consequences for drug therapy. Patients who receive the same standard dosage of a CYP2D6 substrate show marked differences in drug plasma concentrations according to their constitutive *CYP2D6* genotype and consequently may be at increased risk for either drug toxicity (poor metabolizer) or therapeutic failure (ultra-rapid metabolizer).

metabolizers (EM) (see Fig. 5.3).[8] Only three to five alleles account for the majority of mutant *CYP2D6* genotypes such that it is possible to correctly predict the CYP2D6 PM phenotype and thus the lack of catalytic function of the enzyme with a reliability of >99% by CYP2D6 genotyping without the need to phenotype the patient.[8,20,21] In contrast, as of the year 2000, genotyping for the amplified *CYP2D6* alleles identifies only 20–30%[22] of the ultra-rapid phenotype observed in Caucasians.[8,21,22] Recently, the genetic basis of the common CYP2D6 IM phenotype has been elucidated. A promoter polymorphism in the *CYP2D6* 5'-flanking region has been identified which allows the prediction of >60% of CYP2D6 IMs in Caucasian populations.[24]

Significant ethnic differences exist in the frequencies of the PM as well the UM phenotype, which may have clinical consequences for drug therapy with CYP2D6 substrates in different ethnic populations. Thus, it is interesting to note that a much higher proportion (up to 29%) of northern African populations demonstrate the *CYP2D6* gene duplication.[25] This fact may – from an evolutionary perspective – point to a possible survival benefit in 'animal–plant warfare' (as it is frequently called) by permitting the rapid metabolism of food-borne xenobiotics.[26]

As discussed below, knowledge of the metabolic capacity of each patient clearly offers the possibility of adjustment of drug dosage.[27] In addition, awareness of the *CYP2D6* genotype may influence the selection of drugs. For example, codeine is routinely administered as an analgesic drug for the treatment of cancer pain. Approximately 10% of orally administered codeine is O-demethylated by CYP2D6 to morphine, the sole mediator of the analgesic action of codeine. Patients with the CYP2D6 PM phenotype (up to 10% of Caucasians) will not metabolize codeine to morphine efficiently and will not benefit from its analgesic effect. Additionally, codeine cannot be recommended as an analgesic for the subgroup of patients with ultra-rapid CYP2D6 activity, since rapid generation of morphine can produce severe opioid side-effects.[28,29]

3.1.2.2 CYP2C9 and CYP2C19

The polymorphic expression of other important CYP isozymes, particularly CYP2C9 and CYP2C19, has been investigated in recent years. As shown in Table 5.2, these enzymes are involved in the metabolism of many widely prescribed drugs, some of them with narrow therapeutic indices. For CYP2C9, polymorphisms have been identified that lead to two common alleles associated with decreased, albeit not absent, activity. About 2% of the Caucasian population has substantially decreased 2C9 activity, and about 24% display intermediate activity for CY2C9. For CYP2C19 only one inactive allele is of significant importance in Caucasians. In this population, about 4% exhibit diminished activity, while about 32% are intermediate metabolizers for CYP2C19.[25,30–32]

3.1.3 Thiopurine S-methyltransferase (TPMT)

The best-characterized polymorphic enzyme of Phase II drug metabolism is thiopurine S-methyltransferase (TPMT), which is involved in the catabolic inactivation of thiopurine drugs such as azathioprine, 6-mercaptopurine and 6-thioguanine. Patients deficient for TPMT who are treated with standard doses of these drugs have an increased risk of developing severe and sometimes fatal haematopoietic toxicity.[33,34]

A prime example is the case of a 65-year-old heart transplant recipient, who attracted tragic notoriety in transplantation medicine. As part of his immunosuppressive regimen this patient received azathioprine in standard doses and soon suffered from severe leukopenia, which resolved after the discontinuation of the drug. After a second similar course with leukopenia, the patient received a third course with a somewhat reduced dosage. However, agranulocytosis ensued and the patient finally died of sepsis. The clinical course of the patient was easily explainable after post hoc diagnosis of TPMT deficiency.[35]

TPMT activity is affected by genetic polymorphism. In Caucasians, about 90% display high TPMT activity, about 9–10% intermediate activity and about 1 in every 300, very low to absent TPMT activity. By the end of 2000, eight variant

Table 5.3 Suggested adjustments in drug dose according to patient genotype

Drug	Reference dose (mg)	CYP2D6 genotype			
		PM	IM	EM	UM
Propafenone	450	40%	(80%)	130%	
Amitriptyline	150	50%*	(90%)*	120%*	
Tropisetron	10	30%	(80%)	130%	(150%)
Haloperidol	5	80%*	100%*	110%*	
Zuclopenthixol	25	70%*	80%*	120%*	
Metoprolol	100	30%*	60%*	140%*	

PM, poor metabolizer; IM, intermediate metabolizer; EM, extensive metabolizer; UM, ultra-rapid metabolizer.
*Recommended percentage dose adjustments are derived from steady-state data. Unmarked recommendations are derived from single-dose studies. Recommendations in brackets are estimations based on analogy. All data are according to Bröckmoller et al.[25]
Caution: These data are preliminary and are currently not intended as medical advice for individual patients; they await confirmation by prospective clinical studies (see text). Drug dosage must be adapted by the physician to each individual patient, after consideration of all relevant parameters.

alleles associated with low TPMT activity had been reported. However, the ethnic distribution of these alleles varies significantly among Caucasians, Asians, Africans and African-Americans. The TPMT *3A allele, for example, accounts for >80% of mutant alleles in Caucasians, but for only about 17% in African-Americans.[33,36] TPMT status can be determined by measurement of the enzyme activity and by determination of the patient's TPMT genotype. Since TPMT erythrocyte enzyme activity correlates well with hepatic activity, phenotype can be determined in peripheral blood samples by various established methods (e.g. radiochemical or HPLC analysis).

However, there are a number of limitations with respect to the measurement of constitutive TPMT enzyme activity in erythrocytes. For example, if a deficient or heterozygous patient has received transfusions with red blood cells from a homozygous wild-type individual, TPMT activity cannot be determined reliably within 30–60 days of the transfusion. Furthermore, thiopurine administration itself

may alter TPMT activity in erythrocytes by increasing enzyme activity, resulting in a possible misclassification, especially for heterozygous patients. In principle the limitations of phenotyping can be avoided by genotyping provided that all functionally relevant alleles are known.

For TPMT genotyping, various methods have been established, including PCR-based RFLP and fluorescence-based methods, as well as screening procedures by direct sequencing or denaturing HPLC.[37] It has become possible to detect the presence of TPMT deficiency with up to 95% concordance between genotype and phenotype in different populations by screening of the most relevant clinical mutations (TPMT *2, *3A, *3C).[33,38,39] The molecular diagnosis of TPMT deficiency thus appears to be a feasible approach to predicting the constitutive TPMT phenotype.

Given the widespread use of thiopurine agents for immunosuppression in solid organ transplantation and in the therapy of autoimmune disorders including inflammatory bowel disease and neurological (e.g. multiple sclerosis) disorders, as well providing maintenance treatment for patients suffering from acute lymphoblastic leukaemia, TPMT genotyping and phenotyping offer the possibility of patient-tailored drug dosing and a substantial reduction of haematopoietic toxicity.

3.2 Drug transport

3.2.1 MDR1/P-glycoprotein (P-gp): structure and function

In recent years it has become increasingly clear that drug transporters play a crucial role in drug absorption, distribution and elimination. The best-studied drug transporter is the *MDR1* gene product: the multi-drug transporter P-glycoprotein (P-gp). This drug transporter was first described in tumour cells, where it contributes to multidrug resistance (MDR) against anticancer agents.[40] Subsequently the gene was cloned from mouse and human cells.

P-gp is a member of the large ATP-binding cassette superfamily of transport proteins. It is composed of two similar halves, each containing six transmembrane domains and one ATP-binding domain. It is an integral membrane protein and is expressed in humans in the epithelial cells of the lower gastrointestinal tract, in the brush border of proximal renal tubule cells, in the liver at the biliary face of hepatocytes, in the apical membrane of pancreatic ductuli, on the luminal surface of capillary endothelial cells in the brain and testes, in the placenta, in the adrenal cortex and in some haematopoietic cells. In brief, P-gp acts as an efflux pump. The function of the protein and the distribution and polarity of P-gp expression suggest that the physiological function of this transporter is as follows: (a) to provide a barrier against the entry of toxic compounds into the body, certain compartments of the body and cells; and (b) to remove xenobiotics from circulation after they have entered (ref. 41, and Delph Y. P-glycoprotein: a tangled web waiting to be unravelled, TAG Basic Science Report 2000, available from: http://www.aidsinfonyc.org/tag/science/pgp.html).

The spectrum of P-gp drug substrates is

Box 5.2	Selected MDR1 substrates	
Amiodarone	Fluphenazine	Ondansetron
Cefazolin	Gallopamil	Perphenazine
Chinidin	Hydrocortisone	Phenytoin
Cyclosporin A	Ivermectin	Tamoxifen
Dexamethasone	Loperamide	Terfenadine
Digoxin	Methadone	Thioridazine
FK506	Morphine	Verapamil

wide, most of them lipophilic and amphipathic (Box 5.2).[54] They usually contain at least one aromatic ring. It is noteworthy that there is a broad substrate overlap between P-gp and CYP3A4.

3.2.2 MDR1 and the pharmacokinetics of drugs

Experiments with the mouse *mdr1 -/-* knockout model have provided further insights into the role of P-gp in drug therapy. Mice that lack the *mdr1a* gene (the homologue to the human *MDR1*) demonstrate a 100-fold higher concentration of ivermectin in the brain after a given dose than *mdr1a* wild-type mice.[42] Further experiments in this mouse model have shown that the lack of this transporter gene has effects on the bioavailability, pharmacokinetics and distribution, as well as drug effects and side-effects of other therapeutic drugs (e.g. vinblastine, dexamethasone, digoxin and cyclosporin A).[43,44]

In humans, clinical studies have showed that P-gp limits oral bioavailability of many of its substrates, including the immunosuppressant drugs cyclosporin A and tacrolimus, and HIV protease inhibitors.[45–47] Furthermore, the co-administration of P-gp inhibitors (sometimes called 'reversal agents' for historical reasons) such as verapamil, cyclosporin A and PSC833 (a non-immunosuppressive analogue of cyclosporin A) has been shown to increase the bioavailability of drugs whose absorption is normally limited by P-gp activity.[41,48] The overall clinical consequences of this approach remain to be elucidated more thoroughly, since not only bioavailability but also tissue distribution in key compartments such as the CNS will change and may cause undesired effects.

3.2.3 MDR1 polymorphisms

The *MDR1* gene has recently been found to be highly polymorphic and *MDR1* polymorphisms may account for individual differences in the bioavailability and tissue distribution of P-gp substrates. Preliminary data suggest that one polymorphism in exon 26 of the *MDR1* gene ($C^{3435}T$) influences the intestinal expression of P-gp and affects the pharmacokinetics of digoxin. About 24–29% of Caucasians demonstrate the homozygous TT genotype, which is associated with significantly lower P-gp expression in the small intestine in comparison with subjects with the CC genotype and higher plasma concentrations of digoxin (e.g. maximum plasma concentration, area under curve, AUC) after oral administration of the drug. At least 14 additional polymorphisms in this gene have been reported, and their functional and clinical consequences await elucidation.[49,50]

More recently it has become apparent that some drug interactions can take place at the level of the drug transporter.[51] It is interesting to speculate that genetic factors may contribute to inter-individual variability in propensity to drug interactions at this level.

3.3 Drug action targets

Over the past 10 years, great effort has been expended on elucidating the role of hereditary factors in the susceptibility to, and the natural history of, many complex diseases. An early phase of euphoria prevailed in this field, owing largely to results from small case-control studies that provided positive associations of single polymorphisms with the course of complex diseases and patients' susceptibility to them. Since then the publication of conflicting reports has indicated that proof of an association between single gene polymorphisms and disease susceptibility is not straightforward and requires careful study design, often involving large numbers of patients.

Given that many of the genes examined in the course of these studies encode drug targets (e.g. receptors, transporters, ion channels, lipoproteins, coagulation factors, and genes involved in cell cycle control, immune system and cell development) it is not surprising that there has been keen interest in the effect of polymorphisms in these genes on the pharmacodynamic action of drugs. While this is a complex field, examples of associations between particular polymorphisms and drug response are increasing. Two are discussed below.

3.3.1 ALOX5

A randomized, placebo-controlled trial involving the lipoxygenase inhibitor ABT-761, a derivative of zileuton, recently showed that treatment response was dependent on the 5-lipoxygenase (ALOX5) genotype. The study focused on a tandem repeat polymorphism in the *ALOX5* promoter, which is known to be associated with the level of gene transcription. About 6% of the study population ($n = 114$) were carriers of a variant of the promoter that was easily recognized by appropriate genotyping techniques. At the end of the study period, none of the patients with the promoter variant showed improvement in FEV_1, which was in strong contrast to the patients with the wild-type allele, all of whom exhibited a clinically significant improvement in FEV_1.[52] Since no significant differences in drug metabolism of ABT-761 were observed between the two groups, it has been assumed that the group of patients carrying the variant genotype suffered from a distinct subtype of asthma that do not benefit from this treatment and require alternative therapy. If true, prospective genotyping in this context could be used to predict which patients would benefit from this expensive drug and which patients should be spared exposure to the compound.

3.3.2 Beta₂-adrenergic receptor

A second pioneering study in the field of asthma therapy emphasized the important fact that responsiveness to therapy could in all likelihood be predicted even more effectively if not only single polymorphisms but complex haplotypes were also considered. This elegant investigation clearly revealed marked differences in in vivo bronchodilatatory response to the beta-adrenergic agonist albuterol in a cohort of asthmatics, based on the beta$_2$-adrenergic receptor haplotypes. In contrast to the results derived using haplotypes (comprising 13 polymorphisms), an additional analysis disclosed that no single polymorphism demonstrated any predictive utility in this study.[53]

4. CLINICAL APPLICATION OF PHARMACOGENETICS

4.1 Current dose recommendations are not appropriate for all patients

Traditionally, clinicians treating patients suffering from renal insufficiency use pocket-dosing tables for the administration of drugs eliminated by the kidneys. From these tables, the required dose adjustment can be read according to the patient's creatinine clearance. We anticipate that in future the dose of certain drugs may also take into account the patient's genotype to individually maximize therapeutic benefit and minimize risk.

Figure 5.4 shows a representative result from a phenotyping experiment. To test enzyme activity, patients are given a probe drug (for CYP2D6 phenotyping, debrisoquine, sparteine or dextrometorphan may be used). The metabolic capacity for this drug can be calculated from the ratio of drug metabolites to parent drug. In this figure, the group on the right represents patients with low enzyme activity due to inactive alleles, and the very small group on the left comprises patients with very high enzyme activity. In order to achieve comparable plasma concentrations in the three patient groups, the dose of drugs metabolized by this enzyme should be adjusted to the individual's enzyme activity. The manufacturer's dose recommendations are based on an unselected patient population and the therapeutic response of that population. In the example, the manufacturer recommends a dose (in the example, two capsules) that has the desired effect in as many patients as possible. However, this

represents the optimal dosage for only a fraction of all patients (shown shaded in grey in the figure). It would most probably be too high for patients whose enzyme activity is low, and too low for the group of patients situated on the left. Thus dose recommendations usually represent only the best fit for the average patient, while in many cases the dosage is suboptimal for a significant number of other patients. This is particularly important for drugs with a steep dose–response curve and a low therapeutic index, i.e. the plasma level necessary for therapeutic effect lies close to that producing side-effects. For drugs metabolized by certain drug-metabolizing enzymes, this problem can be solved by considering the individual phenotype of the patient – which may be predicted from their genotype – and by adjusting the dose accordingly.

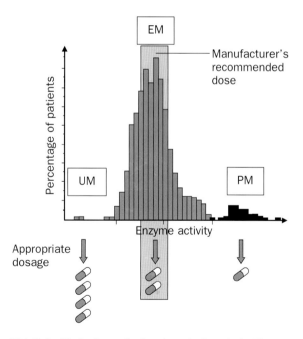

Fig. 5.4 Typical result of a phenotyping study. The three distinct groups comprise patients with very high (UM), normally high (EM) and low (PM) enzyme activity. The figure shows the appropriate dosage according to enzyme activity, and the dose recommendation typically given in a drug instruction leaflet.

4.2 Genotype-based dose recommendations

Preliminary genotype-based dose recommendations for key drugs have recently been derived and calculated from the literature.[25] This has been possible because – in addition to molecular and genetic research in the field – a large volume of clinical studies has been conducted, mostly on healthy volunteers, on the clinical and pharmacokinetic consequences of functional polymorphisms in drug-metabolizing enzymes. From these data, together with the known distribution of the relevant alleles in the population, tentative recommendations have been tabulated. Table 5.3 shows how such genotype-based dose adjustments could appear for a number of drugs. If genotyping alone is used to predict the patient's constitutive phenotype, phenotype–genotype correlation studies are required to show the predictive power of the genotyping strategy, as has been performed for CYP2D6 and TPMT (discussed above). For these enzymes, the PM status can reliably be predicted by DNA-based methods with an accuracy of 95–99%.

The limitations of the current data and experience must be recognized.[27] Most important is the fact that the published recommendations are derived from small-scale studies, conducted mostly on healthy young volunteers. Before such genotype-based dosing rules can be applied routinely in clinical practice, it is necessary for these recommendations to be verified in appropriate prospective clinical trials in patients and to confirm that this type of dose adjustment offers true benefits to the patients without additional harm.

5. CONCLUSIONS AND FUTURE PROSPECTS FOR DRUG THERAPY

This chapter outlines the major hereditary factors that determine an individual patient's response to drugs. Consideration is given to the effects of these factors on pharmacokinetic and pharmacodynamic processes. It is known that crucial enzymes of Phase I (e.g. CYP2C9, CYP2C19 and CYP2D6) and Phase II (e.g. TPMT) drug metabolism are subject to genetic polymorphism, which may in turn lead to reduced or totally absent enzyme activity, and that these differences in enzyme activity may make a significant contribution to inter-individual differences in drug concentrations. Additionally, polymorphic drug transporters must also be taken into account in explaining observed inter-individual differences in drug kinetics. In parallel with the ongoing elucidation of the genetic basis of diseases, there is an increasing awareness of the possible uses of genetic information to subdivide previously homogeneous conditions into subgroups that respond differently to drugs or to identify individuals at risk of 'idiosyncratic' adverse responses, not predictable on the basis of the known pharmacology of the drug. This chapter covers some salient examples of polymorphic drug targets and the consequences for drug selection. The first examples of genotype-based dosing tables are given (Table 5.3) to demonstrate how the results from basic and clinical research could be incorporated favourably into drug prescribing.

Despite a number of promising examples, the use of genotype information in drug prescribing is still in its infancy. The implementation of pharmacogenetics into clinical practice, like other new procedures, must be subject to clinical trials. Increasingly, the clinical trials that form part of drug development are designed by pharmaceutical companies with the collection and analysis of genotype information in mind. It may be possible to identify genotype-response relationships at an early stage such that the drug is marketed with appropriate recommendations. Typically, however, the number of patients included in these early studies is small and may not be sufficient to detect more subtle interactions. There is a need, therefore, for well-conducted studies after licensing of a drug and as part of post-marketing surveillance to detect associations as well as to establish and test the validity and usefulness of the pharmacogenetic approach.

By necessity, the tailoring of drug treatment in this way requires the collection of sensitive information from the patient. In a manner analogous to the documentation given to patients receiving chronic anticoagulation treatment, a 'genetic passport' has been suggested, which would carry a genetic fingerprint and indicate to a physician which drugs are safe and which should be avoided in a particular patient. There has been and continues to be widespread discussion on the social and legal consequences of the collateral information produced by such a practice, especially in the context of predicting susceptibility to hitherto incurable diseases. This topic cannot be treated lightly but the potential benefits from prospective genotyping means that every effort to ensure that genetic data is collected and used appropriately should be explored.

In conclusion, pharmacogenetics offers the perspective of profound improvement in drug therapy. However, before this knowledge can be adopted routinely in clinical practice, convincing prospective clinical trials demonstrating the benefits of pharmacogenetic-guided drug therapy must be performed.

GLOSSARY OF TERMS

Cytochrome P450 (CYP) enzyme
Superfamily of major drug-metabolizing enzymes

CYP2C9, CYP2C19, CYP2D6, CYP3A4	Significant members of the CYP family
Genotyping	Determination of the genetic make-up of a patient to predict the patient's phenotype
HPLC	High-performance liquid chromatography
MDR1	Multi-drug resistance gene 1: coding for the multi-drug transporter P-glycoprotein
PCR/RFLP	Polymerase chain reaction/restriction fragment length polymorphism – still one of the most widely used genotyping methods
Phenotyping	Measuring the activity of a drug-metabolizing enzyme by application of a probe drug and determination of the ratio of parent drug to metabolite
TPMT	Thiopurine-S-methyltransferase: polymorphic phase II enzyme, crucial for the metabolism of thioguanine drugs

ACKNOWLEDGEMENTS

This work was supported by the German Ministry of Education, and Research grants 031U209B, and 01 GG 9845/5, and the Robert Bosch Foundation.

REFERENCES

Further reading

Brockmöller J, Kirchheiner J, Meisel C, Roots, I. Pharmacogenetic diagnostics of cytochrome P450 polymorphisms in clinical drug development and in drug treatment. *Pharmacogenomics* 2000; **1:** 125–51.

Evans WE, Relling MV. Pharmacogenomics: translating functional genomics into rational therapeutics. *Science* 1999; **286:** 487–91.

Ingelman-Sundberg M, Oscarson M, McLellan RA. Polymorphic human cytochrome P450 enzymes: an opportunity for individualized drug treatment. *TIPs* 1999; **20:** 342–9.

Meisel C, Roots I, Cascorbi I, Brinkmann U, Brockmöller J. How to manage individualized drug therapy: application of pharmacogenetic knowledge of drug metabolism and transport. *Clin Chem Lab Med* 2000; **38:** 869–76.

Roses AD. Pharmacogenetics and the practice of medicine. *Nature* 2000; **405:** 857–65.

Wolf RC, Smith G, Smith RL. Pharmacogenetics. *BMJ* 2000; **320:** 987–90.

Web-sites

■ http://drnelson.utmem.edu/cytochrome P450.html

Very frequently updated CYP home page.

- http://medicine.iupui.edu/flockhart
Extensive and up-to-date resource for CYP-specific drug metabolism.

- http://www.imm.ki.se/cypalleles/
Comprehensive overview of CYP alleles. The home page is run by the CYP allele nomenclature committee.

- http://humanabc.4t.com/humanabc.htm
Comprehensive human ABC transporters home page.

Scientific papers

1. Lazarou J, Pomeranz BH, Corey PN. Incidence of adverse drug reactions in hospitalized patients: a meta-analysis of prospective studies. *JAMA* 1998; **279**: 1200–5.
2. Vogel F. Moderne Probleme der Humangenetik. *Erge Inn Med Kinderheilkd* 1959; **12**: 52–125.
3. Kalow W. Familial incidence of low pseudocholinesterase level. *Lancet* 1956; **2**: 576–7.
4. Bönicke R, Losboa BP. Über die Erbbedingtheit der intraindividuellen Konstanz der Isoniazidausscheidung beim Menschen (Untersuchungen an eineiigen Zwillingen). *Naturwissenschaften* 1957; **44**: 314.
5. Harmer D, Evans DA, Eze LC, Jolly M, Whibley EJ. The relationship between the acetylator and the sparteine hydroxylation polymorphisms. *J Med Genet* 1986; **23**: 155–6.
6. Mahgoub A, Idle JR, Dring LG, Lancaster R, Smith RL. Polymorphic hydroxylation of Debrisoquine in man. *Lancet* 1977; **2**: 584–6.
7. Eichelbaum M, Spannbrucker N, Steincke B, Dengler HJ. Defective N-oxidation of sparteine in man: a new pharmacogenetic defect. *Eur J Clin Pharmacol* 1979; **16**: 183–7.
8. Sachse C, Brockmöller J, Bauer S, Roots I. Cytochrome P450 2D6 variants in a Caucasian population: allele frequencies and phenotypic consequences. *Am J Hum Genet* 1997; **60**: 284–95.
9. Gonzalez FJ, Skoda RC, Kimura S et al. Characterization of the common genetic defect in humans deficient in debrisoquine metabolism. *Nature* 1988; **331**: 442–6.
10. Heim, M, Meyer UA. Genotyping of poor metabolizers of debrisoquine by allele-specific PCR amplification. *Lancet* 1990; **336**: 529–32.
11. Liggett SB. Pharmacogenetic applications of the Human Genome project. *Nat Med* 2001; **7**: 281–3.
12. Rao VV, Dahlheimer JL, Bardgett ME et al. Choroid plexus epithelial expression of MDR1 P glycoprotein and multidrug resistance-associated protein contribute to the blood-cerebro-spinal-fluid drug-permeability barrier. *Proc Natl Acad Sci USA* 1999; **96**: 3900–5.
13. Meisel C, Roots I, Cascorbi I, Brinkmann U, Brockmöller J. How to manage individualized drug therapy: application of pharmacogenetic knowledge of drug metabolism and transport. *Clin Chem Lab Med* 2000; **38**: 869–76.
14. Evans WE, Relling MV. Pharmacogenomics: translating functional genomics into rational therapeutics. *Science* 1999; **286**: 487–91.
15. Eichelbaum M, Burk O. CYP3A genetics in drug metabolism. *Nat Med* 2001; **7**: 285–7.
16. Meyer UA, Zanger UM. Molecular mechanisms of genetic polymorphisms of drug metabolism. *Annu Rev Pharmacol Toxicol* 1997; **37**: 269–96.
17. Hammer W, Sjoqvist F. Plasma levels of monomethylated tricyclic antidepressants during treatment with imipramine-like compounds. *Life Sci* 1967; **6**: 1895–903.
18. Bertilsson L, Dahl ML, Sjoqvist F et al. Molecular basis for rational megaprescribing in ultrarapid hydroxylators of debrisoquine. *Lancet* 1993; **341**: 63.
19. Dalen P, Dahl ML, Ruiz ML, Nordin J, Bertilsson L. 10-Hydroxylation of nortriptyline in white persons with 0, 1, 2, 3, and 13 functional CYP2D6 genes. *Clin Pharmacol Ther* 1998; **63**: 444–52.
20. Marez D, Legrand M, Sabbagh N et al. Polymorphism of the cytochrome P450 CYP2D6 gene in a European population: characterization of 48 mutations and 53 alleles, their frequencies and evolution. *Pharmacogenetics* 1997; **7**: 193–202.
21. Griese EU, Zanger UM, Brudermanns U et al. Assessment of the predictive power of genotypes for the in-vivo catalytic function of CYP2D6 in a German population. *Pharmacogenetics* 1998; **8**: 15–26.
22. Lovlie R, Daly A, Matre G, Molven A, Steen V. Polymorphisms in CYP2D6 duplication-negative individuals with the ultrarapid metabolizer phenotype: a role for the CYP2D6*35 allele in ultrarapid metabolism? *Pharmacogenetics* 2001; **11**: 45–55.
23. Dahl ML, Johansson I, Bertilsson L, Ingelman-Sundberg M, Sjoqvist F. Ultrarapid hydroxylation of debrisoquine in a Swedish population.

Analysis of the molecular genetic basis. *J Pharmacol Exp Ther* 1995; **274:** 516–20.

24. Raimundo S, Fischer J, Eichelbaum M, Griese EU, Schwab M, Zanger UM. Elucidation of the genetic basis of the common 'intermediate metabolizer' phenotype for drug oxidation by CYP2D6. *Pharmacogenetics* 2000; **10:** 577–81.

25. Aklillu E, Persson I, Bertilsson L, Johansson I, Rodrigues F, Ingelman-Sundberg M. Frequent distribution of ultrarapid metabolizers of debrisoquine in an Ethiopian population carrying duplicated and multiduplicated functional CYP2D6 alleles. *J Pharmacol Exp Ther* 1996; **278:** 441–6.

26. Kalow W. Pharmacogenetics in biological perspective. *Pharmacol Rev* 1997; **49:** 369–79.

27. Brockmöller J, Kirchheiner J, Meisel C, Roots I. Pharmacogenetic diagnostics of cytochrome P450 polymorphisms in clinical drug development and in drug treatment. *Pharmacogenomics* 2000; **1:** 125–51.

28. Dalen P, Frengell C, Dahl ML, Sjöqvist F. Quick onset of severe abdominal pain after codeine in an ultrarapid metabolizer of debrisoquine. *Ther Drug Monit* 1997; **19:** 543–4.

29. Poulsen L, Brosen K, Arendt-Nielsen L, Gram LF, Elbaek K, Sindrup SH. Codeine and morphine in extensive and poor metabolizers of sparteine: pharmacokinetics, analgesic effect and side effects. *Eur J Clin Pharmacol* 1996; **51:** 289–95.

30. Ingelman-Sundberg M, Oscarson M, McLellan RA. Polymorphic human cytochrome P450 enzymes: an opportunity for individualized drug treatment. *TIPs* 1999; **20:** 342–9.

31. Miners JO, Birkett DJ. Cytochrome P4502C9: an enzyme of major importance in human drug metabolism. *Br J Clin Pharmacol* 1998; **45:** 525–38.

32. Wedlund PJ. The CYP2C19 enzyme polymorphism. *Pharmacology* 2000; **61:** 174–83.

33. McLeod HL, Krynetski EY, Relling MV, Evans WE. Genetic polymorphism of thiopurine methyltransferase and its clinical relevance for childhood acute lymphoblastic leukemia. *Leukemia* 2000; **14:** 567–72.

34. Weinshilboum R. Thiopurine pharmacogenetics: clinical and molecular studies of thiopurine methyltransferase. *Drug Metab Dispos* 2001; **29:** 601–5.

35. Schütz E, Gummert J, Mohr F, Oellerich M. Azathioprine-induced myelosuppression in thiopurine methyltransferase deficient heart transplant recipient [letter]. *Lancet* 1993; **341:** 436.

36. Krynetski EY, Evans WE. Pharmacogenetics as a molecular basis for individualized drug therapy:

the thiopurine S-methyltransferase paradigm. *Pharm Res* 1999; **16:** 342–9.

37. Schaeffeler E, Lang T, Zanger UM, Eichelbaum M, Schwab M. High-throughput genotyping of thiopurine S-methyltransferase by denaturing HPLC. *Clin Chem* 2001; **47:** 548–55.

38. Coulthard SA, Rabello C, Robson J et al. A comparison of molecular and enzyme-based assays for the detection of thiopurine methyltransferase mutations. *Br J Haematol* 2000; **110:** 599–604.

39. Yates CR, Krynetski EY, Loennechen T et al. Molecular diagnosis of thiopurine S-methyltransferase deficiency: genetic basis for azathioprine and mercaptopurine intolerance. *Ann Intern Med* 1997; **126:** 608–14.

40. Juliano RL, Ling V. A surface glycoprotein modulating drug permeability in Chinese hamster ovary cell mutants. *Biochim Biophys Acta* 1976; **455:** 152–62.

41. Ambudkar SV, Dey S, Hrycyna CA, Ramachandra M, Pastan I, Gottesman MM. Biochemical, cellular, and pharmacological aspects of the multidrug transporter. *Annu Rev Pharmacol Toxicol* 1999; **39:** 361–98.

42. Schinkel AH, Smit JJ, van Tellingen O et al. Disruption of the mouse mdr1a P-glycoprotein gene leads to a deficiency in the blood-brain barrier and to increased sensitivity to drugs. *Cell* 1994; **77:** 491–502.

43. Schinkel AH, Wagenaar E, van Deemter L, Mol CA, Borst P. Absence of the mdr1a P-Glycoprotein in mice affects tissue distribution and pharmacokinetics of dexamethasone, digoxin, and cyclosporin A. *J Clin Invest* 1995; **96:** 1698–705.

44. Schinkel AH, Mayer U, Wagenaar E et al. Normal viability and altered pharmacokinetics in mice lacking mdr1-type (drug-transporting) P-glycoproteins. *Proc Natl Acad Sci USA* 1997; **94:** 4028–33.

45. Fricker G, Drewe J, Huwyler J, Gutmann H, Beglinger C. Relevance of p-glycoprotein for the enteral absorption of cyclosporin A: in vitro-in vivo correlation. *Br J Pharmacol* 1996; **118:** 1841–7.

46. Floren LC, Bekersky I, Benet LZ et al. Tacrolimus oral bioavailability doubles with coadministration of ketoconazole. *Clin Pharmacol Ther* 1997; **62:** 41–9.

47. Kim RB, Fromm MF, Wandel C et al. The drug transporter P-glycoprotein limits oral absorption and brain entry of HIV-1 protease inhibitors. *J Clin Invest* 1998; **101:** 289–94.

48. Fromm MF. P-glycoprotein: a defense mechan-

ism limiting oral bioavailability and CNS accumulation of drugs. *Int J Clin Pharmacol Ther* 2000; **38:** 69–74.

49. Hoffmeyer S, Burk O, von Richter O et al. Functional polymorphisms of the human multidrug-resistance gene: multiple sequence variations and correlation of one allele with P-glycoprotein expression and activity in vivo. *Proc Natl Acad Sci USA* 2000; **97:** 3473–8.

50. Cascorbi I, Gerloff T, Johne A et al. Frequency of single nucleotide polymorphisms in the P-glycoprotein drug transporter MDR1 gene in white subjects. *Clin Pharmacol Ther* 2000; **69:** 169–74.

51. Greiner B, Eichelbaum M, Fritz P et al. The role of intestinal P-glycoprotein in the interaction of digoxin and rifampin. *J Clin Invest* 1999; **104:** 147–53.

52. Drazen JM, Yandava CN, Dube L et al. Pharmacogenetic association between ALOX5 promoter genotype and the response to anti-asthma treatment. *Nat Genet* 1999; **22:** 168–70.

53. Drysdale CM, McGraw DW, Stack CB et al. Complex promoter and coding region beta 2-adrenergic receptor haplotypes alter receptor expression and predict in vivo responsiveness. *Proc Natl Acad Sci USA* 2000; **97:** 10483–8.

54. Seelig A. A general pattern for substrate recognition by P-glycoprotein. *Eur J Biochem* 1998; **251:** 252–61.

6

Drug chirality: pharmacology in three dimensions

Andrew J Hutt

SUMMARY

One in four of all prescribed drugs are used as mixtures rather than as single chemical entities. These mixtures are not drugs coformulated for some perceived therapeutic advantage but combinations of stereoisomers, most frequently racemic mixtures of synthetic chiral drugs. It has been known since the early years of the last century that the individual stereoisomers (enantiomers) present in such mixtures may differ in terms of their pharmacological activity. However, it is only relatively recently, with advances in stereochemical technologies, that the potential significance of stereochemistry in pharmacology has been appreciated and drug stereopurity has become a topic of concern. The aims of this chapter are to provide the reader with a background to stereochemistry (particularly with respect to the terminology and nomenclature used), to illustrate the significance of stereochemical considerations in pharmacology and to describe briefly the current regulatory position concerning chiral drugs.

1. INTRODUCTION

The British pharmacologist, Cushny, demonstrated differences in the pharmacological activity of atropine and $(-)$-hyoscyamine and $(-)$- and $(+)$-adrenaline in the early part of the last century.[1] However, it is only relatively recently that the stereochemical nature of drug molecules has become a topic of concern and pharmacology has moved from a 'flatland' two-dimensional science to one of three-dimensional spatial awareness. This change in philosophy with respect to chiral pharmaceuticals, the majority of which are used as racemic mixtures, has been brought about largely as a result of advances in chemical technologies for the analysis, synthesis and preparation of single stereoisomers. The ability to produce and determine the stereochemical purity of single stereoisomers has facilitated an evaluation of their pharmacological properties. As a result there has been an increased appreciation of the potential significance of the differential pharmacological properties of the enantiomers present in a racemate and the problems that may arise from the use of such mixtures.

As pointed out above the majority of synthetic chiral drugs are used as racemic mixtures. A survey of 1675 drugs carried out in the 1980s indicated that 25% of the agents examined were used as racemic mixtures rather than single stereoisomers.[2] Such figures indicate that drug stereochemistry is not restricted to particular therapeutic groups but is an across-the-board problem.

To the prescribing physician the complexities of stereochemistry, and the intricacies of stereochemical nomenclature, are probably of little interest. This view is not surprising as physicians could reasonably expect the pharmaceutical industry and regulatory authorities to resolve chemical problems and provide them with drugs of proven quality, safety and efficacy. However, it is obviously important that physicians are aware of the nature of the material they are prescribing, i.e. mixture or single chemical entity, particularly with the development of the so-called racemic or chiral switch (see section 5.1) and the possibility that both single stereoisomer and racemic mixture products of some drugs either are, or will be, available concurrently. Thus an appreciation of stereochemical considerations in pharmacology and the nomenclature employed is of significance.

2. TERMINOLOGY

Stereoisomers are compounds that differ in the three-dimensional spatial arrangement of their constituent atoms and may be divided into two groups, enantiomers and diastereoisomers. Enantiomers are stereoisomers that are non-superimposable mirror images of one another and are therefore pairs of compounds related as an object to its mirror image in the same way that the left and right hands (or feet) are related. Such molecules are said to be chiral – from the Greek *chiros* meaning 'handed' (see Box 6.1). Such isomers are also referred to as optical isomers because of their ability to rotate the plane of plane polarized light, which is equal in magnitude but opposite in direction (Box 6.1).

In terms of the compounds of interest in pharmacology the most frequent, but not the

only, cause of chirality results from the presence of a tetracoordinate carbon atom in a molecule to which four different atoms or groups are attached (Figs 6.1 and 6.2). The presence of one such centre of chirality in a molecule gives rise to a pair of enantiomers, the presence of **n** such different centres yields 2^n stereoisomers and half that number of pairs of enantiomers.

Fig. 6.1 Three-dimensional representation of a pair of enantiomers. The structure on the right is a non-superimposable mirror image of that on the left. In this type of projection formula the bonds drawn as solid lines are in the plane of the paper, those represented by the wedge project above the plane, towards the reader, and those represented by the dashed lines project back into the plane, away from the reader. An alternative representation of stereoisomeric structures is shown in Fig. 6.6.

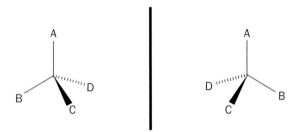

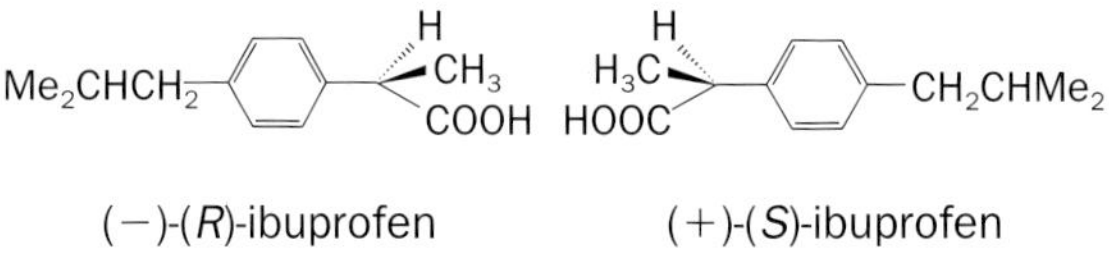

(−)-(*R*)-ibuprofen   (+)-(*S*)-ibuprofen

Fig. 6.2 The enantiomers of the nonsteriodal anti-inflammatory drug ibuprofen. The major pharmacological activity of ibuprofen, inhibition of cyclooxygenase, resides in the enantiomer of the *S*-absolute configuration, which is dextrorotatory as the free acid. The disposition of ibuprofen is complicated, as following administration of the racemate to man the relatively inactive *R*-enantiomer undergoes partial metabolic chiral inversion to (*S*)-ibuprofen. The drug is currently marketed in the UK as the racemate but ibuprofen was one of the first compounds to undergo the so-called chiral switch (see section 5.1) and the single enantiomer, dexibuprofen, was marketed in Austria in 1994 and more recently in Switzerland.

Box 6.1   Stereochemical terminology

Isomers	Compounds that have identical molecular formulae but differ in the ways in which the atoms are bonded to one another.
Stereoisomers	Structural isomers that have identical chemical constitutions but differ in the spatial arrangement of their atoms or groups.
Enantiomers	Stereoisomers which are non-superimposable mirror images of one another (Fig. 6.1), which are identical in all their physicochemical properties other than their rotation of the plane of plane polarized light, which is equal in magnitude but opposite in direction.
Racemate	A mixture of enantiomers in a 1:1 ratio which is not optically active.
Diastereoisomers	Stereoisomers which are not enantiomeric irrespective of their ability to rotate the plane of plane polarized light. The definition therefore also includes geometrical isomers or *cis/trans* isomers.
Epimers	Diastereoisomers which differ in configuration at one centre of chirality only.
Chirality	A term used to describe molecules (or any other objects, e.g. hands, feet) that cannot be superimposed on their mirror images. From the Greek word *chiros* meaning handed.
Achiral	A molecule (or object) that has a plane of symmetry and is therefore superimposable on its mirror image.
Dextrorotatory	Stereoisomers which rotate the plane of plane polarized light to the right (clockwise), indicated by a (+)- sign as a prefix to the chemical name.
Laevorotatory	Stereoisomers which rotate the plane of plane polarized light to the left (anticlockwise), indicated by a (−)- sign as a prefix to the chemical name.
Absolute configuration	The three-dimensional spatial arrangement of the atoms and/or groups bonded to a centre of chirality.
Relative configuration	The configuration of a centre of chirality determined in relation to a compound of known absolute configuration, e.g. the carbohydrate D-glyceraldehyde or the amino acid L-serine.

Those stereoisomers that are not enantiomeric, i.e. not mirror-image related, are said to be diastereomeric (Box 6.1; Fig. 6.3).

In a pair of enantiomers the relative positions, and interactions, between the individual atoms are identical as is the energy content and therefore, other than the direction of rotation of plane polarized light, their physicochemical properties are also identical. In contrast, the relative positions of the individual atoms, and their interactions, in a pair of diastereoisomers differ as do their physicochemical properties. As a result of their identical properties the separation, or resolution, of a pair of enantiomers

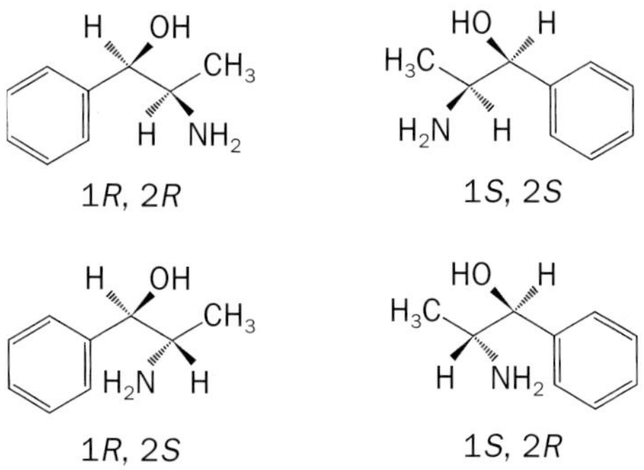

Fig. 6.3 Stereoisomers of norpseudoephedrine (upper pair) and norephedrine (lower pair). These molecules are also known as stereoisomers of phenylpropanolamine (and chemically as 2-amino-1-phenylpropanol). As the structure contains two centres of chirality four stereoisomers, two pairs of enantiomers, are possible; those stereoisomers that are not enantiomeric being diastereoisomeric. In this figure those compounds related horizontally (i.e. the upper and lower pairs) are enantiomeric, whereas those related vertically are diastereomeric. Thus the enantiomers of norpseudoephedrine are diastereoisomers of the enantiomers of norephedrine. Racemic norephedrine (phenylpropanolamine) was withdrawn in the USA (October 2000) following a report associating the drug with risk of haemorrhagic stroke. Some confusion was caused in the UK following a statement, subsequently found to be incorrect, that European products contained the single enantiomer (+)-norpseudoephedrine. UK products do in fact contain racemic norephedrine.

was (until recently) fairly difficult, whereas diastereoisomers may, in principle at least, be separated relatively easily.

As enantiomers differ with respect to the direction of rotation of the plane of plane polarized light, this property is frequently used in their designation. Those enantiomers that rotate light to the right are said to be dextrorotatory, indicated by a (+)- sign before the name of the compound or alternatively the prefix dex or dextro, whereas those which rotate light to the left are said to be laevorotatory, indicated by a (−)- sign or the prefix lev or levo. A racemic mixture is indicated by a (±)- prefix to the name. It is important to appreciate that this designation yields information concerning a physical property of the material but does not provide information regarding the three-dimensional spatial arrangement, or absolute configuration, of the molecule – the significant feature in pharmacology.

Once the three-dimensional structure of a stereoisomer has been determined (e.g. by X-ray crystallography), then the configuration of the molecule may be indicated by the use of a prefix letter to the name of the compound. Two systems are in use, the sequence rule or *R/S* notation or the older D/L system. The D/L system relates the stereochemistry of a molecule to that of a standard reference compound, either the carbohydrate D-glyceraldehyde or the amino acid L-serine. The use of this system has resulted in ambiguities and confusion, as the lower case letters may also be used to indicate the direction of rotation of light. Problems also arise as journal editors frequently alter the lower case letters to upper case in the titles of articles. Thus a defined, correct physicochemical property is transformed into a configurational designation that may well be incorrect. The D/L system is now outdated and should be restricted to the designation of carbohydrates and amino acids.

The sequence rule notation employs a 'ranking' approach for the designation of configuration. The substituent atoms bonded to the centre of chirality are placed in an order of priority based on their atomic number, the higher the atomic number the greater the priority. The molecule is then 'viewed' from the side opposite the group of lowest priority and if the remaining highest to lowest priorities are in a clockwise direction (to the right) the molecule is assigned the *Rectus* or R- configuration, and if anticlockwise (to the left) the *Sinister* or S- configuration (Figs 6.2 and 6.3). A racemic mixture is indicated by the prefix *R,S-* to the name of the compound.

These designations are defined by a set of arbitary rules and with respect to biological activity the significant feature is the three-dimensional spatial arrangement of the functionalities in the molecule. For example, the β-adrenoceptor blocking agents may be divided into two series of compounds, the arylethanolamines (e.g. sotalol, labetalol) and the aryloxypropanolamines (e.g. propranolol, metoprolol, etc.). In the case of the former agents the β-blocking activity resides in the enantiomers of the *R*- configuration, whereas in the latter series the active agents are those of the *S*- configuration. Examination of the structures presented in Fig. 6.4 indicates that the spatial orientation of the aromatic ring, hydroxyl and secondary amino functions are the same in both series of compounds even though their configurational designation is

reversed. This alteration in designation arises as a result of the introduction of the oxygen atom in the aryloxypropanolamine series causing an alteration in the ranking of the groups about the centre of chirality. Without a knowledge of the sequence rules and their application it could be assumed that the stereochemical requirements for activity within the two series of compounds were for some reason reversed.

2.1 Nomenclature and generic names

The dex/levo approach to nomenclature does provide information with respect to a physical property of the material and does indicate to the clinician the stereochemical nature, i.e. single enantiomer or mixture, of the drug he is prescribing. However, the situation here is not as straightforward as it first appears, as both the magnitude and direction of rotation may vary with the conditions used to make the determination, e.g. with solvent and form of the analyte (either free acid or base or as a salt).

The use of the dex/levo prefixes has been adopted for the approved names of a number of agents and a list of the agents indexed in this form in the current editions of the *British National Formulary* (No. 44) and *British Pharmacopoeia* (2002) are presented in Box 6.2. This approach has also been employed in a number of instances where both single enantiomer and racemic mixtures are, or were, available at the same time as a result of the chiral switch (see section 5.1), e.g. dexfenfluramine and fenfluramine, dexibuprofen and ibuprofen. An alternative approach that was introduced recently incorporates the configurational designation into the names of some agents previously available only as racemates. Thus the single enantiomer forms of the proton pump inhibitor (*S*)-omeprazole and the selective serotonin reuptake inhibitor (*S*)-citalopram have been designated as esomeprazole and escitalopram respectively. In some instances a completely different name has been used for a single isomer product, e.g. dilevalol for the β-blocking stereoisomer of the combined α- and β-blocking agent labetalol.

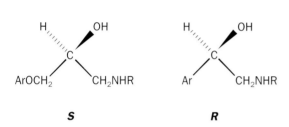

Fig. 6.4 Three-dimensional spatial arrangements of the functionalities in the stereoisomers of the β-adrenoreceptor blockers. The commercially available β-blockers fall into two chemical groups, aryloxypropanolamine (left) and arylethanolamine (right) derivatives. The β-blocking activity resides predominantly in the enantiomers of the *S*-absolute configuration in the aryloxypropanolamine series and the *R*-enantiomers of the arylethanolamine series. From a cursory consideration of this information it would appear that the stereoselectivity in action within the two series of compounds is reversed. However, this reversal is artificial, as the three-dimensional spatial arrangement of the functionalities of the active isomers in each series is identical, i.e. the relative orientations of the aromatic ring (Ar), the hydroxyl group and the alkyl (R) substituted secondary amino groups about the centres of chirality are identical. The alteration in configurational designation arises because of the introduction of the ether oxygen atom in the aryloxypropanolamine series, resulting in a change in group priority on application of the sequence rules.

Box 6.2   Single stereoisomer compounds indexed using the Dex/Lev prefix in the *British National Formulary (BNF)* and *British Pharmacopoeia (BP)*

Levamisole (hydrochloride)[‡]	Dexamethasone (plus esters)
Levetiracetam*	Dexamfetamine (sulphate; Dexamphetamine sulphate)[‡]
Levobunolol (hydrochloride)[‡]	Dexchlorpheniramine maleate[†]
Levobupivacaine*	Dexfenfluramine*
Levocabastine (hydrochloride)[‡]	Dexketoprofen*
Levocarnitine[†]	Dexpanthenol[†]
Levocetirizine*	Dextromethorphan (hydrobromide)[‡]
Levodopa	Dextromoramide (tartrate)[‡]
Levodropropizine[†]	Dextropropoxyphene (hydrochloride, napsilate)[‡]
Levofloxacin*	
Levofolinic acid* (calcium levofolinate)	
Levomenthol[†]	
Levomepromazine (hydrochloride, maleate)[‡]	
Levonorgestrel	
Levothyroxine (sodium)[‡]	

*BNF (No. 44, September 2002) only; [†]BP (2002) only; [‡]BP, salt form indexed.

---

3. BIOLOGICAL DISCRIMINATION OF STEREOISOMERS

At a molecular level biological environments are highly chiral, being composed of 'handed' biopolymers (e.g. proteins, glycolipids and polynucleotides) from the chiral precursors of L- series amino acids and D- series carbohydrates. The macromolecular structures of such biopolymers also give rise to chirality as a result of helicity. Helical structures may have either a left- or right-handed turn in the same way that a spiral staircase, or corkscrew, may be left- or right-handed. In the case of the DNA double-helix and the protein α-helix the molecules have a right-handed turn.

Since many of the processes of drug action and disposition involve an interaction with chiral biological macromolecules it should not be surprising that enzymes and receptors frequently show a stereochemical preference for one of a pair of enantiomers. Indeed many of the natural ligands for such systems, e.g. neuro-transmitters, hormones, endogenous opiods, etc., are single stereoisomers and as Lehmann (1982; Further reading) stated 'the stereoselectivity displayed by pharmacological systems constitutes the best evidence that receptors exist and that they incorporate concrete molecular entities as integral components of their active sites'.

The possibility that a pair of enantiomers could exhibit different biological activities was established in the early years of the last century.[1] In order to rationalize these observed differences in pharmacodynamic activity between enantiomers Easson and Stedman[4] proposed their so-called 'three point-fit' model for the drug receptor interaction (Fig. 6.5). According to this model the more potent enantiomer is involved with a minimum of three intermolecular interactions with complementary sites on the receptor, whereas the less potent enantiomer may interact at two sites only. This model is a useful but obviously relatively simplistic representation of the drug–receptor interaction, since it assumes that

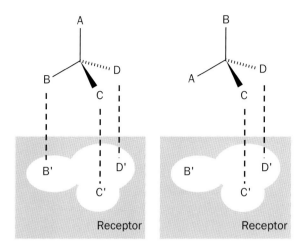

Fig. 6.5 Biological discrimination of a pair of enantiomers on interaction with a biological macromolecule (Easson–Stedman model). The enantiomer on the left takes part in three bonding interactions with complementary functionalities on the receptor, whereas that on the right interacts at two sites only. Alternative orientations of the enantiomer on the right to the receptor surface are possible but only two interactions may take place at one time.

the drug adopts a particular orientation in relation to the receptor site. In addition, conformational changes in both the drug and receptor may take place during the interaction such that the final 'model' may be highly complex.

The differential pharmacodynamic activity of drug stereoisomers has given rise to additional terminology, which is summarized in Box 6.3.

The magnitude of the eudismic ratio varies with the compounds under investigation, and between receptor systems for compounds that interact with more than one receptor, values of eudismic ratio between 100- and 1000-fold are not uncommon.

The Eutomer/Distomer designations of stereoisomers refer to a single activity of the drug, and for dual action compounds the eutomer for one activity may be the distomer for the other, or the stereoisomers may be equipotent. For example, the β-blocking activity of propranolol resides in the enantiomer of the S- absolute configuration, whereas the two isomers are equipotent with respect to their membrane-stabilizing properties.

Differentiation between stereoisomers also occurs in drug disposition and may be significant for those processes that depend on a direct interaction with a chiral macromolecule, i.e. an enzyme during metabolism or a transporter system during absorption and distribution. Stereochemistry has little impact on enantioselectivity of passive processes that are dependent on the physicochemical properties of a molecule (i.e. pK_a, lipid solubility, molecular size), such as diffusion across biological membranes – the major mechanism associated with absorption, distribution and renal excretion. In contrast, differentiation may occur between diastereoisomers as a result of their differential solubility.

With respect to the parameters used in pharmacokinetics the magnitude of the differences

Box 6.3 Stereochemical terminology and biological activity

Eutomer	Stereoisomer with the greater receptor affinity or activity.
Distomer	Stereoisomer with the lower receptor affinity or activity.
Eudismic ratio	Ratio of the affinities, or activities, of the eutomer to the distomer.
Eudismic index	Logarithm of the eudismic ratio.
Eudismic affinity quotient	Slope of a plot of eudismic index versus pK_{Eu}. A quantitative measure of the stereoselectivity within a compound series for a particular biological effect.

between enantiomers (generally 1–3-fold) (Table 6.1), tend to be much smaller than those observed in their pharmacodynamic properties.[5] This is particularly the case for parameters that represent the whole body level of organization such as systemic clearance, volume of distribution and half-life. Larger differences may be observed in parameters representing organ levels of organization, e.g. hepatic metabolic clearance and renal clearance, and larger still at the macromolecular level, e.g. intrinsic metabolite formation clearance.[6] Those parameters that represent the whole body are determined by multiple organ parameters which in turn are a reflection of multiple macromolecular interactions which may show opposite stereoselectivities. Thus, stereoselectivity may be either amplified or attenuated with each level of organization.

As a result of stereoselectivity in drug disposition the plasma profiles of the enantiomers of a drug administered as a racemate frequently differ, and an examination of plasma concentration–effect relationships, or the determination of pharmacokinetic parameters based on 'total' drug present in biological samples is essentially meaningless or 'sophisticated nonsense'.[7]

4. PHARMACODYNAMIC COMPLEXITIES

A number of possible scenarios may arise with respect to the pharmacodynamic properties of a pair of enantiomers and these are summarized in Box 6.4. There are relatively few examples of drugs in which the pharmacodynamic activity is restricted to a single enantiomer with the other being totally devoid of activity. In the majority of cases a pair of enantiomers will differ either quantitatively or qualitatively in terms of their activity. Similarly, there are few examples where the beneficial activity resides in a single enantiomer and the adverse effects, or toxicity, are associated with the other. In some cases the activity of a pair of enantiomers may be so different that both are marketed with specific therapeutic indications. For example, in the case of propoxyphene the dextrorotatory isomer is used as an analgesic, whereas levopropoxyphene is marketed as an antitussive

---

Box 6.4 Enantiomers and pharmacodynamic complexity

- Activity resides in a single enantiomer
- Both enantiomers have similar pharmacodynamic profiles
- Both enantiomers are marketed with different therapeutic indications
- Enantiomers have opposite effects at the same biological target
- One enantiomer antagonizes the adverse effects of the other
- The required activity resides in both with the adverse effects predominantly associated with one enantiomer
- The required activity resides in a single enantiomer with the adverse effects associated with both

---

(Fig. 6.6). In this example not only are the molecules mirror image-related but so are their trade names, Darvon and Novrad. A similar situation occurs with other opiate derivatives, e.g. dextromethorphan (antitussive) and levomethorphan (analgesic).

Examples are also known where a pair of enantiomers have opposite effects and interactions occur such that the observed activity of the racemate does not provide a clear indication of what in fact is occurring. Racemic picenadol, a phenylpiperidine derivative with analgesic activity, is a partial agonist at the μ receptor. Examination of the properties of the individual enantiomers indicates that the analgesic activity resides in the (+)-3S, 4R-stereoisomer whereas (−)-(3R, 4S)-picenadol is a μ receptor antagonist, the partial agonist activity of the racemate arising from the greater agonist potency of the (+)-stereoisomer.[8]

Similarly, the enantiomers of a number of the 1,4-dihydropyridine calcium channel-blocking agents, used in the treatment of angina and hypertension, have opposite actions on channel

Table 6.1   Stereoselectivity in pharmacokinetic parameters following the oral administration of racemic drugs to man

Drug	Enantiomer	Clearance (units)	Renal clearance (units)	Volume of distribution (units)	Half-life (h)	Fraction unbound (%)
Bupivacaine*	R	0.40 l/min	–	117 l	3.5	6.6
	S	0.32 l/min	–	71 l	2.6	4.5
Carvedilol	R	0.87 l/min	–	302 l	5.3	0.45
	S	1.26 l/min	–	487 l	5.1	0.63
Etodolac	R	22 ml/h/kg	–	0.21 l/kg	6.6	0.47
	S	288 ml/h/kg	–	1.6 l/kg	4.3	0.85
Hexobarbitone	R	136 l/h	1.47 L/h	–	6.7	–
	S	21 l/h	0.13 L/h	–	2.8	–
Ketorolac[†]	R	19.0 ml/h/kg	–	0.075 l/kg	3.6	–
	S	45.9 ml/h/kg	–	0.135 l/kg	2.4	–
Mephobarbitone	R	170 l/h	–	716 l	3.1	36.5
	S	1.5 l/h	–	105 l	50.5	43.9
Metoprolol	R	1.7 l/h/kg	74.8 ml/min	7.6 l/kg	2.7	–
	S	1.2 l/h/kg	69.7 ml/min	5.5 l/kg	3.0	–
Mexiletine	R	8.6 ml/min/kg	0.61 ml/min/kg	6.6 l/kg	9.1	19.8
	S	8.1 ml/min/kg	0.72 ml/min/kg	7.3 l/kg	11.0	28.3
Nitrendipine	R	6.6 l/min	–	–	7.5	–
	S	3.1 l/min	–	–	7.7	–
Nivaldipine	R	110 ml/min/kg	–	–	2.1	–
	S	39.5 ml/min/kg	–	–	1.5	–
Prenylamine	R	4.0 l/min	1.3 ml/min	–	8.2	–
	S	20.5 l/min	4.0 ml/min	–	24.0	–
Propranolol*	R	1.21 l/min	–	4.82 l/kg	3.5	–
	S	1.03 l/min	–	4.08 l/kg	3.6	–
Propranolol	R	6.9 l/min	–	–	4.3	20.3
	S	4.6 l/min	–	–	4.8	17.6
Verapamil	R	1.72 l/min	–	2.74 l/kg	4.1	6.3
	S	7.46 l/min	–	6.42 l/kg	4.8	11.5
Warfarin	R	1.9 ml/h/kg	–	129 ml/kg	47.1	3.6
	S	2.0 ml/h/kg	–	70.5 ml/kg	24.4	2.2

*Intravenous administration, [†]intramuscular administration.
Average values only provided.
Data from Eichelbaum and Gross (1996; Further reading), and references 5 and 6.

Propoxyphene

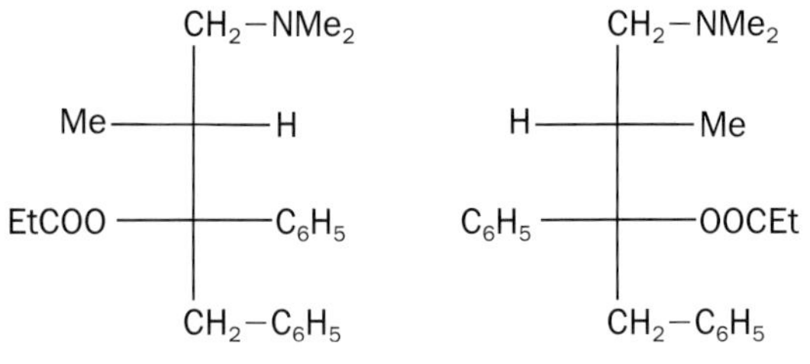

	CH$_2$-NMe$_2$			CH$_2$-NMe$_2$	
Me	—	H	H	—	Me
EtCOO	—	C$_6$H$_5$	C$_6$H$_5$	—	OOCEt
	CH$_2$-C$_6$H$_5$			CH$_2$-C$_6$H$_5$	

(+)-2R,3S
Analgesic
Darvon

(−)-2S,3R
Antitussive
Novrad

Fig. 6.6 Stereoisomers of propoxyphene. Propoxyphene contains two centres of chirality in its structure and therefore four stereoisomers, two pairs of enantiomers, are possible. In the pair of enantiomers shown the dextrorotatory isomer (left), dextropropoxyphene, is marketed as an analgesic whereas the laevorotatory isomer (right), levopropoxyphene, is marketed in the USA as an antitussive. The trade names of the two products, Darvon and Novrad, are also mirror image-related. The structures are presented in an alternative three-dimensional representation to the wedge diagrams used in the previous figures, known as a Fischer projection. In a projection of this type all bonds are represented by plain lines and the chiral centre under examination lies in the plane of the paper. Those groups that are vertically linked to the chiral centre project back away from the reader, i.e. below the plane of the paper, whereas those linked horizontally project towards the reader, i.e. above the plane of the paper.

function; the S-enantiomers are activators, whereas the R-enantiomers are antagonists at L-type calcium channels. At one time it was thought that the enantiomers acted at different sites, however, it is now thought that conformational differences between the open and inactivated states of the channels account for the observed stereoselectivity. The situation is further complicated as the S-enantiomers of some of these agents are antagonists under depolarizing conditions. Indeed, as a result of the complexity of action of these agents Triggle[9] has described them as 'molecular chameleons'.

The inotropic sympathomimetic agent dobut-amine is a racemic drug reported to increase the force of myocardial contraction without increasing either heart rate or blood pressure. Examination of the pharmacodynamic properties of the individual enantiomers in vitro indicates that they are both active but at different receptors. (+)-Dobutamine acts as a relatively potent agonist at β$_1$- and β$_2$-adrenoceptors and has weak α-antagonist properties, whereas the (−)-enantiomer is a potent α$_1$-adrenoceptor agonist. Thus it appears that both enantiomers contribute to the positive inotropic effects of the drug and that the peripheral vasoconstrictor and vasodilation effects of the (−)- and (+)-enantiomers respectively, essentially cancel each other out. In the case of dobutamine it would appear that the use of the racemate has advantages over the individual enantiomers.[10]

Differences in pharmacodynamic activity between enantiomers may also be exploited to yield a product with an improved therapeutic profile. Administration to man of the loop diuretic racemic indacrinone, evaluated for the treatment of hypertension and congestive heart failure, results in the elevation of serum uric acid. Examination of the properties of the individual enantiomers indicated that the diuretic and natriuretic activity resides in the R-enantiomer (half-life 10–12 h), whereas the S-enantiomer (half-life 2–5 h) possesses uricosuric activity. Following administration of the racemate the half-life of (S)-indacrinone, and hence its uricosuric activity, is too short to prevent the observed increase in serum uric acid.[11] Alteration of the enantiomeric composition of the drug from the 1:1 ratio of the racemate by increasing the content of the S-enantiomer to S:R:4:1 results in a mixture which is isouricaemic and a further increase to 8:1 yields a hypouricaemic product.[12] Hence in the case of indacrinone the evaluation and exploitation of the properties of the individual enantiomers resulted in an agent with an improved therapeutic profile. The development of indacrinone was stopped in the mid-1980s but from the investigations reported the principle of manipulation of stereoisomer composition for an improved therapeutic profile of a product was established.

There are also examples of compounds currently available as single stereoisomers where the enantiomer may offer a potential advantage. The β-blocker timolol is used as the single *S*-enantiomer for the treatment of angina, hypertension and glaucoma. Following local administration to the eye significant amounts of the drug are systemically absorbed and cardiovascular and pulmonary effects have been observed.[13] Such effects are obviously of significance in patients for whom β-blockers are contraindicated, e.g. asthmatics, and cases of severe bronchoconstriction and deaths have been reported.[14] Evaluation of the activity of (*R*)-timolol has indicated a 3–4-fold reduction in potency in comparison with the *S*-enantiomer in terms of reducing intraocular pressure but a 50–90-fold reduction in terms of β-blockade. Thus timolol probably represents an example of an agent where both enantiomers could be marketed with their own indications, with the advantage of reduced systemic effects of the *R*-enantiomer for the treatment of glaucoma.

In addition to the possible pharmacodynamic complexities outlined above, relatively little information is available with respect to the influence of route of administration, formulation and biological factors on the disposition and action of the enantiomers of the large number of agents currently available as racemates. Examples of what may occur are summarized in Table 6.2.[15-24] As a result of such considerations, together with potential adverse reaction and drug safety issues,[25] drug stereochemistry became the subject of considerable debate and an issue for both the pharmaceutical industry and regulatory agencies.

5. RACEMATES VERSUS ENANTIOMERS

With the realization of the potential significance of the pharmacological differences between enantiomers in the late 1980s and early 1990s, drug stereochemistry and racemates versus enantiomers became topics of considerable debate. Advocates of the use of single stereoisomers regarded racemates as drugs containing 50% impurity, while others stated that the use of racemates is essentially polypharmacy with the proportions in the mixture being dictated by chemical rather than therapeutic or pharmacological criteria.

A compound frequently cited, particularly in the popular scientific and lay press, as an example where the use of a single stereoisomer would have prevented a tragedy is the hypnotic teratogen thalidomide. A study in the late 1970s reported that following administration of the individual enantiomers to mice the teratogenic activity resided in the *S*-enantiomer. However, previous studies in a more sensitive test species, New Zealand White rabbits, indicated that both enantiomers are teratogenic and additional investigations have indicated that the drug readily undergoes racemization in biological media.[26-28] Therefore even if a product containing the single *R*-enantiomer had been available patients would still have been exposed to both stereoisomers. Thus, taken together the available data indicate that the situation with thalidomide is by no means as clear-cut as implied by the secondary literature and the compound is not a useful example to cite in favour of single stereoisomer products.

There are a number of potential advantages associated with the use of single enantiomers (Box 6.5) and the majority of the major regulatory authorities have examined the issues associated with drug chirality and have either published policy statements or issued guidelines.[29] To date none of the regulatory agencies

---

Box 6.5 Potential advantages of single enantiomer products

- Less complex more selective pharmacodynamic profile
- Potential for an improved therapeutic index
- Less complex pharmacokinetic profile
- Reduced potential for complex drug interactions
- Less complex relationship between plasma concentration and effect

Table 6.2 Factors influencing the stereoselectivity of drug action and disposition

Factor	Drug	Comment
Route of administration	Verapamil	Concentration–effect relationships based on 'total' drug plasma concentrations indicate an enhanced effect following intravenous compared with oral administration; associated with stereoselective first-pass metabolism of the more active S-enantiomer.[15]
	Propranolol	Appears to be less potent following intravenous compared with oral administration; due to stereoselective first-pass metabolism of the less active R-enantiomer.[16]
Formulation	Verapamil	Enantiomeric ratio (R/S) of the maximum plasma concentrations (Cmax) and area under the plasma concentration versus time curves (AUC) significantly lower following immediate-release (IR) than sustained-release (SR) formulations (Cmax, IR, 4.52; SR, 5.83; AUC, IR, 5.04; SR, 7.75); variation associated with concentration and/or input rate-related saturable first-pass metabolism of (S)-verapamil.[17]
Drug interactions	Warfarin	Extensively examined drug with respect to stereoselectivity in drug interactions, some agents (e.g. phenylbutazone, sulphinpyrazone, metronidazole, cotrimoxazole, ticrynafen and quinalbarbitone) selective for the more active S-enantiomer; others (e.g. cimetidine, enoxacin, rifampicin and clofibrate) selective for (R)-warfarin, whereas others show no selectivity (e.g. amiodarone).[5]
	Verapamil	Stereoselective reduction in clearance of the S-enantiomer following administration with cimetidine, resulting in an increased negative dromotropic effect on atrioventricular conduction.[18]
	Hexobarbitone	Stereoselective increase in clearance following administration with rifampicin; S-enantiomer, 6-fold increase; R-enantiomer, 89-fold increase.[19]
Ageing	Hexobarbitone	Stereoselective decrease in clearance with age; S-enantiomer twofold greater clearance in young compared with elderly subjects; R-enantiomer, no age effect.[20]
Disease	Ibuprofen	Plasma concentrations of (S)-ibuprofen lower than those of the R-enantiomer in cirrhotic patients; ratio of area under the plasma concentration time curve (S/R) 0.94 in cirrhotic patients compared with 1.3 in healthy volunteers.[21]

Table 6.2 Continued

Factor	Drug	Comment
Gender	Mephobarbital	Oral clearance of *R*-enantiomer significantly greater in young men compared with young or elderly women, or elderly men; *S*-enantiomer no significant differences between groups.[22]
Pharmacogenetics	Metoprolol	Enantiomeric ratio (*S/R*) of the area under the plasma concentration versus time curve decreases from 1.37 in extensive metabolizers (EMs) to 0.90 in poor metabolizers (PMs) of debrisoquine; the 'total' plasma concentration–effect relationship shifts to the right in poor compared with extensive metabolizers.[23]
	Mephenytoin	Oral clearance of (*S*)-mephenytoin reduced from 4.7 l/min in EMs to 0.029 l/min in PMs; *R*-enantiomer clearance 0.03 and 0.02 l/min in EMs and PMs respectively.[6]
Race	Propranolol	Oral clearance of both enantiomers greater in black compared with white subjects; stereoselective for the *R*-enantiomer.[24]

have an absolute requirement for the development of single stereoisomer products. The decision on the stereochemical form, i.e. single stereoisomer or racemic mixture, to be developed resides with the compound sponsor, but this decision should be scientifically justified on quality, safety and efficacy criteria, together with the risk-benefit ratio.[29] Some of the arguments that could be used to support the submission of a racemic mixture are presented in Box 6.6.

As a result of regulatory attitudes the number of chiral 'new chemical entities' (NCEs) submitted for approval as single stereoisomers over the last 10 years has increased. In 1998 some 40 synthetic agents were granted generic and proprietary names in the USA, which may be used as an indication of the number of agents at an advanced stage of development. Of these, 20 were single stereoisomers, 9 were racemic mixtures and the remainder were

achiral.[30] The most recent information from the Medicines Control Agency, for the years 1996–1999, indicates that of 37 synthetic chiral NCEs submitted for evaluation 24 were single stereoisomers.[29] The trend toward single stereoisomer products is obvious and in the future single isomer products are likely to be the norm and mixtures the exception.

5.1 Chiral switch

In addition to NCEs a number of agents currently marketed as racemic mixtures have been re-examined as potential single enantiomer products. The concept of investigating single stereoisomers following either the observation of unacceptable adverse effects or developments in technology that enable the production of a single enantiomer is not new. Penicillamine, used as a synthetic racemate in the USA, was withdrawn as a result of optic neuritis; however, D-penicillamine was used in the UK and the adverse effect was not observed at that time.[31,32] Similarly the initial use of racemic dopa for the treatment of Parkinson's disease resulted in a number of adverse effects which on administration of L-dopa were either reduced or abolished.[33,34] The oral contraceptive agent norgestrel, the hormonal activity of which resides in the laevorotatory enantiomer, was initially marketed in the UK in 1974 as a racemic mixture. Subsequently, following developments in the synthetic process, levonorgestrel was marketed in 1979. Both the single enantiomer and the racemate are commercially available and the subject of separate monographs in the *British Pharmacopoeia* (2002).

The so-called racemic or chiral switches have resulted in a number of compounds being remarketed as single stereoisomers and several others are at an advanced stage of development (Table 6.3).[35–60] Such re-introductions, as pointed out above, may result in products containing the single stereoisomer and racemic mixture being available at the same time and therefore there is a requirement for physicians to have some knowledge of stereochemical nomenclature to ensure that they know what they have prescribed.

Box 6.6   Possible arguments for the justification of racemates

- The individual enantiomers are stereochemically unstable and readily racemize in vitro and/or in vivo
- The preparation of the drug as a single isomer on a commercial scale is not technically feasible
- The individual enantiomers have similar pharmacological and toxicological profiles
- One enantiomer is known to be totally inactive and does not provide an additional body burden or influence the pharmacokinetic properties of the other
- The use of a racemate produces a superior therapeutic effect to either individual enantiomer
- The therapeutic significance of the compound in relation to the disease state and adverse reaction profile

Table 6.3   Racemate to single enantiomer: chiral switch

Drug	Action/indication	Comment
Dexfenfluramine	Anoretic	Both single enantiomer and racemate withdrawn following reports of valvular heart disease and pulmonary hypertension.[35]
Levofloxacin	Antimicrobial agent	Activity resides in the $(-)$-S-enantiomer and slight differences in enantiomeric disposition favour the single enantiomer.[36,37]
Dilevalol	β-Blocker	R,R-stereoisomer of labetalol marketed in Japan and Portugal, approved in several other countries, but rapidly withdrawn due to hepatotoxicity.[25]
Dexibuprofen	NSAID	Following administration of the racemate (R)-ibuprofen undergoes partial chiral inversion to the active S-enantiomer. The mean daily dose of (S)-ibuprofen in patients with rheumatoid arthritis reduced by approximately one third compared with the racemate.[38] Available in Austria and Switzerland.
Dexketoprofen	NSAID	Reduced dose requirement; formulation as the water-soluble trometamol salt results in more rapid absorption and onset of action compared with administration of the racemic free acid; reduced potential for gastric ulceration in animals.[39]
Levobupivacaine	Local anaesthetic	Clinical profile similar to that of racemic bupivacaine but with a reduction in cardiotoxicity.[40,41]
(S)-Ketamine	Anaesthetic	(S)-Ketamine 3–4-fold more potent, with approximately twice the affinity for opiate receptors compared with the R-enantiomer; emergence reactions (hallucinations and agitation) and abuse potential of the drug reduced.[42] Licensed in Germany.
(R)-Fluoxetine	Antidepressant	Development stopped because of a significant increase in QTc prolongation at higher doses.[43]
(S)-Fluoxetine	Migraine prophylaxis	Phase II placebo-controlled study indicated decreased attack frequency earlier and greater in the treatment compared with the placebo group; authors concluded that the data support progression to a Phase III evaluation.[44]
Esomeprazole	Proton pump inhibitor	Lower first-pass metabolism, slower plasma clearance and greater systemic availability than (R)-omeprazole. Metabolism mediated by cytochrome P450 2C19, plasma clearance in EMs and PMs of the S-enantiomer are 1.04 and 0.22 l/h/kg, respectively, corresponding values for (R)-omeprazole being 1.44 and 0.13 l/h/kg.[45] Evidence that esomeprazole maintains intragastric pH in patients with gastro-oesophageal reflux disease more effectively than other proton pump inhibitors.[46]

continued

Table 6.3 Continued		
Drug	**Action/indication**	**Comment**
Cisatracurium	Neuromuscular blocker	Developed from atracurium, a compound containing four chiral centres in its structure, that owing to its symmetrical nature exists as a mixture of 10 stereoisomeric forms, with cisatracurium (the $1R, 2R, 1'R, 2'R$-stereoisomer) comprising approximately 15% of the mixture. Cisatracurium is approximately threefold more potent than the mixture, with a slightly slower onset of action and reduced histamine-releasing properties. As a result of the lower dose requirement of cisatracurium the formation of laudanosine (a metabolite reported to induce seizures in animals) is reduced compared with atracurium.[47]
(R)-Salbutamol	β_2-Agonist	Racemic and (S)-salbutamol induce airway hyperresponsiveness in sensitized animals; use of the racemate associated with some loss of bronchodilator potency, decreased protection against bronchoprovocation and increased sensitivity to allergen challenge and some bronchoconstrictor stimuli.[48] Studies in both children and adults have indicated that inhalation of (R)-salbutamol produces significantly greater bronchodilation than the equivalent dose of the racemate.[49] Licensed in the USA.
Escitalopram	Selective serotonin reuptake inhibitor	(S)-Citalopram, which is between 130- and 160-fold more potent than the R-enantiomer in in vitro test systems.[50] Clinical studies indicate a faster onset of action, a reduction in side-effects and improved tolerability profile, compared with the racemate.[51,52]
Levocetirizine	H_1-Antihistamine	(R)-Cetirizine; K_i values against H_1-receptors 3.2 and 6.3 nM for the R-enantiomer and racemate, respectively. Clinical studies indicate the equivalence of a 2.5 mg oral dose of the enantiomer and 5 mg of the racemate, (S)-cetirizine being essentially inactive.[53,54]
(R,R)-Methylphenidate	Attention-deficit hyperactivity disorder	The R,R-enantiomer is approximately 10-fold more potent than (S,S)-methylphenidate in the inhibition of dopamine and noradrenaline uptake into striatal and hypothalamic synaptosomes, respectively.[55] The drug undergoes stereoselective presystemic metabolism, the bioavailability of the R,R- and S,S-enantiomers being approx. 0.23 and approx. 0.05, respectively.[56] The single enantiomer is reported to be equally effective as the racemate at half the dose, with a more rapid onset of action and possible improved side-effect profile. Licensed in the USA.[57]

In addition to the agents cited above a number of other compounds, some of which are at an advanced stage of development, are undergoing evaluation as single stereoisomer products including: (drug (indication; proposed advantage)): (R, R)-formoterol (asthma; decreased development of airway hyperreactivity), (S)-oxybutinin (urinary incontinence; decreased anticholinergic side-effects); (S)-doxazosin (benign prostatic hyperplasia: decreased orthostatic hypotension); (S)-lansoprazole, (−)-pantoprazole (gastro-oesophageal reflux); (+)-norcisapride (nocturnal heartburn; reduced cardiotoxicity).[58–60]

Such re-evaluations are not without problems and in some instances unexpected findings may result. For example, the development of the single β-blocking stereoisomer dilevalol, from the combined α- and β-blocking drug labetalol was terminated due to hepatotoxicity; the SWORD trial (Survival With Oral d-Sotalol) was terminated prematurely because of increased mortality in patients treated with the drug compared with those in the placebo group;[61] both dex- and racemic fenfluramine were withdrawn following an association with valvular heart disease;[35] and more recently the development of (R)-fluoxetine was terminated because of a small but significant increase in QTc prolongation at the highest dose tested.[43] The above examples indicate that the removal of the 'isomeric ballast' from a mixture is not a trivial matter and may have significant financial consequences.

5.2 Economic considerations

In some instances it could be argued that the development of a single isomer product from a previously marketed racemate would not provide a genuine therapeutic benefit.[62] However, the global market for pharmaceuticals is enormous, approximately $300 billion in 1997, and with a number of commercially highly successful drugs marketed as racemates the economic significance of drug stereochemistry is obvious. For example, omeprazole was the biggest selling drug worldwide in 1997 with US sales in excess of $5 billion.[62] Replacement of such agents with single stereoisomer products could result in an extension of patent protection for the innovator and also protection against generic competition with the racemate. There are instances of agents where the individual enantiomers were not patented by the innovators and companies specializing in chiral technologies have entered into licensing agreements. However, the development of single stereoisomers from marketed racemates is not without financial risk. For example, it has been estimated that the research and development costs of dilevalol represented an investment of $100 million[63,64] and the recent termination of the licensing agreement between Lilly and Sepracor for (R)-fluoxetine resulted in the latter company receiving only $23 million of what was to have been a $90 million deal, and a fall in stock value of 28%.[43]

6. CONCLUDING COMMENTS

The above brief discussion has attempted to highlight the significance of stereochemical considerations in pharmacology and to indicate the advantages of 'chiral pharmacology' in terms of providing additional insight into drug action. For many agents currently available as racemates relatively little is known with respect to the pharmacodynamic, toxicological and pharmacokinetic properties of the individual enantiomers, or on the influence of disease state, ageing, gender, race or genetic factors on enantiomeric disposition and/or response. Additional investigations on the enantiomers of marketed racemates may result in new indications for 'old' compounds, in improved clinical use of these agents with an increase in safety and efficacy, and the re-marketing of established compounds for hopefully sound therapeutic as well as commercial reasons.

In the future single stereoisomer products will be the norm and racemates the exception, and in the not too distant future we will wonder what the stereochemical 'fuss' was all about.

REFERENCES

Further reading

Aboul-Enein HY, Wainer IW, eds. *The Impact of Stereochemistry on Drug Development and Use*. New York: John Wiley, 1997.

Ariëns EJ, Soudijn W, Timmermans PBMWM, eds. *Stereochemistry and Biological Activity of Drugs*. Oxford: Blackwell Scientific, 1983.

Crossley R. *Chirality and the Biological Activity of Drugs*. Boca Raton, FL: CRC Press, 1995.

Eichelbaum M, Gross AS. Stereochemical aspects of drug action and disposition. In: Testa B, Meyer UA, eds. *Advances in Drug Research*, Vol 28. London: Academic Press, 1996: 1–64.

Eichelbaum M, Testa B, Somogi A, eds.

Stereochemical Aspects of Drug Action. Heidelberg: Springer, 2002.

Lehmann PAF. Quantifying stereoselectivity or how to choose a pair of shoes when you have two left feet. *Trend Pharmacol Sci* 1982; **3**: 103–6.

Lough WJ, Wainer IW, eds. *Chirality in Natural and Applied Sciences.* Oxford: Blackwell, 2002.

Smith DF, ed. *CRC Handbook of Stereoisomers: Drugs in psychopharmacology.* Boca Raton, FL: CRC Press, 1984.

Smith DF, ed. *Handbook of Stereoisomers: Therapeutic drugs.* Boca Raton, FL: CRC Press, 1989.

Wainer IW, ed. *Drug Stereochemistry. Analytical methods and pharmacology*, 2nd edn. New York: Marcel Dekker, 1993.

Wainer IW, Drayer DE, eds. *Drug Stereochemistry. Analytical methods and pharmacology.* New York: Marcel Dekker, 1988.

Web-sites

■ http://www.nobel.se/chemistry/laureates/2001/public.html
Nobel Prize in Chemistry 2001. Three scientists shared the 2001 Nobel Prize in Chemistry: William S. Knowles, previously at Monsanto Company, St Louis, MO, USA; Ryoji Noyori, Nagoya University, Chikusa, Nagoya, Japan; and K. Barry Sharpless, Scripps Research Institute, La Jolla, CA, USA. The Royal Swedish Academy of Sciences has awarded the Prize for their development of catalytic asymmetric synthesis. The achievements of these three chemists are of great importance for academic research, for the development of new drugs and materials, and are being used in many industrial syntheses of pharmaceutical products and other biologically active substances. This provides a description and background information about the scientists' award-winning discoveries.

■ http://www.nobel.se/chemistry/educational/poster/2001/index.html
Illustrated presentation.

Scientific papers

1. Cushny AR. *Biological Relations of Optically Isomeric Substances.* London: Baillière, Tindall and Cox, 1926.

2. Ariëns EJ, Wuis EW, Veringa EJ. Stereoselec-

tivity of bioactive xenobiotics. A pre-Pasteur attitude in medicinal chemistry, pharmacokinetics and clinical pharmacology. *Biochem Pharmacol* 1988: **37**: 9–18.

3. Lehmann PAF, Rodrigues de Miranda JF, Ariëns EJ. Stereoselectivity and affinity in molecular pharmacology. In: Jucker E, ed. *Progress in Drug Research*, Vol 20. Basel: Birkhäuser Verlag, 1976: 101–42.

4. Easson LH, Stedman E. Studies on the relationship between chemical constitution and physiological action. V. Molecular dissymmetry and physiological activity. *Biochem J* 1933; **27**: 1257–66.

5. Tucker GT, Lennard MS. Enantiomer specific pharmacokinetics. *Pharmacol Ther* 1990; **45**: 309–29.

6. Levy RH, Boddy AV. Stereoselectivity in pharmacokinetics: a general theory. *Pharm Res* 1991; **8**: 551–6.

7. Ariëns EJ. Stereochemistry, a basis for sophisticated nonsense in pharmacokinetics and clinical pharmacology. *Eur J Clin Pharmacol* 1984; **26**: 663–8.

8. Carter RB, Dykstra LA. Quantitative analysis of the interaction between the agonist and antagonist isomers of picenadol (LY 150720) on electric shock titration in the squirrel monkey. *Eur J Pharmacol* 1985; **106**: 469–76.

9. Triggle DJ. Ion channels. In: Krogsgaard P, Bundgaard H, eds. *A Textbook of Drug Design and Development.* Reading: Harwood Academic, 1991: 357–86.

10. Ruffolo RR. Chirality in α- and β-adrenoceptor agonists and antagonists. *Tetrahedron* 1991; **47**: 9953–80.

11. Vlasses PH, Irvin JD, Huber PB et al. Pharmacology of enantiomers and (−)-p-OH metabolite of indacrinone. *Clin Pharmacol Ther* 1981; **29**: 798–807.

12. Tobert JA, Cirillo VJ, Hitzenberger G et al. Enhancement of uricosuric properties of indacrinone by manipulation of the enantiomer ratio. *Clin Pharmacol Ther* 1981; **29**: 344–50.

13. Richards R, Tattersfield AE. Bronchial β-adrenoceptor blockade following eyedrops of timolol and its isomer L-714, 465 in normal subjects. *Br J Clin Pharmacol* 1985; **20**: 459–62.

14. Fraunfelder FT, Barker AF. Respiratory effects of timolol. *N Engl J Med* 1985; **311**: 1441.

15. Echizen H, Vogelgesang B, Eichelbaum M. Effects of d,l-verapamil on atrioventricular con-

duction in relation to its stereoselective first-pass metabolism. *Clin Pharmacol Ther* 1985; **38:** 71–6.

16. Walle T, Webb JG, Bagwell EE, Walle UK, Daniell HB, Gaffney TE. Stereoselective delivery and actions of beta receptor antagonists. *Biochem Pharmacol* 1988; **37:** 115–24.

17. Karim A, Piergies A. Verapamil stereoisomerism: enantiomeric ratios in plasma dependent on peak concentrations, oral input rate, or both. *Clin Pharmacol Ther* 1995; **58:** 174–84.

18. Mikus G, Eichelbaum M, Fischer C, Gumulka S, Klotz U, Kroemer HK. Interaction of verapamil and cimetidine: stereochemical aspects of drug metabolism, drug disposition and drug action. *J Pharmacol Exp Ther* 1990; **253:** 1042–8.

19. Smith DA, Chandler MHH, Shedlofsky SI, Wedlund PJ, Blouin RA. Age-dependent stereoselective increase in the oral clearance of hexobarbitone isomers caused by rifampicin. *Br J Clin Pharmacol* 1991; **32:** 735–9.

20. Chandler MHH, Scott SR, Blouin RA. Age associated stereoselective alterations in hexobarbital metabolism. *Clin Pharmacol Ther* 1988; **43:** 436–41.

21. Li G, Treiber G, Maier K, Walker S, Klotz U. Disposition of ibuprofen in patients with liver cirrhosis. Stereochemical considerations. *Clin Pharmacokin* 1993; **25:** 154–63.

22. Hooper WD, Qing MS. The influence of age and gender on the stereoselective metabolism and pharmacokinetics of mephobarbital in humans. *Clin Pharmacol Ther* 1990; **48:** 633–40.

23. Lennard MS, Tucker GT, Silas JH, Freestone S, Ramsay LE, Woods HF. Differential stereoselective metabolism of metoprolol in extensive and poor debrisoquin metabolisers. *Clin Pharmacol Ther* 1983; **34:** 732–7.

24. Johnson JA, Burlew BS. Racial differences in propranolol pharmacokinetics. *Clin Pharmacol Ther* 1992; **51:** 495–500.

25. Shah RR, Midgley JM, Branch SK. Stereochemical origin of some clinically significant drug safety concerns: lessons for future drug development. *Adverse Drug React Toxicol Rev* 1998; **17:** 145–90.

26. Fabro S, Smith RL, Williams RT. Toxicity and teratogenicity of optical isomers of thalidomide. *Nature* 1967; **215:** 269.

27. Eriksson T, Bjorkman S, Roth B, Fyge A, Hoglund P. Stereospecific determination, chiral inversion *in vitro* and pharmacokinetics in humans of the enantiomers of thalidomide. *Chirality* 1995; **7:** 44–52.

28. Reist M, Carrupt P-A, Francotte E, Testa B. Chiral inversion and hydrolysis of thalidomide: mechanisms and catalysis by bases and serum albumin, and chiral stability of teratogenic metabolites. *Chem Res Toxicol* 1998; **11:** 1521–8.

29. Branch S. International regulation of chiral drugs. In: Subramanian G, ed. *Chiral Separation Techniques A practical approach*, 2nd edn. Weinheim: Wiley–VCH, 2001: 319–42.

30. Caldwell J. Through the looking glass in chiral drug development. *Modern Drug Discovery* 1999; July/August: 51–60.

31. Walshe JM. Penicillamine, a new oral therapy for Wilson's Disease. *Am J Med* 1956; **21:** 487–95.

32. Walshe JM. Chirality of penicillamine. *Lancet* 1992; **339:** 254.

33. Cotzias GC, Van Woert MH, Schiffer LM. Aromatic amino acids and modification of Parkinsonism. *N Engl J Med* 1967; **276:** 374–9.

34. Cotzias GC, Papavasiliou PS, Gellene R. Modification of Parkinsonism – chronic treatment with L-dopa. *N Engl J Med* 1969; **280:** 337–45.

35. Connolly MH, Cary JL, McGoon MD. Valvular heart disease associated with fenfluramine–phentamine. *N Engl J Med* 1997; **337:** 581–8.

36. Hutt AJ, O'Grady J. Drug chirality: a consideration of the significance of the stereochemistry of antimicrobial agents. *J Antimicrob Chemother* 1996; **37:** 7–32.

37. Davies R, Bryson HM. Levofloxacin, a review of its antibacterial activity, pharmacokinetics and therapeutic efficacy. *Drugs* 1994; **47:** 677–700.

38. Stock KP, Geisslinger G, Loew D, Beck WS, Bach GL, Brune K. (S)-Ibuprofen versus ibuprofen-racemate. A randomized double-blind study in patients with rheumatoid arthritis. *Rheumatol Int* 1991; **11:** 199–202.

39. Mauleón D, Artigas R, Garcia ML, Carganico G. Preclinical and clinical development of dexketoprofen. *Drugs* 1996; **52** (Suppl 5): 24–46.

40. Burke D, Bannister J. Left-handed local anaesthetics. *Curr Anaesth Crit Care* 1999; **10:** 262–9.

41. Foster RH, Markham A. Levobupivacaine, a review of its pharmacology and use as a local anaesthetic. *Drugs* 2000; **59:** 551–79.

42. Kohrs R, Durieux ME. Ketamine: teaching an old drug new tricks. *Anesth Analg* 1998; **87:** 1186–93.

43. Thayer A. Eli Lilly pulls the plug on Prozac isomer drug. *Chem Eng News* 2000; 30 October: 8.

44. Steiner TJ, Ahmed F, Findley LJ, MacGregor EA, Wilkinson M. S-Fluoxetine in the prophylaxis of migraine: a phase II double-blind randomized placebo-controlled study. *Cephalagia* 1998; **18:** 283–6.

45. Tybring G, Böttinger Y, Widén J, Bertilsson L. Enantioselective hydroxylation of omeprazole catalyzed by CYP2C19 in Swedish white subjects. *Clin Pharmacol Ther* 1997; **62:** 129–37.

46. Spencer CM, Faulds D. Esomeprazole. *Drugs* 2000; **60:** 321–9.

47. Bryson HM, Faulds D. Cisatracurium besilate. A review of its pharmacology and clinical potential in anaesthetic practice. *Drugs* 1997; **53:** 848–66.

48. Page CP, Morley J. Contrasting properties of albuterol stereoisomers. *J Allergy Clin Immunol* 1999; **104:** S31–S41.

49. Nelson HS. Clinical experience with levalbuterol. *J Allergy Clin Immunol* 1999; **104:** S77–S84.

50. Hyttel J, Bøgesø KP, Perregaard J, Sánchez C. The pharmacological effect of citalopram resides in the (S)-(+)-enantiomer. *J Neural Transm Gen Sect* 1992; **88:** 157–60.

51. Burke, WJ, Gergel I, Bose A. Fixed-dose trial of the single isomer SSRI escitalopram in depressed outpatients. *J Clin Psychiat* 2002; **63:** 331–6.

52. Montgomery SA, Loft H, Sánchez C, Reines EH, Papp M. Escitalopram (S-enantiomer of citalopram): clinical efficacy and onset of action predicted from a rat model. *Pharmacol Toxicol* 2001; **88:** 282–6.

53. Devalia JL, De Vos C, Hanotte F, Baltes E. A randomized, double-blind, crossover comparison among cetirizine, levocetirizine, and ucb 28557 on histamine-induced cutaneous response in healthy adult volunteers. *Allergy* 2001; **56:** 50–7.

54. Wang DY, Hanotte F, De Vos C, Clement P. Effect of cetirizine, levocetirizine, and dextrocetirizine on histamine-induced nasal response in healthy adult volunteers. *Allergy* 2001; **56:** 339–43.

55. Patrick KS, Caldwell RW, Ferris RM, Breese GR. Pharmacology of the enantiomers of *threo*-methylphenidate. *J Pharmacol Exp Ther* 1987; **241:** 152–8.

56. Srinivas NR, Hubbard JW, Korchinski ED, Midha KK. Enantioselective pharmacokinetics of dl-*threo*-methylphenidate in humans. *Pharm Res* 1993; **10:** 14–21.

57. Anon. Focalin approved in the US. *Scrip* 2001; **2698:** 20.

58. Tucker GT. Chiral switches. *Lancet* 2000; **335:** 1085–7.

59. Shah RR. The influence of chirality on drug development. *Future Prescriber* 2000; **1:** 14–17.

60. Agranat I, Caner H, Caldwell J. Putting chirality to work: the strategy of chiral switches. *Nat Rev Drug Discov* 2002; **1:** 753–68.

61. Waldo AL, Camm AJ, de Ruyter H et al. Effect of d-sotalol on mortality in patients with left ventricular dysfunction after recent and remote myocardial infarction. *Lancet* 1996; **348:** 7–12.

62. Maier NM, Franco P, Lindner W. Separation of enantiomers: needs, challenges, perspectives. *J Chromatogr* 2000; **906:** 3–33.

63. Anon. Schering–Plough withdraws dilevalol. *Scrip* 1990; **1540:** 24.

64. Anon. Dilevalol cost Schering $100 million. *Scrip* 1990; **1543:** 19.

7

Surrogate endpoints

James J Oliver, David J Webb

SUMMARY

Surrogate endpoints are substitutes for the clinical endpoints of disease, such as morbidity and mortality. They are commonly used to evaluate the effects of interventions on the outcome of disease. This chapter explores the reasons why surrogate endpoints are used, their ideal characteristics and their limitations. To illustrate some of the principles that are introduced, two common cardiovascular surrogate endpoints, one established (blood pressure), and the other novel (endothelial function), are discussed in detail.

1. INTRODUCTION

The goal of any intervention in medicine, for example the administration of a drug or a change in lifestyle, is to reduce mortality or morbidity, or to improve quality of life. However, establishing whether any given intervention has such effects can be time-consuming and costly. Rather than assess the effects of interventions on outcomes that are relevant to patients, surrogate endpoints are often substituted, in an attempt to improve the efficiency with which interventions are evaluated. The realization that the use of surrogate endpoints is likely to gather pace, as the underlying pathophysiology of different diseases is elucidated and the number of candidate drugs rises, prompted a working party at the National Institutes of Health (NIH) in the USA to formally define the terms biological marker, clinical endpoint and surrogate endpoint (Box 7.1).[1] The term intermediate (or non-ultimate) endpoint is also sometimes used. An intermediate endpoint is a true clinical endpoint, but is not the ultimate endpoint of disease. For example, the main clinical endpoints of ischaemic heart disease are the occurrence of myocardial infarction, heart failure and death. Exercise tolerance might be considered a surrogate endpoint for these, but at the same time may also be considered a clinical endpoint in its own right, given that it is an important determinant of how a patient feels and functions.

The effects that interventions have on surrogate endpoints are commonly accepted by clinicians and regulatory authorities as useful and informative substitutes for the effects on clinical outcomes. However, particular care must be taken when determining the relevance to clinical practice of studies that report effects on surrogate endpoints.

Box 7.1 Definitions	
Biological marker (biomarker)	A characteristic that is objectively measured and evaluated as an indicator of normal biological processes, pathogenic processes, or pharmacological responses to a therapeutic intervention
Clinical endpoint	A characteristic or variable that reflects how a patient feels, functions or survives
Surrogate endpoint	A biomarker that is intended to substitute for a clinical endpoint and is expected to predict clinical benefit (or harm or lack of benefit or harm) based on epidemiological, therapeutic, pathophysiological or other scientific evidence

The terms biological marker, clinical endpoint and surrogate marker, as defined by an NIH working party.[1] Clinical endpoints, for example death, loss of vision or the need for institutional care, are the most credible characteristics used in the assessment of the benefits and risks of a therapeutic intervention. Biomarkers are used in the early assessment of efficacy and safety, to establish the potential of an intervention in early phase clinical trials, as diagnostic tools, in the staging of disease, as indicators of prognosis, and in the prediction and monitoring of clinical response to an intervention. All surrogate endpoints can be considered biomarkers. Indeed, they are the most valuable subset of biomarkers. However, only a minority of biomarkers will become established as surrogate endpoints. Because *surrogate* literally means 'to substitute for', the use of the term surrogate marker was discouraged because it suggests that the substitution is for a clinical marker rather than a clinical endpoint.

2. THE USES OF SURROGATE ENDPOINTS

2.1 To predict delayed clinical events

If a clinical endpoint is relatively easy to assess (e.g. the effect of thrombolytic agents on early survival after acute myocardial infarction), there is little need to employ surrogate endpoints. However, it is often impractical to measure the effect of an intervention on well-defined clinical endpoints, especially when these occur after long periods. Large numbers of patients are needed for such evaluation. Surrogate endpoints have the potential to both reduce the cost and improve the efficiency of clinical trials. The number of patients that are required to demonstrate an effect on a surrogate endpoint should be smaller than the number needed to affect a clinical endpoint. This is because every patient has the surrogate, for example, high blood pressure or cholesterol, whereas far fewer patients will, for example, die or have a myocardial infarction or stroke over a period of a few years. Similarly, the effect of an intervention on a surrogate endpoint can be measured much sooner than the clinical endpoint of interest.

This is particularly relevant for conditions that entail low risk to patients over a prolonged period. For example, in a population of young and middle-aged patients with mild to moderate hypertension there will be few cardiovascular and cerebrovascular events over the course of 5 or 6 years. The MRC trial of treatment of mild hypertension investigated the effects of treating male and female patients aged 35–64 who had a diastolic blood pressure of 90–109 mmHg.[2] From a pool of 515 000 patients screened, 17 354 were recruited and 85 572 patient years were observed. Patients were assigned treatment with bendrofluazide, propranolol or placebo. Although treatment reduced the stroke rate, there were just 60 strokes in the active treatment group and 109 in the placebo group. The number of coronary events was greater, but active treatment had no overall beneficial effect (222 in the treated group and 234 in the placebo group). Active treatment reduced overall mortality in men but appeared to have the opposite effect in women.

Thus, meaningful clinical endpoint data on the effects of antihypertensive treatment require trials that are either very large or last a very long time, even 20 years or longer. Trials of this length are only possible in uncontrolled observational studies. Conventional hypertension treatment trials lasting 5 or 6 years are likely to underestimate the benefits of blood pressure control,[3] a problem that the use of surrogate endpoints has the potential to overcome.

Interventions can be made available to patients sooner if they are assessed by using surrogate endpoints rather than clinical endpoints. In this respect, the use of surrogate endpoints is often considered particularly valuable when there is no established effective treatment for a given disease. Of course, the early availability of an intervention based on its effect on a surrogate endpoint will only result in benefit to patients if the surrogate endpoint is a reliable indicator of clinical outcome. The relationship between a surrogate and clinical endpoint may be well defined in the natural history of a disease. However, when there is no established treatment for the disease there will not have been an opportunity to evaluate the surrogate endpoint in the setting of any intervention. If an intervention is used because of its effects on surrogate endpoints, it is critical that there is confidence in its safety, at both the dose and the duration of treatment proposed, to ensure that any risks are minimized.

2.2 Selecting candidate drugs for further development

The appropriate use of surrogate endpoints early in the drug development process has the potential to significantly improve the efficiency with which drugs are brought to the market place. The genomic revolution and combinatorial chemistry have resulted in a significant increase in the number of candidate compounds with therapeutic potential, based on their biological activity. It is critical that the likelihood for each of these compounds to become commercially successful drugs is assessed as early and as accurately as possible.

Preliminary investigations can be performed in order to determine whether an intervention does what it was designed to do, establishing 'proof-of-concept'. For example, the effects of inhaled intrapulmonary insulin were investigated in 73 patients with type 1 diabetes mellitus in an open-label, proof-of-concept, randomized trial.[4] After 12 weeks glycosylated haemoglobin was no higher in those who received inhaled insulin at mealtimes than in the control group who received insulin by injection. Changes in fasting and postprandial glucose concentrations, and occurrence and severity of hypoglycaemia were also similar between the groups. Furthermore, inhaled insulin was well tolerated and had no adverse effects on pulmonary function.

Although this study investigated the effects of inhaled insulin in a small number of patients using surrogate endpoints, it provided a platform from which larger-scale randomized trials could be performed. If the preparation of inhaled insulin had produced poorer control of diabetes mellitus or had induced bronchospasm, then it is unlikely that it would have been considered either an advance for patients or commercially viable. Instead of progressing to full-scale clinical trials, it is more likely that the pharmaceutical company involved would have attempted to improve the efficacy and safety of the product, before repeating the proof-of-concept study.

Nitric oxide (NO), a potent vasodilator[5] and inhibitor of platelet aggregation,[6] is produced by the vascular endothelium. Endothelial dysfunction results in reduced bioavailability of NO and is considered an important early step in atherogenesis. Although exogenous delivery of NO is an attractive therapeutic option, current drugs that deliver NO do not target areas of endothelial damage and, at least in the case of the organic nitrates, are associated with the development of tolerance to their effects.

The potential of early proof-of-concept studies in drug development can be illustrated by the development of the S-nitrosothiols, novel NO donor compounds that do not appear to engender vascular tolerance.[7,8] S-Nitroso-N-acetyl-D,L-penicillamine (SNAP) is prone to rather unpredictable decomposition. However, N-substituted analogues of SNAP with longer side chains cause prolonged vasodilatation in endothelium-denuded blood vessels, probably because their increased lipophilicity results in their retention in these vessels. For example, whereas SNAP resulted in transient vasodilatation in isolated rat femoral arteries, whether or not the endothelium was intact, the valeryl (SNVP) and hepatanoyl (SNHP) N-substituted analogues of SNAP caused transient vasodilatation in intact vessels, but prolonged vasodilatation in vessels with damaged endothelium.[9] RIG200, an S-nitrosated glyco-amino acid, had previously been shown to cause prolonged NO-mediated dilatation in rat femoral arteries only when the endothelium had been removed, suggesting a selective action of RIG200 in vessels with damaged endothelium.[10] Thus RIG200 might be particularly beneficial in preventing restenosis after coronary angioplasty and reducing the incidence of vasospasm after coronary artery bypass grafting.[11]

A subsequent study of the effects of RIG200 in the dorsal hand veins of healthy volunteers established the compound as a powerful venodilator, with similar efficacy to sodium nitroprusside (SNP). Furthermore, when the endothelium was removed from the hand veins, by perfusing distilled water through them, RIG200 administration resulted in a more prolonged relaxation of the veins. This prolonged effect was not seen before water irrigation or with SNP, either before or after water irrigation.[12] Thus, RIG200 appears to target areas of endothelial damage in vivo in man and an impetus has been provided at an early stage to further develop this compound and others

like it as non-tolerant NO donors with selectivity for at-risk vessels.

3. CHARACTERISTICS OF SURROGATE ENDPOINTS

3.1 Biological plausibility

Surrogate endpoints should have biological plausibility. This means that there should be evidence that the surrogate endpoint is on the causal pathway to the outcome of interest, or is a regular finding associated with that outcome and is plausibly related to a common causal factor. Detailed knowledge of disease pathogenesis and mechanism of drug action can provide a basis for believing that the use of a surrogate endpoint will accurately reflect the ultimate patient outcome. Examples of surrogate endpoints believed to be on the causal pathway of disease include the presence of blood clot in the left atrium associated with atrial fibrillation and the development of embolic stroke, and raised intraocular pressure and the development of visual loss in glaucoma. Alternatively, markers of hepatic synthetic function, such as serum bilirubin concentration and the prothrombin time, might act as surrogate endpoints in chronic liver disease, even though they are the result of impaired liver function, rather than being on the causal pathway of liver disease.

3.2 Correlation with clinical endpoint

The epidemiological relationship between a surrogate endpoint and the clinical endpoint for which it is intended to substitute should be more than simply a correlation. Effects on the surrogate should predict clinical outcome consistently and independently, and the relationship between the magnitude of change in the surrogate and clinical endpoints should be well characterized. It is possible to measure the extent to which a biological marker is a surrogate endpoint for a clinical event.[13,14] Evidently, the ultimate surrogate endpoint would account for all the effects of an intervention on the clinical endpoint.[15] The term *validation* has been used to describe the process by which a surrogate endpoint is established, based on both pathophysiology and its statistical relationship with the clinical endpoint. Assessments of sensitivity, specificity and reproducibility have also been considered part of the validation process. Thus, the validity of a surrogate is seriously weakened by a single well designed and conducted study demonstrating that an intervention results in an overall adverse clinical outcome while having the intended effect on the surrogate.

4. THE LIMITATIONS OF SURROGATE ENDPOINTS

Although reliable surrogate endpoints can be valuable, unfortunately they are rarely, if ever, adequate substitutes for definitive clinical outcomes. Indeed, by definition, judgments on efficacy and safety made on the basis of effects on surrogate endpoints can only be tentative. Thus, care should be exercised when determining the relevance to clinical practice of the effect that an intervention has on a surrogate endpoint, otherwise a misleading assessment of relative risk and benefit may result. In general, there are a number of well-characterized reasons that account for the limitations of surrogate endpoints.

4.1 Lack of a causal relationship

The relationship between a surrogate endpoint and clinical outcome in the natural history of a disease may not be fully defined. A surrogate endpoint may not be causally related to the clinical endpoint as expected, instead it may be coincidental or related to some other factor (Fig. 7.1). For example, prolongation of the prothrombin time might be a useful surrogate endpoint for outcome after paracetamol overdose. Prothrombin time reflects the degree of liver damage and is used to determine whether patients should continue to receive N-acetylcysteine, the antidote for paracetamol poisoning, or whether they should be referred for liver transplantation. However, specifically shortening the prothrombin time, for example with the administration of fresh frozen plasma, may well reduce the risk of serious bleeding in the short term but will have little effect on the underlying liver disease. Thus, although the prothrombin time can be controlled, patients are still likely to die unless they undergo liver transplantation.

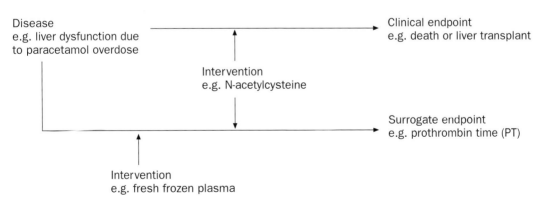

Fig. 7.1 The surrogate endpoint is not causally related to the clinical endpoint, although it may still reflect the activity of the disease process. For example, the prothombin time (PT) is used as an indicator of liver damage in paracetamol overdose. Fresh frozen plasma will shorten the PT but will have no effect on liver necrosis, which results in liver failure and subsequent death unless liver transplantation is performed. In contrast, by preventing liver necrosis N-acetylcysteine can prevent death from liver failure or the need for liver transplantation, and this effect is reflected in a shortening of the PT.

4.2 More than one pathogenic mechanism

There may be multiple disease pathways that influence clinical outcome (Fig. 7.2). An intervention might affect a surrogate endpoint that is on the causal pathway of a disease, but have no influence on any of the other pathways. When this is the case, determining the effect of an intervention on a surrogate endpoint will be of limited value in predicting the effect of the intervention on the clinical endpoint. For example, both bone lesions and hypercalcaemia are of prognostic value in multiple myeloma. The bisphosphonate pamidronate can prevent skeletal events and hypercalcaemia, alleviate bone pain and improve quality of life.[16] However, despite treatment with pamidronate, patients with multiple myeloma still succumb to renal failure, anaemia and bacterial infections.

4.3 More than one therapeutic mode of action

An intervention might influence clinical outcome through a disease pathway other than that represented by the surrogate endpoint (Fig. 7.3). Large randomized controlled trials have established that the LDL cholesterol-lowering statins are effective in reducing important cardiovascular events, including mortality, in both primary[17,18] and secondary[19–21] prevention studies. However, there remains debate as to whether the benefits of these agents can be entirely explained by their effects on LDL cholesterol concentrations. Improved endothelial function, stabilization of atherosclerotic plaque structure, and reduction in thrombosis and inflammation have all been proposed as mechanisms that might mediate their beneficial

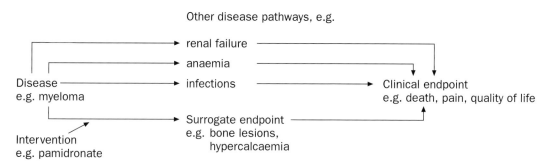

Fig. 7.2 A surrogate endpoint is representative of only one of several causal pathways of disease, illustrated by the use of pamidronate in the treatment of multiple myeloma.

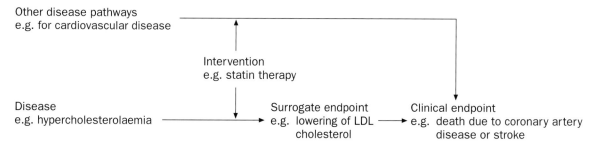

Fig. 7.3 An intervention might have effects on disease pathways other than that involving the surrogate endpoint. For example, statins may be of clinical benefit because of effects on plasma lipoproteins other than LDL cholesterol, endothelial function, plaque architecture and stability, thrombosis and inflammation.

effects. If statins act through mechanisms other than the lowering of LDL cholesterol then measuring the change in plasma LDL cholesterol may not fully predict the benefit of an individual drug.

Specifically, comparison of different statins on the basis of their effects on LDL cholesterol may be flawed if other effects are important. Moreover, the uncertainty surrounding the mechanisms through which the statins exert their beneficial effects means that the lowering of LDL cholesterol should not necessarily be considered a reliable surrogate endpoint when evaluating the effects of other agents that also lower plasma levels of this lipoprotein, including comparison of the effects of such agents with statins.

To illustrate, the HERS study investigated the effect of hormone replacement therapy (HRT) on coronary events in postmenopausal women with established coronary artery disease.[22] Compared to placebo, HRT resulted in an 11% reduction in LDL cholesterol but had no overall effect on coronary heart disease events, including coronary death. When investigating the effects of interventions on clinical endpoints that are the result of multiple disease pathways, the use of more than one surrogate endpoint might provide a more reliable assessment of treatment effects. For example, the overall risk of coronary heart disease can be calculated, based on systolic blood pressure, plasma cholesterol and the presence or absence of diabetes mellitus.[23] However, the benefit, or otherwise, of treating multiple surrogate endpoints representing different disease pathways should be investigated in its own right, rather than calculating the likely clinical outcome on the basis of the effects of interventions on individual surrogate endpoints.

4.4 Generalization of surrogate endpoint data to drugs of the same and different classes

The validation of a surrogate endpoint provides support for its use in the assessment of other interventions that affect it. This is particularly the case for drugs of the same class. Indeed,

over recent years many drugs have entered the market based on their 'class' effects, e.g. β-adrenoceptor blockers, angiotensin-converting enzyme (ACE) inhibitors and statins. However, assuming equivalence, even of drugs in the same class, on the basis of their effects on surrogate endpoints is hazardous. Although different drugs may have a similar mechanism of action, they remain distinct chemical entities. Differences in drug characteristics such as bioavailability, potency, receptor specificity, metabolism and unintended pharmacological actions, might result in important differences between agents of the same class that may, or may not, be associated with effects on the chosen surrogate endpoint.

The use of surrogate endpoints in assessing drugs of the same or different class may be questioned, even for established surrogate endpoints. For example, physicians have become comfortable with the idea that any drug that lowers blood pressure will be of benefit to their patients, so that when new drugs that have been shown to lower blood pressure in small clinical trials become available they are enthusiastically prescribed. However, this generalization of blood pressure as a suitable surrogate endpoint for cardiovascular events has been challenged recently. The ALLHAT study compared the effects of doxazosin and chlorthalidone on patients with hypertension and at least one other coronary heart disease risk factor.[24] The trial was stopped early when an interim analysis showed that treatment with doxazosin resulted in an increased risk of combined cardiovascular disease events, particularly congestive heart failure. Furthermore, a meta-analysis by Pahor et al suggested that calcium antagonists might be inferior to other antihypertensive drugs as first-line agents in reducing the risks of several major complications of hypertension, including acute myocardial infarction and congestive heart failure.[25] It has been proposed that the term *validation* should not be used, but that the process of determining surrogate endpoint status be referred to as *evaluation*.[1]

4.5 Suitability of one surrogate endpoint for several clinical endpoints

A surrogate endpoint might be used as a substitute for a number of clinical endpoints. If an intervention aimed at the surrogate endpoint is shown to be a good predictor of one particular clinical endpoint it should not be assumed that it will be equally predictive of other clinical endpoints, even if they are thought to have a similar pathophysiology. This point is well illustrated by the treatment of risk factors for cardiovascular disease. Coronary artery disease and stroke both result from atherosclerosis and share common risk factors, including hypertension. The treatment of hypertension appears to affect the incidence of myocardial infarction and stroke differently. Thus, the MRC trial of treatment of mild hypertension referred to above[2] found that lowering blood pressure with bendrofluazide or propranolol reduced the incidence of stroke but had no effect on the rate of coronary events. A meta-analysis of outcome trials investigating the effects of treating isolated systolic hypertension in the elderly concluded that treatment prevents stroke more effectively than it prevents coronary events.[26]

4.6 Generalization of surrogate endpoint data to clinical practice

When applying the results of trials that have used surrogate endpoints in clinical practice attention should be paid to the generalizability of the findings. Given that a surrogate endpoint might predict one clinical endpoint more closely than another, it is important that the clinical endpoint being substituted is clearly specified. For example, the efficacy of certain cancer chemotherapy regimens may be evaluated by their effects on tumour size as assessed radiographically. If a reduction in tumour size more accurately relates to quality of life (e.g. as a result of reduced local pressure symptoms) than to survival, it is critical that clinicians are aware of this and that they communicate this to their patients. The characteristics of the population and the disease state in which the substitution is being made should be clarified.

The situation in clinical practice is often complicated by the fact that patients are subjected to multiple interventions. Most commonly, they take a number of different drugs. Thus, after a myocardial infarction, a patient might be taking aspirin, a β-blocker, an ACE inhibitor and a statin. If mild hypertension develops, a further agent (e.g. a thiazide diuretic) might lower the blood pressure. Although we know that, in general, blood pressure reduction in hypertensive patients results in clinical benefit, can this evidence easily be applied in this situation, where the risk reduction associated with treatment may be different and the effects of interactions between these therapies is not known?

4.7 Use of surrogate endpoints as a guide to safety

In general, efforts tend to be concentrated on establishing reliable surrogate endpoints for efficacy. In contrast, the search for surrogate endpoints for safety is relatively neglected. However, an intervention may have effects outside of any of the disease pathways, including that incorporating the surrogate endpoint, such that unfavourable effects might adversely affect the ultimate outcome (Fig. 7.4). There are few drugs on the market to which this principle cannot be applied, to at least some extent. For example, amiodarone is an effective antiarrhythmic agent but can cause serious toxicity, including pulmonary and hepatic fibrosis; β-adrenoceptor blockers can cause bronchoconstriction; and hydralazine can cause systemic lupus erythematosus. Although the chances of detecting adverse events are increased when there is a high level of knowledge of the mechanism, or mechanisms, of action of the intervention, unexpected adverse effects will only be discovered if an adequate patient population is investigated and studies are designed to detect these effects. Of course, even large-scale clinical trials may be inadequate to detect rare but clinically important events, highlighting the importance of post-marketing surveillance programmes for the continual assessment of risk-benefit of individual therapies.

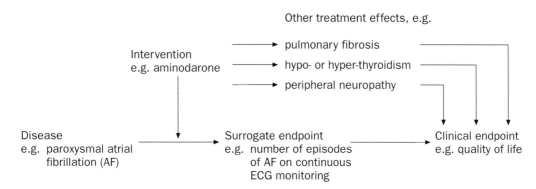

Fig. 7.4 An intervention may have effects on clinical outcome outside of disease pathways, including that of the surrogate endpoint. This is illustrated by the effects of amiodarone on other organ systems.

4.8 Failed surrogate endpoints

A widely cited example of a failed surrogate endpoint is the occurrence of ventricular premature beats (VPBs) after myocardial infarction. It is known that after myocardial infarction there is an increased risk of fatal ventricular arrhythmias and that this risk is associated with the occurrence of frequent VPBs. It had been assumed by many physicians that the use of antiarrhythmic drugs to reduce the frequency of VPBs would, by reducing serious arrhythmias, also result in improved mortality. Indeed, several new drugs were approved on the basis of their ability to suppress arrhythmias, but before there was any evidence that this would result in reduced death rates. The assumption that these drugs were of clinical benefit was shown to be false in a dramatic way with the publication of the Cardiac Arrhythmia Suppression Trial (CAST).[27,28] Patients with a recent myocardial infarction and more than 10 VPBs per hour were randomly assigned either placebo or treatment with encainide, flecainide or moricizine. Treatment with any of these drugs resulted in excess mortality, due to both shock after acute recurrent myocardial infarction and arrhythmia, compared with placebo.

A further example of a failed surrogate concerns the use of quinidine to maintain sinus rhythm in patients who had been cardioverted from atrial fibrillation. A meta-analysis of six trials found that although quinidine was effective in maintaining sinus rhythm it also resulted in a threefold increase in mortality compared with placebo.[29] Box 7.2 summarizes the characteristics and limitations of surrogate endpoints.

Box 7.2   A summary of the characteristics and limitations of surrogate endpoints

Characteristics
- Substitutes for the clinical endpoint of disease
- Of value when the clinical endpoint is rare or delayed
- Has biological plausibility
- Reliably predicts the clinical endpoint
- Facilitates the drug development process
- Accepted by regulatory authorities

Limitations
- Lack of causal relationship between surrogate and clinical endpoints
- Surrogate endpoint represents one of several pathogenic mechanisms
- Intervention has more than one therapeutic mode of action
- Surrogate endpoint substitutes for multiple clinical endpoints
- Intervention has effects outside of disease pathways
- Limited generalizability of surrogate endpoint data to clinical practice

5. BLOOD PRESSURE: THE REFINEMENT OF AN ESTABLISHED SURROGATE ENDPOINT

It is well established that lowering the blood pressure of hypertensive individuals reduces their risk of developing significant coronary artery disease and cerebrovascular disease, and of premature death. Traditionally, diastolic blood pressure (DBP), measured at the brachial artery in a physician's clinic, defined the need for treatment. However, this measurement does not necessarily provide the best surrogate endpoint for cardiovascular events and mortality, and neither does its therapeutic manipulation necessarily provide the best assessment of the overall benefit of treatment. Thus, other blood pressure parameters can be measured or calculated, such as systolic pressure (SBP), mean arterial pressure and pulse pressure (PP, the difference between SBP and DBP). Rather than clinic measurements, blood pressure can be assessed over 24 hours, using ambulatory recording equipment. Furthermore, rather than record the extremes of arterial pressure (SBP and DBP) the entire arterial pulse waveform can be analysed, giving an assessment of both arterial stiffness and blood pressure in the proximal aorta.

5.1 Ambulatory blood pressure monitoring (ABPM)

The blood pressure of any individual varies throughout the day. It is recognized that single blood pressure recordings taken in doctors' consulting rooms might not accurately reflect the real overall blood pressure of an individual, particularly given the anxiety that many patients feel during medical consultations. For this reason, ambulatory blood pressure monitoring (ABPM) readings might relate more closely to clinical outcome than office measurements.

Khattar et al used continuous intra-brachial artery pressure monitoring to investigate the prognostic value of ABPM. They found that patients with 'white-coat hypertension' had a lower risk of developing cardiovascular events than those with sustained mild hypertension[30] and that in refractory hypertension ABPM, but

not clinic blood pressure, further predicted cardiovascular risk.[31] They also found that ABPM, especially ambulatory systolic pressure, but not clinic blood pressure predicted cardiovascular events in a population of patients with essential hypertension.[32] A Japanese study[33] found that ABPM, measured non-invasively, was a stronger predictor of stroke than clinic blood pressure. Average daytime pressure was more closely related to stroke risk than average nighttime blood pressure. A substudy of the Systolic Hypertension in Europe (Syst-Eur) Trial, which recruited elderly patients with isolated systolic hypertension on the basis of clinic measurements, found that ambulatory systolic BP was a significant predictor of cardiovascular risk over and above conventional BP.[34]

On the basis of the recently published data regarding ABPM as an independent predictor of cardiovascular outcome it might be tempting to measure ambulatory blood pressure more widely in the hypertension clinic. However, the role of ABPM in everyday practice is far from fully established. For example, the relative cardiovascular risk of patients with non-sustained (white-coat) hypertension compared to patients who are truly normotensive has not been established; some authors have suggested that there is no increased risk,[35] while others have suggested the contrary.[36] Values for 'normal ranges' for ABPM have yet to be determined. Just because ABPM independently predicts cardiovascular events, it does not automatically follow that the lowering of ambulatory blood pressure values will predict subsequent clinical outcome any more strongly than clinic measurements. There is currently a paucity of data addressing this issue. However, a further substudy of the Syst-Eur trial[37] found that antihypertensive treatment significantly reduced the incidence of cardiovascular events and stroke in those with an average daytime systolic blood pressure of ≥ 160 mmHg, but not in those with systolic pressures lower than this.

5.2 Pulse pressure

Recent data from the Framingham population have shown that diastolic blood pressure tends to rise with age, until around 60 years of age, but then tends to fall. In contrast, systolic pressure and pulse pressure (PP) tend to rise continuously with increasing age.[38] Franklin et al assessed the relative importance of SBP, DBP and PP to coronary heart disease (CHD) risk in more than 6500 Framingham participants.[39] The fascinating results of this study challenge conventional wisdom on the treatment of hypertension. In those younger than 50 years DBP was the strongest predictor of CHD risk. Between the ages of 50 and 59, the risks were comparable for all three BP indexes. In older participants, SBP was directly related and DBP was inversely related to CHD risk, although PP was the strongest predictor. Other studies have also found SBP to be an important independent predictor of cardiovascular morbidity and mortality.[40–42] Data associating the presence of raised SBP with the presence and severity of aortic atherosclerosis[43] and the presence of atherosclerotic plaques in the common carotid artery[44] potentially explain the association of isolated systolic hypertension and thromboembolic events.

The realization of the strength of SBP as a surrogate endpoint for cardiovascular outcome has profound implications for clinical priority setting and the targeting of health-care resources.[45] The major burden of hypertension-related cardiovascular disease occurs in the elderly and raised SBP is by far the most common problem in this population.[46] Furthermore, a number of major trials have established that the treatment of systolic hypertension results in a reduction of both cardiovascular events and overall mortality.[47–49]

It is particularly interesting that the PP was the strongest predictor of coronary risk in older patients.[39] Data from other studies support the hypothesis that PP is an important surrogate endpoint for cardiovascular outcome.[50–52] Earlier data from Framingham indicate that a lower diastolic pressure at any level of systolic pressure >120 mmHg increases coronary risk in older people[53] (Fig. 7.5). While the benefits of treating raised SBP are established, the benefits of specifically lowering the PP are not known. It may be that therapy designed to reduce PP,

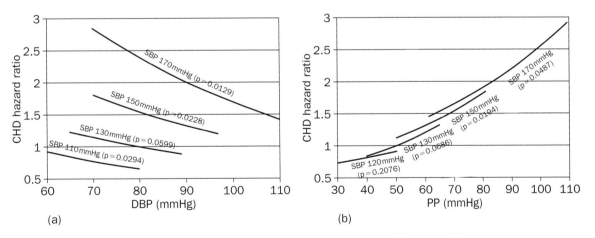

Fig. 7.5 (a) Joint influences of SBP and DBP on coronary heart disease (CHD) risk. CHD hazard ratios were determined from the level of DBP within SBP groups. Hazard ratios were set to a reference value of 1.0 for SBP of 130 mmHg and DBP of 80 mmHg and are plotted for SBP values of 110, 130, 150 and 170 mmHg, respectively. (b) Joint influences of SBP and PP on CHD risk. CHD hazard ratios were determined from the level of PP within SBP groups. Hazard ratios were set to a reference value of 1.0 for SBP of 130 mmHg and PP of 50 mmHg and are plotted for SBP values of 110, 130, 150 and 170 mmHg, respectively. All estimates were adjusted for age, sex, body mass index, cigarettes smoked per day, glucose intolerance and total cholesterol/HDL cholesterol. (Reproduced with permission from Franklin et al[53])

lowering SBP while preserving, or even increasing, DBP, might provide the greatest benefit to patients.[54] Although this hypothesis has not been addressed directly, there is indirect evidence to support it. Some studies have found that reduction of DBP, especially to <70 mmHg,[55] is associated with adverse outcomes.[56] Madhavan et al[57] found that, following treatment for hypertension, those with a high pretreatment PP had a higher subsequent rate of myocardial infarction if their DBP was reduced by ≥18 mmHg, compared with a moderate reduction of 7–17 mmHg. The likely explanation for this observation is that DBP is reduced to such a level that coronary artery blood flow, which occurs predominantly in diastole, is compromised. If this is the case, PP is likely to be a stronger surrogate endpoint for outcome in coronary artery disease than for stroke or peripheral vascular disease.

5.3 ABPM versus PP

The relative predictive power of the various blood pressure parameters that can be obtained from ABPM was investigated by Verdecchia et al,[58] in a study of >2000 patients with essential hypertension, followed up for a mean of 4.7 years. The 24-hour PP was the dominant predictor of both total and fatal cardiac events, but did not independently predict cerebrovascular events. Conversely, 24-hour mean BP independently predicted both total and fatal cerebrovascular events, but was not an independent predictor of cardiac events. Using continuous intra-arterial blood pressure monitoring, Khattar et al[59] found the strongest predictors of cardiovascular events to be DBP in patients younger than 60 years, and PP in patients older than 60 years. This pattern was evident in both patient groups for 24-hour mean, daytime mean or night-time mean measurements. Clinic blood pressures were not of independent prognostic value in either age group.

5.4 Vascular stiffness

The principal cause of increased SBP and PP is large artery stiffness. Stiffening of the large

arteries with increasing age[60–62] directly leads to an increased PP for any given stroke volume. In addition, increased stiffness of the aorta results in a higher pulse wave velocity, so that the arterial wave is reflected back from the peripheral circulation earlier. In younger patients, the reflected arterial wave arrives back at the proximal aorta in diastole, augmenting coronary blood flow. As the arteries stiffen, the reflected wave arrives earlier, augmenting aortic systolic pressure instead of diastolic pressure.[62] Furthermore, an age-related reduction in the cross-section of the peripheral vascular bed results in increased amplitude of wave reflection.[63] As an index of arterial stiffness, the augmentation index (AIx) represents the contribution of wave reflection to central aortic systolic pressure. These age-related changes in the stiffness of the large arteries explain the observation from the Framingham population that, with increasing age, SBP and PP tend to rise continuously, whereas DBP rises until around age 60, but then falls.[38]

As a result of the interaction of incident and reflected waves along the arterial tree each artery is characterized by its own pressure waveform. Although there is a fall in mean arterial pressure between the ascending aorta and the peripheral arteries, the arterial pressure wave is amplified. This amplification is greatest in the young and decreases with age. An important implication of this is that measurement of blood pressure at the brachial artery does not accurately reflect the blood pressure in the more physiologically relevant proximal aorta. Furthermore, age-related changes in brachial blood pressure do not parallel central blood pressure changes, while vasodilating agents may reduce central systolic pressure but have little effect on brachial systolic pressure.[62] Thus, there is a sound pathophysiological basis for believing that measurement of arterial stiffness might constitute a refinement to the measurement of brachial artery SBP or PP as a surrogate endpoint for outcome in cardiovascular disease.

To this end, assessment of AIx, as well as central SBP, DBP and PP, has recently become possible using a simple, non-invasive and reproducible technique, termed pulse wave analysis.[64,65] However, studies on the prognostic value of arterial stiffness measurement are currently awaited. Although pulse wave analysis is presented as a potential advance in the utility of blood pressure as a surrogate endpoint, it is interesting to note that recordings of the arterial pulse waveform were regularly made more than 100 years ago.[66] However, interest in recording the arterial pulse waveform dwindled with the introduction of the cuff sphygmomanometer, which measures just the extremes of blood pressure, but disregards the wealth of information contained within the entire waveform.

5.5 Left ventricular mass

Further stratification of the risk associated with hypertension can be accomplished by measuring the mass of the left ventricle by echocardiography. Left ventricular hypertrophy (LVH) is a strong, independent predictor of cardiovascular complications and death in patients with uncomplicated essential hypertension.[67,68] Indeed, there is a positive association between LV mass and cardiovascular events even when the LV mass is below the current 'upper limits of normal'.[69] Moreover, the reduction of LVH predicts a favourable clinical outcome, and does so independently of blood pressure reduction.[70,71]

5.6 Implications for clinical trials

The story of blood pressure as a surrogate endpoint is a fascinating one. The previous assumptions of the over-riding importance of raised diastolic pressure have been shown to be false. Different blood pressure measurements, e.g. DBP, SBP and PP, have different prognostic values for different populations of patients. When assessment of arterial stiffness, ABPM and LVH are taken into account the use of blood pressure as a surrogate endpoint for clinical outcome becomes rather complex. However, these discoveries are of paramount importance, because the assessment of the benefit of antihypertensive therapies can only be fully evaluated in the appropriate trials when they are performed on the appropriate popu-

lation of patients whose risk of death or cardiovascular events is well characterized.

6. ENDOTHELIAL FUNCTION: A NOVEL SURROGATE ENDPOINT

The vascular endothelium, a monolayer of cells that lines the vascular wall, was once considered little more than a protective barrier. However, research over the last two decades has revealed the endothelium to be metabolically active, producing a number of vasoactive substances. Perhaps the best characterized of these is NO, although the endothelium also produces the vasodilator prostacyclin and the potent vasoconstrictor endothelin-1.

Dysfunction of the endothelium is a common finding in those at risk of cardiovascular disease and is thought to be important in the development of atherosclerosis. Indeed, it has been proposed that endothelial dysfunction is the common pathway through which every cardiovascular risk factor acts to promote atherosclerosis (Fig. 7.6). If this is true, the assessment of endothelial function, by serving as an integrating index of the overall stress on the arterial wall, might be a powerful surrogate endpoint, both for the calculation of cardiovascular risk and the assessment of therapies designed to attenuate this risk.

6.1 Assessment of endothelial function in vivo

There are a number of ways that the function of the endothelium can be assessed in vivo. In the arterial circulation of the forearm vasoactive substances that mediate their effects through the endothelium can be infused and the change in blood flow can be assessed by plethysmography. Acetylcholine (ACh), bradykinin and substance P are commonly used endothelium-dependent vasodilators. The forearm arterial vascular bed undergoes less vasodilatation in response to ACh in patients with coronary artery disease compared with controls.[72] Similarly, endothelial function can be assessed in the coronary circulation at cardiac catheterization. Thus, the local infusion of ACh

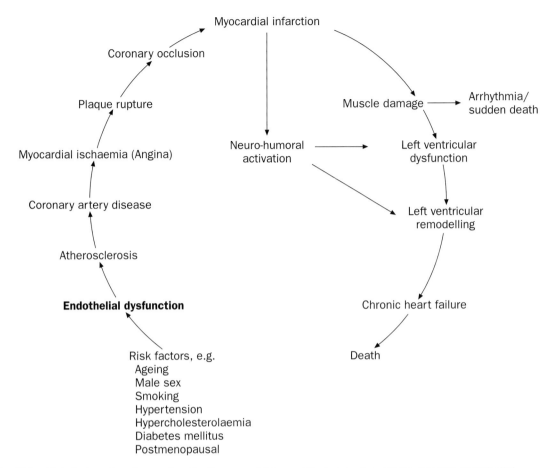

Fig. 7.6 Risk factors for atherosclerotic disease might exert their adverse effects through endothelial dysfunction. If so, the assessment of endothelial function will be a powerful surrogate endpoint for clinical outcome in atherosclerotic disease.

results in vasodilatation of large coronary arteries, while in patients with coronary artery disease a paradoxical vasoconstriction occurs.[73] Although they are useful research tools, the invasive nature of these methods for assessing endothelial function will limit their more general use.

Non-invasive assessment of endothelial function in the brachial artery has recently become possible using flow-mediated dilatation (FMD). While the diameter of the brachial artery is continuously measured by ultrasound, an arterial cuff applied to the forearm is inflated to occlude arterial flow for several minutes. When the cuff pressure is released, reactive hyperaemia occurs, increasing flow through the brachial artery and, consequently, shear stress to the vessel wall. Increased shear stress is a well-characterized stimulus for the release of NO from the endothelium. Thus, when the endothelium is intact, brachial artery vasodilatation occurs, but this response is reduced when the endothelium is dysfunctional. Just as patients with coronary artery disease exhibit impairment of endothelial function in the coronary and forearm circulations, these patients also have reduced FMD of the brachial artery.[74]

6.2 Association of endothelial dysfunction with cardiovascular risk factors

If endothelial dysfunction really was the earliest stage of atherosclerosis, then it could be expected that any patient with cardiovascular risk factors would have impaired endothelial function. Furthermore, it should be possible to demonstrate the presence of endothelial dysfunction associated with each risk factor by any of the techniques that are used to measure endothelial function. In fact, ageing, smoking, essential hypertension and hypercholesterolaemia are all associated with impairment of FMD of the brachial artery,[74–77] and reduced endothelium-dependent vasodilatation in both the forearm[78–80] and coronary circulations.[81–83]

Impairment of FMD of the brachial artery occurs at an earlier age in men than in women.[76] In the forearm circulation, endothelial function is impaired in men with hypercholesterolaemia but not in women.[84] Furthermore, the onset of the menopause is associated with a decline in endothelial function, whether measured by FMD of the brachial artery[76] or plethysmography of the forearm.[85]

The association of type 1 diabetes mellitus with endothelial dysfunction appears to be related to the presence or absence of microalbuminuria. Using FMD of brachial artery, Lambert et al found that normoalbuminuric diabetics had normal endothelial function.[86] In contrast, Dogra et al found that endothelial dysfunction was present in normoalbuminuric diabetics, but that it was more marked in those with microalbuminuria.[87] In the forearm circulation, endothelial function was impaired in patients with microalbuminuria,[88] whereas it was normal in patients who were normoalbuminuric.[89]

To date, studies directly evaluating the relationship of different methods for measuring endothelial function are limited. However, two studies in patients referred for assessment of coronary artery disease have found that coronary artery endothelium-dependent vasomotor responses and FMD in the brachial artery are closely correlated.[90,91]

6.3 The effect of cardiovascular treatments on endothelial dysfunction

Interventions intended to reduce the burden of atherosclerotic disease might act at a number of points in the disease process, e.g. thrombolysis or the modification of left ventricular remodelling after acute myocardial infarction. However, the hypothesis that endothelial dysfunction is a useful surrogate endpoint in atherosclerosis would be further supported by data suggesting that different treatments of established clinical benefit improve endothelial function.

FMD of the brachial artery is improved by both pravastatin within 6 weeks of acute myocardial infarction or unstable angina,[92] and simvastatin given to patients with familial hypercholesterolaemia.[93] The effects on endothelial function of treating hypertension are less clear-cut. In the forearm arterial circulation both nifedipine[94] and isradipine[95] improved ACh-induced vasodilatation, whereas lisinopril improved bradykinin-induced vasodilatation but not ACh-induced vasodilatation.[96] Using FMD of the brachial artery in hypertensive patients, one study found that nifedipine more effectively improved endothelial function than hydrochlorothiazide[97] and a further study found that quinapril improved endothelial function but nitrendipine did not.[98]

An effect on endothelial function might explain the reduction in coronary events associated with oestrogen replacement therapy in postmenopausal women. Brachial artery FMD is impaired in postmenopausal compared with premenopausal women, but is improved in women taking either combined oestrogen and progesterone or oestrogen-only HRT.[99]

6.4 Validation of endothelial dysfunction as a surrogate endpoint

Just because endothelial dysfunction is associated with known cardiovascular risk factors and is improved by therapies of established clinical benefit, it does not necessarily follow that it is valid as a surrogate endpoint. More direct support for the notion that endothelial dysfunction is a valid surrogate endpoint for outcome in atherosclerotic disease has recently been published.

Suwaidi et al investigated the prognostic significance of coronary artery endothelial dysfunction in 157 patients with mildly diseased coronary arteries.[100] Coronary endothelial function was assessed as vasodilatation to intracoronary ACh administration. After an average follow-up of 28 months none of the patients with normal or mildly impaired endothelial function had experienced cardiac events; but 14% of those with severe endothelial dysfunction had experienced cardiac events, including myocardial infarction and cardiac death. Perticone et al investigated the relation between endothelial dysfunction, measured as vasodilatation of the forearm arterial bed to intrabrachial ACh infusion, and cardiovascular events in 225 never-treated hypertensives.[101] Those patients with the worst endothelial function at baseline experienced a greater number of cardiovascular events, including myocardial infarction, angina, stroke and transient cerebral ischaemic attacks.

The hypothesis that endothelial dysfunction is a valid surrogate marker for future cardiovascular events is supported by these prospective studies, particularly given that the findings are similar for both the coronary and forearm circulations. However, for the hypothesis to be proven true there is much work still to be done. The results of the studies by Suwaidi et al[100] and Perticone et al[101] should be reproduced in larger numbers of patients. Studies designed to assess the predictive power of endothelial dysfunction should be performed in groups of patients with each of the known cardiovascular risk factors. It should not be assumed that endothelial dysfunction assessed as FMD is related to clinical outcome in the same way as that assessed by coronary or forearm arterial vasomotion to ACh; separate studies should be performed for FMD. Although it is interesting that interventions known to be clinically effective in atherosclerotic disease appear to improve endothelial function, prospective intervention trials are needed to evaluate the extent to which improvement in endothelial function can inde-

pendently predict improvements in clinical endpoints.

The view that improving endothelial function will necessarily improve atherosclerosis-related clinical endpoints is challenged if interventions known to improve endothelial function do not have significant effects on clinical events. For example, vitamin C improves brachial artery FMD in patients with angina,[102] but evidence that dietary supplementation with this antioxidant has important clinical benefits is lacking. Furthermore, although HRT given to postmenopausal women improves endothelial function, the HERS study found that it had no overall effect on coronary heart disease events, including coronary death, in postmenopausal women with established coronary artery disease.[22] Indeed, there were more events in the HRT group than the placebo group during the first year of therapy, although this trend was reversed after 4–5 years.

Undoubtedly the potential of endothelial dysfunction as a surrogate endpoint in atherosclerotic disease is exciting. Currently, however, it is too early to draw firm conclusions as to its utility in the prediction of clinical events, either in the natural history of disease or following interventions.

7. CONCLUSIONS

Surrogate endpoints are likely to be used increasingly as substitutes for the clinical endpoints that are so pertinent to patients. Although they have valuable roles to play, ultimately they are unable to serve as final proof of clinical efficacy or long-term safety. The effect of an intervention on a surrogate endpoint should be regarded as a provisional evaluation of that intervention. Clinicians should be aware of the limitations associated with surrogate endpoints and, where possible, make use of interventions that have been fully evaluated using clinical endpoints.

REFERENCES

Further reading

Bataille R, Harousseau JL. Multiple myeloma. *N Engl J Med* 1997; **336**: 1657–64.

Celermajer DS. Endothelial dysfunction: does it matter? Is it reversible? *J Am Coll Cardiol* 1997; **30**: 325–33.

Lloyd-Jones DM, Bloch KD. The vascular biology of nitric oxide and its role in atherogenesis. *Annu Rev Med* 1996; **47**: 365–75.

Luscher TF, Noll G. Endothelial function as an endpoint in interventional trials: concepts methods and current data. *J Hypertens* 1996; **14**(Suppl 2): S111–S119.

Maron DJ, Fazio S, Linton MF. Current perspectives on statins. *Circulation* 2000; **101**: 207–13.

Moore TJ. *Deadly Medicine: Why Tens of Thousands of Heart Patients Died in America's Worst Drug Disaster.* New York: Simon & Schuster, 1995.

Nichols WW, O'Rourke MF. *McDonald's Blood Flow in Arteries: Theoretic, Experimental and Critical Principles*, 4th edn. London: Arnold, 1998.

O'Rourke MF, Gallagher DE. Pulse wave analysis. *J Hypertens* 1996; **14**: S147–S157.

Oliver JJ, Webb DJ. Non-invasive assessment of arterial stiffness and risk of atherosclerotic events. *Arterioscler Thromb Vasc Biol* 2003. In press.

Ross R. The pathogenesis of atherosclerosis: a perspective for the 1990s. *Nature* 1993; **362**: 801–9.

Temple R. Are surrogate markers adequate to assess cardiovascular disease drugs? *JAMA* 1999; **282**: 790–5.

Temple RJ. A regulatory authority's opinion about surrogate endpoints. In: Nimmo W, Tucker G, eds. *Clinical Measurement in Drug Evaluation.* Chichester: John Wiley & Sons, 1995: 3–22.

Webb DJ. The pharmacology of human blood vessels in vivo. *J Vasc Res* 1995; **32**: 2–15.

Web-sites

■ http://www.genomicglossaries.com
Glossary of terms – see 'biomarkers'.

■ http://www.cc.nih.gov/ccc/principles
See slide presentation on 'Physiological and laboratory markers of drug effect'.

Scientific papers

1. NIH Working Party. Biomarkers and surrogate endpoints: preferred definitions and conceptual framework. *Clin Pharmacol Ther* 2001;**69**: 89–95.
2. Medical Research Council Working Party. MRC trial of treatment of mild hypertension: principal results. *BMJ* 1985; **291**: 97–104.
3. Zanchetti A, Mancia G. Benefits and cost-effectiveness of antihypertensive therapy. The actuarial versus the intervention trial approach. *J Hypertens* 1996; **14**: 809–11.
4. Skyler JS, Cefalu WT, Kourides IA et al. Efficacy of inhaled human insulin in type 1 diabetes mellitus: a randomised proof-of-concept study. *Lancet* 2001; **357**: 331–5.
5. Palmer RM, Ferrige AG, Moncada S. Nitric oxide release accounts for the biological activity of endothelium-derived relaxing factor. *Nature* 1987; **327**: 524–6.
6. Radomski MW, Palmer RM, Moncada S. An L-arginine/nitric oxide pathway present in human platelets regulates aggregation. *Proc Natl Acad Sci USA* 1990; **87**: 5193–7.
7. Bauer JA, Fung HL. Differential hemodynamic effects and tolerance properties of nitroglycerin and an S-nitrosothiol in experimental heart failure. *J Pharmacol Exp Ther* 1991; **256**: 249–54.
8. Megson IL, Roseberry MJ, Miller MR, Mazzei FA, Butler AR, Webb DJ. S-nitrosothiols are nitric oxide donor drugs that do not engender vascular tolerance and remain effective in glyceryl trinitrate-tolerant rat femoral arteries. *Br J Clin Pharmacol* 1999; **126**: 78P.
9. Megson IL, Morton S, Greig IR et al. N-Substituted analogues of S-nitroso-N-acetyl-D,L-penicillamine: chemical stability and prolonged nitric oxide mediated vasodilatation in isolated rat femoral arteries. *Br J Pharmacol* 1999; **126**: 639–48.
10. Megson IL, Greig IR, Gray GA, Webb DJ, Butler AR. Prolonged effect of a novel S-nitrosated glyco-amino acid in endothelium-denuded rat femoral arteries: potential as a slow release nitric oxide donor drug. *Br J Pharmacol* 1997; **122**: 1617–24.
11. Megson IL, Greig IR, Butler AR, Gray GA, Webb DJ. Therapeutic potential of S-nitrosothiols as nitric oxide donor drugs. *Scott Med J* 1997; **42**: 88–9.
12. Sogo N, Wilkinson IB, MacCallum H et al. A novel S-nitrosothiol (RIG200) causes prolonged relaxation in dorsal hand veins with damaged endothelium. *Clin Pharmacol Ther* 2000; **68**: 75–81.
13. Freedman LS, Graubard BI, Schatzkin A.

Statistical validation of intermediate endpoints for chronic diseases. *Stat Med* 1992; **11**: 167–78.

14. Lin DY, Fleming TR, De Gruttola V. Estimating the proportion of treatment effect explained by a surrogate marker. *Stat Med* 1997; **16**: 1515–27.

15. Prentice RL. Surrogate endpoints in clinical trials: definition and operational criteria. *Stat Med* 1989; **8**: 431–40.

16. Berenson JR, Lichtenstein A, Porter L et al. Efficacy of pamidronate in reducing skeletal events in patients with advanced multiple myeloma. Myeloma Aredia Study Group. *N Engl J Med* 1996; **334**: 488–93.

17. Shepherd J, Cobbe SM, Ford I et al. Prevention of coronary heart disease with pravastatin in men with hypercholesterolemia. West of Scotland Coronary Prevention Study Group. *N Engl J Med* 1995; **333**: 1301–7.

18. Downs JR, Clearfield M, Weis S et al. Primary prevention of acute coronary events with lovastatin in men and women with average cholesterol levels: results of AFCAPS/TexCAPS. Air Force/Texas Coronary Atherosclerosis Prevention Study. *JAMA* 1998; **279**: 1615–22.

19. The 4S Investigators. Randomised trial of cholesterol lowering in 4444 patients with coronary heart disease: the Scandinavian Simvastatin Survival Study (4S). *Lancet* 1994; **344**: 1383–9.

20. Sacks FM, Pfeffer MA, Moye LA et al. The effect of pravastatin on coronary events after myocardial infarction in patients with average cholesterol levels. Cholesterol and Recurrent Events Trial Investigators. *N Engl J Med* 1996; **335**: 1001–9.

21. The Long-Term Intervention with Pravastatin in Ischaemic Disease (LIPID) Study Group. Prevention of cardiovascular events and death with pravastatin in patients with coronary heart disease and a broad range of initial cholesterol levels. *N Engl J Med* 1998; **339**: 1349–57.

22. Hulley S, Grady D, Bush T et al. Randomized trial of estrogen plus progestin for secondary prevention of coronary heart disease in postmenopausal women. Heart and Estrogen/progestin Replacement Study (HERS) Research Group. *JAMA* 1998; **280**: 605–13.

23. Joint British recommendations on prevention of coronary heart disease in clinical practice. British Cardiac Society, British Hyperlipidaemia Association, British Hypertension Society, endorsed by the British Diabetic Association. *Heart* 1998; **80**(Suppl 2): S1–S29.

24. ALLHAT Collaborative Research Group. Major cardiovascular events in hypertensive patients randomized to doxazosin vs chlorthalidone: the antihypertensive and lipid-lowering treatment to prevent heart attack trial (ALLHAT). *JAMA* 2000; **283**: 1967–75.

25. Pahor M, Psaty BM, Alderman MH et al. Health outcomes associated with calcium antagonists compared with other first-line antihypertensive therapies: a meta-analysis of randomised controlled trials. *Lancet* 2000; **356**: 1949–54.

26. Staessen JA, Gasowski J, Wang JG et al. Risks of untreated and treated isolated systolic hypertension in the elderly: meta-analysis of outcome trials. *Lancet* 2000; **355**: 865–72.

27. Echt DS, Liebson PR, Mitchell LB et al. Mortality and morbidity in patients receiving encainide, flecainide, or placebo. The Cardiac Arrhythmia Suppression Trial. *N Engl J Med* 1991; **324**: 781–8.

28. The Cardiac Arrhythmia Suppression Trial II Investigators. Effect of the antiarrhythmic agent moricizine on survival after myocardial infarction. *N Engl J Med* 1992; **327**: 227–33.

29. Coplen SE, Antman EM, Berlin JA, Hewitt P, Chalmers TC. Efficacy and safety of quinidine therapy for maintenance of sinus rhythm after cardioversion. A meta-analysis of randomized control trials. *Circulation* 1990; **82**: 1106–16.

30. Khattar RS, Senior R, Lahiri A. Cardiovascular outcome in white-coat versus sustained mild hypertension: a 10-year follow-up study. *Circulation* 1998; **98**: 1892–7.

31. Khattar RS, Swales JD, Banfield A, Dore C, Senior R, Lahiri A. Prediction of coronary and cerebrovascular morbidity and mortality by direct continuous ambulatory blood pressure monitoring in essential hypertension. *Circulation* 1999; **100**: 1071–6.

32. Khattar RS, Swales JD, Senior R, Lahiri A. Racial variation in cardiovascular morbidity and mortality in essential hypertension. *Heart* 2000; **83**: 267–71.

33. Ohkubo T, Hozawa A, Nagai K et al. Prediction of stroke by ambulatory blood pressure monitoring versus screening blood pressure measurements in a general population: the Ohasama study. *J Hypertens* 2000; **18**: 847–54.

34. Staessen JA, Thijs L, Fagard R et al. Predicting cardiovascular risk using conventional vs ambulatory blood pressure in older patients with systolic hypertension. Systolic Hypertension in Europe Trial Investigators. *JAMA* 1999; **282**: 539–46.

35. Verdecchia P, Schillaci G, Borgioni C et al. White coat hypertension and white coat effect. Similarities and differences. *Am J Hypertens* 1995; **8**: 790–8.

36. Palatini P, Mormino P, Santonastaso M et al. Target-organ damage in stage I hypertensive subjects with white coat and sustained hypertension: results from the HARVEST study. *Hypertension* 1998; **31**: 57–63.

37. Fagard RH, Staessen JA, Thijs L et al. Response to antihypertensive therapy in older patients with sustained and nonsustained systolic hypertension. Systolic Hypertension in Europe (Syst-Eur) Trial Investigators. *Circulation* 2000; **102**: 1139–44.

38. Franklin SS, Gustin WT, Wong ND et al. Hemodynamic patterns of age-related changes in blood pressure. The Framingham Heart Study. *Circulation* 1997; **96**: 308–15.

39. Franklin SS, Larson MG, Khan SA et al. Does the relation of blood pressure to coronary heart disease risk change with aging? The Framingham Heart Study. *Circulation* 2001; **103**: 1245–9.

40. Kannel WB, Gordon T, Schwartz MJ. Systolic versus diastolic blood pressure and risk of coronary heart disease. The Framingham study. *Am J Cardiol* 1971; **27**: 335–46.

41. Antikainen R, Jousilahti P, Tuomilehto J. Systolic blood pressure, isolated systolic hypertension and risk of coronary heart disease, strokes, cardiovascular disease and all-cause mortality in the middle-aged population. *J Hypertens* 1998; **16**: 577–83.

42. Alli C, Avanzini F, Bettelli G, Colombo F, Torri V, Tognoni G. The long-term prognostic significance of repeated blood pressure measurements in the elderly: SPAA (Studio sulla Pressione Arteriosa nell'Anziano) 10-year follow-up. *Arch Intern Med* 1999; **159**: 1205–12.

43. Agmon Y, Khandheria BK, Meissner I et al. Independent association of high blood pressure and aortic atherosclerosis: a population-based study. *Circulation* 2000; **102**: 2087–93.

44. Ebrahim S, Papacosta O, Whincup P et al. Carotid plaque, intima media thickness, cardiovascular risk factors, and prevalent cardiovascular disease in men and women: the British Regional Heart Study. *Stroke* 1999; **30**: 841–50.

45. Wilkinson IB, Cockcroft JR. Isolated systolic hypertension: a radical rethink. It's a risk factor that needs treatment, especially in the over 50s. *BMJ* 2000; **320**: 1685.

46. Izzo JL, Jr, Levy D, Black HR. Clinical Advisory Statement. Importance of systolic blood pressure in older Americans. *Hypertension* 2000; **35**: 1021–4.

47. SHEP Cooperative Research Group. Prevention of stroke by antihypertensive drug treatment in older persons with isolated systolic hypertension. Final results of the Systolic Hypertension in the Elderly Program (SHEP). *JAMA* 1991; **265**: 3255–64.

48. Staessen JA, Fagard R, Thijs L et al. Randomised double-blind comparison of placebo and active treatment for older patients with isolated systolic hypertension. The Systolic Hypertension in Europe (Syst-Eur) Trial Investigators. *Lancet* 1997; **350**: 757–64.

49. Liu L, Wang JG, Gong L, Liu G, Staessen JA. Comparison of active treatment and placebo in older Chinese patients with isolated systolic hypertension. Systolic Hypertension in China (Syst-China) Collaborative Group. *J Hypertension* 1998; **16**: 1823–9.

50. Benetos A, Safar M, Rudnichi A et al. Pulse pressure: a predictor of long-term cardiovascular mortality in a French male population. *Hypertension* 1997; **30**: 1410–15.

51. Domanski MJ, Davis BR, Pfeffer MA, Kastantin M, Mitchell GF. Isolated systolic hypertension: prognostic information provided by pulse pressure. *Hypertension* 1999; **34**: 375–80.

52. Millar JA, Lever AF, Burke V. Pulse pressure as a risk factor for cardiovascular events in the MRC Mild Hypertension Trial. *J Hypertens* 1999; **17**: 1065–72.

53. Franklin SS, Khan SA, Wong ND, Larson MG, Levy D. Is pulse pressure useful in predicting risk for coronary heart disease? The Framingham Heart Study. *Circulation* 1999; **100**: 354–60.

54. Safar ME, Rudnichi A, Asmar R. Drug treatment of hypertension: the reduction of pulse pressure does not necessarily parallel that of systolic and diastolic blood pressure. *J Hypertens* 2000; **18**: 1159–63.

55. Somes GW, Pahor M, Shorr RI, Cushman WC, Applegate WB. The role of diastolic blood pressure when treating isolated systolic hypertension. *Arch Intern Med* 1999; **159**: 2004–9.

56. Smulyan H, Safar ME. The diastolic blood pressure in systolic hypertension. *Ann Intern Med* 2000; **132**: 233–7.

57. Madhavan S, Ooi WL, Cohen H, Alderman MH. Relation of pulse pressure and blood pres-

sure reduction to the incidence of myocardial infarction. *Hypertension* 1994; **23:** 395–401.

58. Verdecchia P, Schillaci G, Reboldi G, Franklin SS, Porcellati C. Different prognostic impact of 24-hour mean blood pressure and pulse pressure on stroke and coronary artery disease in essential hypertension. *Circulation* 2001; **103:** 2579–84.

59. Khattar RS, Swales JD, Dore C, Senior R, Lahiri A. Effect of aging on the prognostic significance of ambulatory systolic, diastolic, and pulse pressure in essential hypertension. *Circulation* 2001; **104:** 783–9.

60. Van Bortel LM, Spek JJ. Influence of aging on arterial compliance. *J Hum Hypertens* 1998; **12:** 583–6.

61. McVeigh GE, Bratteli CW, Morgan DJ et al. Age-related abnormalities in arterial compliance identified by pressure pulse contour analysis: aging and arterial compliance. *Hypertension* 1999; **33:** 1392–8.

62. O'Rourke MF. Isolated systolic hypertension, pulse pressure, and arterial stiffness as risk factors for cardiovascular disease. *Curr Hypertens Rep* 1999; **1:** 204–11.

63. Nichols WW, O'Rourke MF, Avolio AP et al. Effects of age on ventricular-vascular coupling. *Am J Cardiol* 1985; **55:** 1179–84.

64. O'Rourke MF, Gallagher DE. Pulse wave analysis. *J Hypertens* 1996; **14**(Suppl): S147–S157.

65. Wilkinson IB, Fuchs SA, Jansen IM et al. Reproducibility of pulse wave velocity and augmentation index measured by pulse wave analysis. *J Hypertens* 1998; **16:** 2079–84.

66. Mahomed FA. The physiology and clinical use of the sphygmograph. *Med Times Gazette* 1872; **1:** 62.

67. Levy D, Garrison RJ, Savage DD, Kannel WB, Castelli WP. Prognostic implications of echocardiographically determined left ventricular mass in the Framingham Heart Study. *N Engl J Med* 1990; **322:** 1561–6.

68. Koren MJ, Devereux RB, Casale PN, Savage DD, Laragh JH. Relation of left ventricular mass and geometry to morbidity and mortality in uncomplicated essential hypertension. *Ann Intern Med* 1991; **114:** 345–52.

69. Schillaci G, Verdecchia P, Porcellati C, Cuccurullo O, Cosco C, Perticone F. Continuous relation between left ventricular mass and cardiovascular risk in essential hypertension. *Hypertension* 2000; **35:** 580–6.

70. Muiesan ML, Salvetti M, Rizzoni D, Castellano

M, Donato F, Agabiti-Rosei E. Association of change in left ventricular mass with prognosis during long-term antihypertensive treatment. *J Hypertens* 1995; **13:** 1091–5.

71. Verdecchia P, Schillaci G, Borgioni C et al. Prognostic significance of serial changes in left ventricular mass in essential hypertension. *Circulation* 1998; **97:** 48–54.

72. Sinisalo J, Vanhanen H, Pajunen P, Vapaatalo H, Nieminen MS. Ursodeoxycholic acid and endothelial-dependent, nitric oxide-independent vasodilatation of forearm resistance arteries in patients with coronary heart disease. *Br J Clin Pharmacol* 1999; **47:** 661–5.

73. Ludmer PL, Selwyn AP, Shook TL et al. Paradoxical vasoconstriction induced by acetylcholine in atherosclerotic coronary arteries. *N Engl J Med* 1986; **315:** 1046–51.

74. Celermajer DS, Sorensen KE, Gooch VM et al. Non-invasive detection of endothelial dysfunction in children and adults at risk of atherosclerosis. *Lancet* 1992; **340:** 1111–15.

75. Celermajer DS, Sorensen KE, Georgakopoulos D et al. Cigarette smoking is associated with dose-related and potentially reversible impairment of endothelium-dependent dilation in healthy young adults. *Circulation* 1993; **88:** 2149–55.

76. Celermajer DS, Sorensen KE, Spiegelhalter DJ, Georgakopoulos D, Robinson J, Deanfield JE. Aging is associated with endothelial dysfunction in healthy men years before the age-related decline in women. *J Am Coll Cardiol* 1994; **24:** 471–6.

77. Li J, Zhao SP, Li XP, Zhuo QC, Gao M, Lu SK. Non-invasive detection of endothelial dysfunction in patients with essential hypertension. *Int J Cardiol* 1997; **61:** 165–9.

78. Panza JA, Quyyumi AA, Brush JE, Jr, Epstein SE. Abnormal endothelium-dependent vascular relaxation in patients with essential hypertension. *N Engl J Med* 1990; **323:** 22–7.

79. Taddei S, Virdis A, Mattei P et al. Aging and endothelial function in normotensive subjects and patients with essential hypertension. *Circulation* 1995; **91:** 1981–7.

80. Noon JP, Walker BR, Hand MF, Webb DJ. Impairment of forearm vasodilatation to acetylcholine in hypercholesterolemia is reversed by aspirin. *Cardiovasc Res* 1998; **38:** 480–4.

81. Nitenberg A, Antony I, Foult JM. Acetylcholine-induced coronary vasoconstriction in young,

heavy smokers with normal coronary arterio-graphic findings. *Am J Med* 1993; **95:** 71–7.

82. Chauhan A, More RS, Mullins PA, Taylor G, Petch C, Schofield PM. Aging-associated endothelial dysfunction in humans is reversed by L-arginine. *J Am Coll Cardiol* 1996; **28:** 1796–804.

83. Shiode N, Kato M, Hiraoka A, Yamagata T, Matsuura H, Kajiyama G. Impaired endothe-lium-dependent vasodilation of coronary resis-tance vessels in hypercholesterolemic patients. *Intern Med* 1996; **35:** 89–93.

84. Chowienczyk PJ, Watts GF, Cockcroft JR, Brett SE, Ritter JM. Sex differences in endothelial function in normal and hypercholesterolaemic subjects. *Lancet* 1994; **344:** 305–6.

85. Taddei S, Virdis A, Ghiadoni L et al. Menopause is associated with endothelial dys-function in women. *Hypertension* 1996; **28:** 576–82.

86. Lambert J, Aarsen M, Donker AJ, Stehouwer CD. Endothelium-dependent and -independent vasodilation of large arteries in normoalbumin-uric insulin-dependent diabetes mellitus. *Arterioscler Thromb Vasc Biol* 1996; **16:** 705–11.

87. Dogra G, Rich L, Stanton K, Watts GF. Endothelium-dependent and independent vasodilation studies at normoglycaemia in type I diabetes mellitus with and without microalbu-minuria. *Diabetologia* 2001; **44:** 593–601.

88. Elliott TG, Cockcroft JR, Groop PH, Viberti GC, Ritter JM. Inhibition of nitric oxide synthesis in forearm vasculature of insulin-dependent dia-betic patients: blunted vasoconstriction in patients with microalbuminuria. *Clin Sci* 1993; **85:** 687–93.

89. Meeking DR, Allard S, Munday J, Chowienczyk PJ, Shaw KM, Cummings MH. Comparison of vasodilator effects of substance P in human forearm vessels of normoalbuminuric Type 1 diabetic and non-diabetic subjects. *Diabetic Med* 2000; **17:** 243–6.

90. Anderson TJ, Uehata A, Gerhard MD et al. Close relation of endothelial function in the human coronary and peripheral circulations. *J Am Coll Cardiol* 1995; **26:** 1235–41.

91. Takase B, Uehata A, Akima T et al. Endothelium-dependent flow-mediated vasodi-lation in coronary and brachial arteries in sus-pected coronary artery disease. *Am J Cardiol* 1998; **82:** 1535–9, A7–8.

92. Dupuis J, Tardif JC, Cernacek P, Theroux P. Cholesterol reduction rapidly improves endothelial function after acute coronary syn-dromes. The RECIFE (reduction of cholesterol in ischemia and function of the endothelium) trial. *Circulation* 1999; **99:** 3227–33.

93. Alonso R, Mata P, De Andres R, Villacastin BP, Martinez-Gonzalez J, Badimon L. Sustained long-term improvement of arterial endothelial function in heterozygous familial hypercholes-terolemia patients treated with simvastatin. *Atherosclerosis* 2001; **157:** 423–9.

94. Taddei S, Virdis A, Ghiadoni L et al. Restoration of nitric oxide availability after cal-cium antagonist treatment in essential hyper-tension. *Hypertension* 2001; **37:** 943–8.

95. Perticone F, Ceravolo R, Maio R et al. Calcium antagonist isradipine improves abnormal endothelium-dependent vasodilation in never treated hypertensive patients. *Cardiovasc Res* 1999; **41:** 299–306.

96. Taddei S, Virdis A, Ghiadoni L, Mattei P, Salvetti A. Effects of angiotensin converting enzyme inhibition on endothelium-dependent vasodilatation in essential hypertensive patients. *J Hypertens* 1998; **16:** 447–56.

97. Muiesan ML, Salvetti M, Monteduro C et al. Effect of treatment on flow-dependent vasodila-tion of the brachial artery in essential hyperten-sion. *Hypertension* 1999; **33:** 575–80.

98. Uehata A, Takase B, Nishioka T et al. Effect of quinapril versus nitrendipine on endothelial dysfunction in patients with systemic hyperten-sion. *Am J Cardiol* 2001; **87:** 1414–16.

99. McCrohon JA, Adams MR, McCredie RJ et al. Hormone replacement therapy is associated with improved arterial physiology in healthy post-menopausal women. *Clin Endocrinol* 1996; **45:** 435–41.

100. Suwaidi JA, Hamasaki S, Higano ST, Nishimura RA, Holmes DR, Jr, Lerman A. Long-term fol-low-up of patients with mild coronary artery disease and endothelial dysfunction. *Circulation* 2000; **101:** 948–54.

101. Perticone F, Ceravolo R, Pujia A et al. Prognostic significance of endothelial dysfunc-tion in hypertensive patients. *Circulation* 2001; **104:** 191–6.

102. Hamabe A, Takase B, Uehata A, Kurita A, Ohsuzu F, Tamai S. Impaired endothelium-dependent vasodilation in the brachial artery in variant angina pectoris and the effect of intra-venous administration of vitamin C. *Am J Cardiol* 2001; **87:** 1154–9.

8

Positron emission tomography as a tool in pharmacology: examples from neuroscience

Eugenii A Rabiner, Paul M Grasby

Summary • Introduction • Principles of PET • Types of studies • Conclusions • References

SUMMARY

Positron emission tomography (PET) has become a valuable tool in the evaluation of drug kinetics and action in humans. The aim of this chapter is to introduce the fundamentals of PET and explore the opportunities that PET offers in translational pharmacological research.

1. INTRODUCTION

Positron emission tomography (PET) is a minimally invasive technique, developed to use radiotracers labelled with short-lived positron-emitting isotopes, as molecular probes to image and measure biological processes in vivo. PET allows a detailed 3-D reconstruction of the anatomical distribution of the radiotracer's target site in the body, and absolute quantification of the target. In a typical study, a positron-labelled radiotracer is injected intravenously, and PET scans provide tissue concentrations of the radiotracer, and its labelled products, over time. These data are processed with a mathematical model containing a description of the transport and reactions undergone by the radiotracer, combined with a measure of delivery of the radiotracer to the brain, to derive images of the rate of process under study. PET is extremely sensitive, with common tissue concentrations of the radiotracer being in the pico- to femtomole per gram range. Over 500 radiotracers have been developed, ranging from enzymes to transporter substrates, receptor ligands, hormones, antibodies, peptides, drugs and oligonucleotides. Radiolabelled enzyme substrates can provide information about the synthesis of neurotransmitters; receptor-binding ligands can help determine receptor density and binding kinetics; radiolabelled analogues of glucose can inform on brain metabolism; while radiolabelled water can be used to estimate regional blood flow. PET images represent an endpoint of an integrated system from the cyclotron to the resultant image, and require the input of a team of specialists: physicists, radiochemists, radiographers and clinicians and/or biologists. PET has found applications in oncology,[1,2] and cardiology;[3] however, this chapter will concentrate on the use of PET in psychopharmacology.

2. PRINCIPLES OF PET

2.1 Physics

Positron emitters used for PET are nuclides with an excess of protons. Positron emission occurs when a proton is converted into a neutron. The energy liberated by this transformation is shared between the positron (β^+ or e^+) and the neutrino. The positron loses kinetic energy by colliding with the surrounding matter and eventually combines with an electron (β^- or e^-) when both particles are annihilated. Two photons of the same energy (511 keV, resting mass of the electron) are emitted, and travel at almost exactly 180° to each other. Because of their high energy these photons undergo relatively little interaction with surrounding tissue, and thus can be detected externally by dense scintillators (such as BGO) coupled to photomultipliers. The emission of two photons following β^+/β^- annihilation gives the additional advantage of registering only those photons, which are detected at the same time at approximately 180° to each other (coincidence detection). The original annihilation event will lie on the line joining the two detectors involved in coincidence detection. A PET scanner will contain thousands of such detectors. Coincidences are recorded and used to make an image of regional concentrations of positron-emitting material using reconstruction algorithms. The resulting image is a series of tomographic slices, which can be acquired as a time series. The accurate compensation of count loss and random coincidence detection (mainly owing to photon interactions with the surrounding tissue) via attenuation and scatter correction algorithms, as well as correction of differences in detector efficiency, allows absolute quantification of radioactive tracer in selected regions of interest. The spatial resolution of a PET image is fairly coarse (typically 5–10 mm with current PET scanners), because of factors such as positron travel between emission and annihilation, detector size and the angulation of the photon pair, away from 180°, because of residual positron motion.

Because of the coarse spatial resolution of PET, animal studies have traditionally been conducted in larger species such as primates. However, the development of dedicated small animal scanners[4,5] has allowed the use of smaller mammals (such as rats and mice) in pharmacological PET research (see Myers et al, 1999; Further reading). The improvement in resolution required for small animal scanning has often been achieved at the expense of sensitivity, and the trade-off between the two remains an issue in most dedicated small-animal systems.

2.2 Radiochemistry

The purpose of radiochemistry is to incorporate the positron-emitting nuclides, manufactured by the bombardment of suitable targets in a cyclotron, into organic molecules of clinical interest for use in PET imaging.

Most commonly used positron emitters (Table 8.1) have the advantage of being isotopes of normal constituents of organic molecules,

---

Table 8.1 Commonly used positron emitters		
β^+-emitting nuclide	Half-life (min)	Specific radioactivity (GBq/μmol)
^{11}C	20.40	110–260 (up to 340×10^3 in theory)
^{13}N	9.96	700×10^3
^{15}O	2.04	3400×10^3
^{18}F	109.80	185–370 (up to 60×10^3 in theory)

and as such can be substituted into these molecules without a change in the compound's pharmacological activity. Thus, a large number of biologically active compounds can be labelled with positron emitters and used for non-invasive in vivo studies. The total mass of the radioligand injected is usually in the low microgram range. The PET radioligands are therefore often referred to as radiotracers, since they are used in concentrations that are too low to induce biochemical or physiological effects.

The short half-lives of the positron emitters (see Table 8.1) present a number of difficulties in radiolabelling compounds for clinical PET studies. All radiosyntheses start with fundamental molecules (e.g. $[^{11}C]$carbon dioxide and $[^{11}C]$methane for $[^{11}C]$ synthesis) obtained from the bombardment of targets in the cyclotron. The fundamental molecules must then be converted into suitable radiolabelling agents, which react with suitable organic precursor molecules to produce the radiotracer of clinical interest. The choice of precursor for use in radiosynthetic process is very important, as the short half-lives of the radionuclides limit the number of possible reaction steps. Therefore speed and reproducibility must be achieved in radiosynthesis, as well as in quality control of the synthesized radiotracer.

An important consideration in the preparation of radiotracers is their specific activity, expressed as radioactivity per mass of compound (GBq/μmol). Specific activity provides a measure of the dilution of the radiotracer by the non-radiolabelled compound, the carrier. To prevent the loss of PET signal caused by the saturation of the biological target system by the carrier, specific radioactivity of the radiotracer needs to be high (typically 40–550 GBq/μmol). Because of the high specific activity required of the end product radiotracer, and because of the short half-life of the radionuclides, the radiation exposure during radiosynthesis is too high for repeated exposure by the radiochemists. Thus automation of radiosynthesis is a necessity.

2.3 Mathematical models

The purpose of PET data modelling is to convert the acquired emission dynamic data (counts/voxel) to useful physiological parameters. The amount of acquired radiation per voxel of image depends on variables such as the amount of radioactive tracer injected, radiotracer delivery to the target tissue and metabolism of the tracer. Raw PET images can be processed by applying tracer kinetic principles to derive absolute regional measurements or physiological parameters such as receptor number (B_{max}) or radiotracer affinity for the receptor (K_d). However, since multiple scans are often required to derive B_{max} or K_d, which is often impractical in human subjects, composite parameters such as binding potential (BP = B_{max}/K_d) are often used instead, and interpretation of PET scan results needs to bear in mind the assumptions inherent in using such composite parameters. An appropriate tracer needs to be chosen, and tracer biochemical and physiological properties need to be known a priori. A mathematical model is then developed and tested using numerical simulations and animal and human experiments. The model used will depend on the particular characteristics of the radiotracer, such as specificity of binding, reversibility of binding and rate of metabolism. The modelling approaches range from the data-led (such as spectral analysis) to the model-led (such as compartmental analysis).

Compartmental models divide the total body distribution of the radiotracer into one or more kinetically distinct compartments. The solutions to these models tend to be exponential, which corresponds to the physiological behaviour of radiotracers in the body. In addition, compartments are easily translated into physiological concepts such as specifically bound tracer, unbound tracer, etc. For these reasons compartmental models have traditionally enjoyed a central role in the analysis of PET data (Fig. 8.1).

Non-compartmental models such as graphical analysis have been useful in the examination of certain radiotracers.[6] The practical utility of PET has been enhanced by the development of reference region approaches, which obviates the need for arterial cannulation to estimate the input function.[7,8]

In developing models for the analysis of PET data, there is always a trade-off between bias and

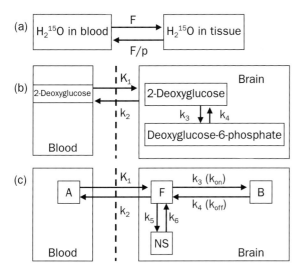

Fig. 8.1 Compartmental models describing radiotracer distribution in tissue. (a) One-tissue compartment model. The distribution of $H_2^{15}O$ in the brain. F = flow, p = partition ratio between the blood and the brain. (b) Two-tissue compartment model. The distribution of ^{18}F-deoxy-glucose (^{18}FDG) in the brain. K_1 and k_2 are constants relating to ^{18}FDG transport between the blood and the 'free tracer' compartment, k_3 and k_4 are the constants relating to ^{18}FDG transport between the 'free' tracer in the tissue and the specific binding compartment. (c) Three-tissue compartment model. The distribution of $[^{11}C]WAY$-100635 in the brain. K_1 and k_2 are constants relating to $[^{11}C]WAY$-100635 transport between the blood and the 'free tracer compartment', k_3 and k_4 are the constants relating to $[^{11}C]WAY$-100635 transport between the 'free tracer compartment' in the tissue and the specific binding compartment, and k_5 and k_6 are the constants relating to the $[^{11}C]WAY$-100635 transport between the 'free tracer compartment' and the non-specific binding compartment.

variance. It may be necessary to reduce the complexity of a model (by fixing some of the parameters at a constant value), at the risk of introducing bias, but with a view to reducing the variance on the estimate of the remaining parameters.

3. TYPES OF STUDIES

Pharmacological PET studies can be divided into two broad categories: studies aimed at determining the distribution of the drug to the receptor or enzyme target (pharmacokinetic studies) and studies determining the action of the drug at the receptor or enzyme (pharmacodynamic studies). The most common types of study and the questions they are designed to answer are summarized in Table 8.2.

3.1 Assessment of drug availability at the receptor (pharmacokinetics)

3.1.1 Drug distribution

By labelling a drug with a positron-emitting radiotracer an in vivo assessment of the drug pharmacokinetics may be achieved. Following the injection of the labelled drug, serial PET images (time frames) are acquired, and the regional tissue concentration of radioactivity is assessed. Dividing the radioactivity concentration by the specific activity of the injected drug will give the tissue concentration of the drug examined, as long as no metabolism of the drug has occurred. If metabolism of the drug has occurred, a specific mathematical model will need to be constructed to take into account the contribution of radioactive metabolites to the total signal. By considering the time-dependent distribution of the drug in specific organs, organ-specific pharmacokinetic parameters (relative to blood) such as peak concentration (C_{max}), time to peak concentration (t_{max}) and total amount of drug absorbed by the organ (AUC, area under the concentration-time curve) can be calculated. However, it should be noted that the pharmacokinetics of a labelled drug given in tracer amounts may differ from the kinetics of the same drug given in pharmacological amounts. Knowledge of organ-specific in vivo pharmacokinetic parameters in humans can be extremely valuable in the development of novel pharmaceuticals. For drugs acting on the central nervous system an important consideration is whether the drug crosses the blood–brain barrier, and the relative blood and brain concentrations. Examples of compounds examined include nicotine,[9] the anticancer agent 5-fluorouracil, and the antifungal agent fluconazole (for discussion see ref. 2).

Table 8.2 Common types of PET study	
Research question	**Type of study**
Pharmacokinetics	
What is the distribution of a drug in the body?	Radiolabel the drug
Does the drug bind to a particular target (receptor, enzyme, etc.)?	Radiolabel a radiotracer specific for the target
Pharmacodynamics	
What are the functional consequences of a drug's interaction with a target?	Change in blood flow ($H_2{}^{15}O$)
	Change in metabolism (^{18}FDG)
	Change in neurotransmitter release
	Change in gene expression

3.1.2 Drug–receptor interactions

Drugs usually produce their effects by interacting with specific receptors or enzymes (e.g. paroxetine and the 5-HT transporter, L-dopa and aromatic acid decarboxylase). Drug–receptor interactions can be studied directly (by labelling the drug of interest with a positron-emitting isotope) or indirectly (by examining the interaction of a drug with a receptor in the presence of a radiotracer specific for the receptor of interest). The direct examination of drug–receptor interaction, while simplest in theory, is hampered by the fact that the vast majority of drugs used in clinical neuroscience are not specific for a single receptor, and/or have unacceptably high levels of non-specific binding. In practice therefore, most interactions are examined in the presence of a radiotracer specific for the receptor or enzyme of interest. Studies involve the derivation of parameters such as receptor number (B_{max}), affinity (K_d), binding potential (B_{max}/K_d), or radiotracer influx into the cell (K_I, assumed to be related to enzyme activity). The occupancy of a receptor or enzyme by a drug is inferred as the change in the parameter examined in the presence of a drug (Fig. 8.2). Drug–receptor interactions may be useful in predicting response from the assessment of receptor occupancy, and in calcu-

lation of an optimal dosing regime to achieve a desired level of receptor occupancy.

3.1.3 Examples of receptor occupancy studies

3.1.3.1 Antipsychotic occupancy at the dopamine 2 (D_2) receptor

The assessment of optimal receptor occupancy associated with clinical response has been demonstrated for the D_2 receptor and antipsychotic medication. [^{11}C]Raclopride was used to examine the D_2 receptor occupancy in patients with schizophrenia who were on antipsychotic medication.[10–12] These studies established the

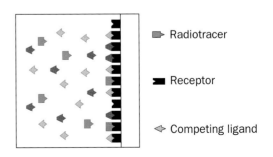

Fig. 8.2 Radiotracer binding to a receptor of interest before and after the addition of a competing ligand.

threshold receptor occupancy required for antipsychotic effects of standard antipsychotic medication (65%), as well as the threshold occupancy above which extra-pyramidal side-effects become pronounced (80%).

3.1.3.2 Pindolol occupancy of the serotonin 1A (5-HT$_{1A}$) receptor

PET has been used to evaluate the mechanism of action for a novel antidepressant strategy, the augmentation of selective serotonin reuptake inhibitors (SSRIs) by the β-adrenergic/5-HT$_{1A}$ partial agonist pindolol. This strategy has been proposed to accelerate the onset of antidepressant effect via the blockade of the inhibitory somatodendritic 5-HT$_{1A}$ autoreceptor by pindolol; however, clinical studies have produced mixed results.[13] One of the possible drawbacks of the clinical studies is the fact that since the effective dose of pindolol for the occupancy of the 5-HT$_{1A}$ receptor was unknown, the dose used in clinical trials (7.5 mg/day) was chosen mainly with a view to avoiding the β-adrenergic side-effects, rather than providing an adequate dose for action at the 5-HT$_{1A}$ site. The use of the specific 5-HT$_{1A}$ radiotracer [^{11}C]WAY-100635 allowed the examination of 5-HT$_{1A}$ receptor occupancy by pindolol in healthy volunteers,[14,15] and the conclusion that the dose used in clinical studies was inadequate was subsequently confirmed by an independent study.[16] An examination of depressed patients on combined SSRI/pindolol treatment confirmed that the doses of pindolol used in clinical trials were not sufficient to produce a consistent occupancy of the 5-HT$_{1A}$ autoreceptor.[17] These findings provide a putative explanation for the mixed results of clinical studies, and suggest that a thorough examination of the concept of pindolol augmentation of SSRIs will require clinical studies with higher doses of pindolol.

3.1.3.3 DU 125530 occupancy of the 5-HT$_{1A}$ receptor

DU 125530 is a novel silent antagonist at the 5-HT$_{1A}$ receptor with potential applications in the treatment of psychiatric disorders. PET with [^{11}C]WAY-100635 was used to evaluate the occupancy of the 5-HT$_{1A}$ receptor by DU 125530, and the relationship of plasma levels to receptor occupancy levels (Fig. 8.3).[18] As well as the effective dose required, the time course of a drug's occupancy of a receptor can be assessed. [^{11}C]WAY-100635 has been used to evaluate the time course of brain 5-HT$_{1A}$ receptor occupancy by the novel compound DU 125530.[18] Although DU 125530 has a half-life of ~12 hours in plasma, its occupancy of the 5-HT$_{1A}$ receptor at 24 hours was ~50% of its peak occupancy, indicating that it can be administered in a once-daily regime (Fig. 8.4).

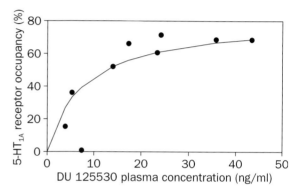

Fig. 8.3 Results of a PET occupancy study. 5-HT$_{1A}$ receptor occupancy by DU 125530 2 hours after the last dose. A best fit curve plotted to fit a single site model, Occupancy = [DU 125530]B$_{max}$/(ED50+ [DU 125530]), allowing the estimation of B$_{max}$ and ED50.[36]

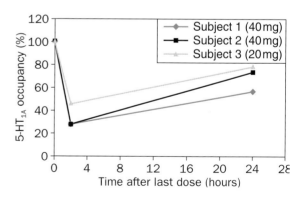

Fig. 8.4 The time course of 5-HT$_{1A}$ receptor occupancy by DU 125530 in three subjects. Occupancy was assessed at 2 hours (~t$_{max}$) and 24 hours after the last dose. The occupancy at 24 hours is ~50% of that at 2 hours.[36]

3.2 Assessment of drug action at the receptor (pharmacodynamics)

3.2.1 Combined pharmacokinetic/pharmacodynamic study

The most direct method of examining drug action at a receptor is to examine the clinical effects of a range of drug doses and simultaneously examine the receptor occupancy by the drug in the same individuals. This approach has been used in the study of the effects of antipsychotic medication in schizophrenic patients, as well as in the evaluation of the proconvulsant effects of benzodiazepine inverse agonists. On the basis of PET studies it has been suggested that the therapeutic range between the presence of antipsychotic effects and the emergence of unacceptable extra-pyramidal side-effects lies between 70% and 80% occupancy of the striatal D_2 receptor.[19,20]

3.2.2 Changes in metabolism

The response to a pharmacological intervention may often lead to a change in neural activity, which can be indexed by changes of glucose metabolism of the brain. This change in metabolism following a pharmacological or a non-pharmacological intervention can be assessed by PET with a metabolic indicator such as tissue glucose utilization. This approach is particularly suitable for the examination of the brain, where glucose represents the sole energy source. An alternative approach has been to examine regional cerebral blood flow, which is tightly coupled to regional cerebral glucose metabolism, and has been used to detect changes in neural activity occurring over a time course of 30–60 seconds.

The ^{18}F-labelled deoxyglucose analogue of glucose, ^{18}FDG, is initially phosphorylated by hexokinase to ^{18}FDG-6-PO$_4$, in a manner analogous to glucose, but does not undergo further glycolysis. The accumulation of ^{18}FDG-6-PO$_4$ in the brain allows the estimation of brain glucose metabolism in the baseline state, as well as following drug administration (for an introduction to ^{18}FDG modelling see Cunningham and Cremer, 1985; Further reading). H$_2$^{15}O is used as a radiotracer to index regional blood flow changes in response to a pharmacological intervention. The ^{18}FDG approach benefits from a good signal-to-noise ratio, as well as being a more direct measure of neural activity. On the other hand, because of the extremely short half-life of ^{15}O (2 minutes) the H$_2$^{15}O technique benefits from the possibility of performing several studies (up to 16) in each PET session, thus maximizing statistical power. The disadvantage of H$_2$^{15}O is the low signal-to-noise ratio, and the possible dissociation of blood flow and metabolism under certain conditions.

A particular problem in conducting studies of brain metabolism is the achievement of a stable baseline. Since a state of 'rest' is very ill defined and poorly reproducible (phenomena such as daydreaming being difficult to control) brain metabolism is likely to vary both between sessions and between subjects. To standardize 'resting' brain metabolism the examination of pharmacological modification of a psychological task has become a standard approach. Therefore, a crucial factor to be considered in assessing changes in metabolic response is the disentangling of the expected metabolic consequences of the experimental drug, from the metabolic changes induced by the psychological paradigm and the unintended physiological side-effects of the drug examined.

Activation studies in healthy volunteers using the psychological paradigm of auditory-verbal word-list memory task examined the effects of the non-selective dopamine agonist apomorphine, compared to the 5-HT$_{1A}$ partial agonist buspirone, on cerebral blood flow.[21] Differential patterns of task-related changes in cerebral blood flow were found, confirming the utility of H$_2$^{15}O PET in detecting pharmacological effects in the brain. A similar approach has been used to assess the influence of cholinergic stimulation on blood flow changes during a working memory task.[22] In schizophrenic patients, studies of tasks requiring executive processing and/or working memory revealed decreased regional blood flow compared with healthy subjects (hypofrontality),[23] which can be corrected by the administration of dopamine agonist drugs.[24]

Changes in regional glucose metabolism

have been demonstrated in patients with various neuropsychiatric disorders, including Alzheimer's disease,[25] epilepsy[26] and Parkinson's disease.[27] The effects of neuroleptic treatment on striatal metabolism have been assessed in schizophrenic patients using [18]FDG.[28]

3.2.3 Changes in neurotransmitter synthesis

One of the novel strategies utilized in overcoming the effects of the degeneration of dopaminergic neurons in Parkinson's disease involves the transplantation of embryonic mesencephalic tissue. Viability of the transplanted tissue has been demonstrated with the radiotracer [^{18}F]-dopa, which is a substrate for aromatic acid decarboxylase, and thus allows the estimation of the integrity of dopaminergic terminals, which contain this enzyme.[29]

3.2.4 Endogenous neurotransmitter release

The assessment of endogenous neurotransmitter release is a valuable tool in elucidating the pathophysiology of neuropsychiatric conditions. The change in the occupancy of a receptor by a radiotracer following an intervention designed to alter the levels of an endogenous neurotransmitter will provide an index of neurotransmitter release. This technique depends on the availability of radiotracers, such as the D_2 antagonists [^{11}C]raclopride and the structurally related single photon emission (SPECT) radiotracer [123]IBZM, the binding of which to receptors is sensitive to competition by endogenously released dopamine. [^{11}C]Raclopride and [123]IBZM have been used to assess dopamine release in healthy volunteers following administration of methylphenidate[30] or amphetamine,[31] and following a behavioural manipulation.[32] Dopamine release was found to be increased in patients with schizophrenia compared with healthy volunteers.[33,34] The release of dopamine from human embryonic cell transplant used to treat Parkinson's disease has been demonstrated following amphetamine administration.[29]

3.2.5 Gene expression

Gene expression can be a target of PET probes seeking to investigate the regulation of gene expression by normal and pathological processes, as well as by pharmacological therapy. In vivo imaging of gene expression is possible with PET, to visualize effects of drug treatment and to assess the results of gene therapy (see Phelps, 2000; Further reading). The imaging of gene expression can be directed either at genes externally transferred into cells (transgenes) or at endogenous genes. Imaging of endogenous gene expression can be used to study the expression of genes in normal biological processes such as ageing, as well as the expression of genes in response to therapy. One approach to imaging endogenous genes is the use of ^{18}F-labelled oligodeoxynucleotides.[35]

The imaging of transgene expression employs the transfection of a PET reporter gene (PRG) into a subject via one of the established methods (e.g. an adenovirus). The PRG is linked to a therapeutic gene by a common promoter, which initiates the transcription of the PRG mRNA at the same time as the transcription of the therapeutic gene mRNA. The mRNA of the PRG is then translated into a protein product (such as a D_2 receptor), which is a target for the PET radiotracer. The PRG approach can also be used to image endogenous gene expression by transferring a PRG with the same promoter as the endogenous gene of interest into cells.

The imaging of gene expression has been conducted mainly in animal models, but its employment in humans is bound to increase over the next few years, as demand for systems to monitor gene expression in vivo grows.

4. CONCLUSIONS

Over the past decade PET has become an increasingly important tool in pharmacological research. PET provides the opportunity to assess drug–receptor interactions in a physiologically valid context, as well as follow the time course of drug distribution in the same organism on multiple occasions. Indeed, in some areas, such as the development of novel antipsychotic agents, PET studies demonstrating adequate occupancy of the D_2 receptor are now considered an essential part of drug development. PET has an exciting future as the only technique currently available for the direct examination of in vivo brain neurochemistry, but it does require a considerable investment, both financial and scientific. The role of PET as a significant methodology in pharmacological research is likely to continue to grow.

REFERENCES

Further reading

Cunningham VJ, Cremer JE. Current assumptions behind the use of PET scanning for measuring glucose utilization in brain. *Trends Neurosci* 1985; **8:** 96–9.

Myers R, Hume S, Bloomfield P, Jones T. Radioimaging in small animals. *J Psychopharmacol* 1999; **13:** 352–7.

Phelps M. Positron emission tomography provides molecular imaging of biological processes. *Proc Natl Acad Sci USA* 2000; **97:** 9226–33.

Web-sites

■ http://www.crump.ucla.edu/software
Let's Play PET – an educational slide show (and CDROM) that lets the user explore all aspects of PET, from the principles of cyclotron operation to the clinical application of PET in cardiology, neurology and oncology.

■ http://www.cu.mrc.ac.uk/cyclotron_unit
MRC Cyclotron Unit web-site – Hammersmith is the location of the first hospital-based cyclotron, which was commissioned in 1955. Today, the focus of the unit's work is the clinical research applications of positron-emitting tracers and positron emission tomography.

■ http://www.ami-imaging.org
Academy of Molecular Imaging web-site.

Scientific papers

1. Aboagye EO, Price PM, Jones T. *In vivo* pharmacokinetics and pharmacodynamics in drug development using positron-emission tomography. *Drug Discov Today* 2001; **6:** 293–302.
2. Saleem A, Aboagye EO, Price PM. In vivo monitoring of drugs using radiotracer techniques. *Adv Drug Deliv Rev* 2000; **41:** 21–39.
3. Schelbert HR. PET contributions to understanding normal and abnormal cardiac perfusion and metabolism. *Ann Biomed Eng* 2000; **28:** 922–9.
4. Bloomfield PM, Rajeswaran S, Spinks TJ et al. Design and physical characteristics of a small animal positron emission tomograph. *Phys Med Biol* 1995; **40:** 1105–26.
5. Jeavons AP. Small-animal PET cameras. *J Nucl Med* 2000; **41:** 1442–3.
6. Logan J, Fowler JS, Volkow ND et al. Graphical analysis of reversible radioligand binding from time-activity measurements applied to [N-^{11}C methyl]-cocaine PET studies in human subjects. *J Cereb Blood Flow Metab* 1990; **10:** 740–7.
7. Cunningham VJ, Lammertsma AA. Radioligand studies in brain: kinetic analysis of PET data. *Med Chem Res* 1994; **5:** 79–96.
8. Lammertsma AA, Hume SP. Simplified reference tissue model for PET receptor studies. *Neuroimage* 1996; **4:** 153–8.
9. Hartvig P, Lindner KJ, Tedroff J, Langstrom B. Positron emission tomography illuminating in vivo drug disposition. *Eur J Pharmaceutical Sci,* 1994: 44–6.
10. Farde L, Wiesel FA, Halldin C, Sedvall G. Central D$_2$-dopamine receptor occupancy in schizophrenic patients treated with antipsychotic drugs. *Arch Gen Psychiatry* 1988; **45:** 71–6.
11. Nordstrom AL, Farde L, Wiesel FA et al. Central D2-dopamine receptor occupancy in relation to antipsychotic drug effects: a double-blind PET study of schizophrenic patients. *Biol Psychiatry* 1993; **33:** 227–35.
12. Wiesel FA, Farde L, Nordstrom LA, Sedvall G. Central D1 and D2 receptor occupancy during antipsychotic drug treatment. *Prog Neuropsychopharmacol Biol Psychiatry* 1990; **14:** 759–67.
13. Artigas F, Celada P, Laruelle M, Adell, A. How does pindolol improve antidepressant action? *Trends Pharmacol Sci* 2001; **22:** 224–8.
14. Rabiner EA, Gunn RN, Castro ME et al. β-blocker binding to human 5-HT$_{1A}$ receptors *in vivo* and *in vitro*: implications for antidepressant therapy. *Neuropsychopharmacology* 2000; **23:** 285–93.
15. Rabiner EA, Sargent PA, Gunn RN, Bench CJ, Cowen PJ, Grasby PM. Imaging pindolol binding to 5-HT$_{1A}$ receptors in man using PET. *Int J Neuropsychopharmacol* 1998; **1:** S65–S66.
16. Martinez D, Broft A, Laruelle M. Pindolol augmentation of antidepressant treatment: recent contributions from brain imaging studies. *Biol Psychiatry* 2000; **48:** 844–53.

17. Rabiner EA, Bhagwagar Z, Gunn RN et al. Pindolol augmentation of SSRI antidepressant efficacy: PET evidence suggests the dose used in clinical trials is too low. *Am J Psychiatry* 2001; **158:** 2080–2.

18. Rabiner EA, Wilkins MR, Turkheimer F et al. *In vivo* human receptor occupancy by DU 125530: a selective 5-HT$_{1A}$ antagonist. *J Psychopharmacol* 2001; **15:** A17.

19. Farde L, Nordstrom AL, Wiesel FA, Pauli S, Halldin C, Sedvall G. Positron emission tomographic analysis of central D1 and D2 dopamine receptor occupancy in patients treated with classical neuroleptics and clozapine. Relation to extrapyramidal side effects. *Arch Gen Psychiatry* 1992; **49:** 538–44.

20. Farde L, Wiesel FA, Nordstrom A-L, Sedvall G. D1- and D2-dopamine receptor occupancy during treatment with conventional and atypical neuroleptics. *Psychopharmacology (Berl)* 1989; **99:** 28–31.

21. Grasby PM, Friston KJ, Bench CJ et al. The effect of apomorphine and buspirone on regional cerebral blood flow during the performance of a cognitive task – Measuring neuromodulatory effects of psychotropic drugs in man. *Eur J Neurosci* 1992; **4:** 1203–12.

22. Furey ML, Pietrini P, Haxby JV et al. Cholinergic stimulation alters performance and task-specific regional cerebral blood flow during working memory. *Proc Natl Acad Sci USA* 1997; **94:** 6512–16.

23. Weinberger DR, Berman KF, Zec RF. Physiologic dysfunction of dorsolateral prefrontal cortex in schizophrenia. I Regional cerebral blood flow evidence. *Arch Gen Psychiatry* 1986; **43:** 114–24.

24. Daniel DG, Berman KF, Weinberger DR. The effect of apomorphine on regional cerebral blood flow in schizophrenia. *J Neuropsychiatry Clin Neurosci* 1989; **1:** 377–84.

25. Ibanez V, Pietrini P, Alexander GE et al. Regional glucose metabolic abnormalities are not the result of atrophy in Alzheimer's disease. *Neurology* 1998; **50:** 1585–93.

26. Henry TR. PET: cerebral blood flow and glucose metabolism – presurgical localisation. In: Henry TR, Duncan JS, Berkovic SF, eds. *Functional Imaging in the Epilepsies*, Vol 83. Philadelphia: Lippincott Williams & Wilkins, 2000.

27. Hu MT, Taylor-Robinson SD, Chaudhuri KR et al. Cortical dysfunction in non-demented Parkinson's disease patients: a combined (31)P-MRS and (18)FDG-PET study. *Brain* 2000; **123:** 340–52.

28. Buchsbaum MS, Potkin SG, Siegel BV et al. Striatal metabolic rate and clinical response to neuroleptics in schizophrenia. *Arch Gen Psychiatry* 1992; **49:** 966–74.

29. Piccini P, Brooks DJ, Bjorklund A et al. Dopamine release from nigral transplants visualized in vivo in a Parkinson's patient. *Nat Neurosci* 1999; **2:** 1137–40.

30. Volkow ND, Wang GJ, Fowler JS et al. Imaging endogenous dopamine competition with [^{11}C]raclopride in the human brain. *Synapse* 1994; **16:** 255–62.

31. Laruelle M, Abi-Dargham A, van Dyck CH et al. SPECT imaging of striatal dopamine release after amphetamine challenge. *J Nucl Med* 1995; **36:** 1182–90.

32. Koepp MJ, Gunn RN, Lawrence AD et al. Evidence for striatal dopamine release during a videogame. *Nature* 1998; **393:** 266–8.

33. Breier A, Su TP, Saunders R et al. Schizophrenia is associated with elevated amphetamine-induced synaptic dopamine concentrations: evidence from a novel positron emission tomography method. *Proc Natl Acad Sci USA* 1997; **94:** 2569–74.

34. Laruelle M, Abi-Dargham A, Gil R, Kegeles L, Innis R. Increased dopamine transmission in schizophrenia: relationship to illness phases. *Biol Psychiatry* 1999; **46:** 56–72.

35. Tavitian B, Terrazzino S, Kuhnast B et al. *In vivo* imaging of oligonucleotides with positron emission tomography. *Nat Med* 1998; **4:** 467–71.

36. Rabiner EA, Wilkins MR, Turkheimer F *et al.* 5-Hydroxytryptamine1A receptor occupancy by novel full antagonist 2-[4- [4-(7-chloro-2,3-dihydro-1,4-benzdioxyn-5-yl)-1-piperazinyl]butyl]-1,2- benzisothiazol-3-(2H)-one-1,1-dioxide: a[11C][O-methyl-3H]-N-(2(4-(2- methoxyphenyl)-1-piperazinyl)ethyl)-N-(2-pyridinyl)cyclohexanecarboxamide trihydrochloride (WAY-100635) positron emission tomography study in humans. *J Pharmacol Exp Ther* 2002; **301:** 1144–50.

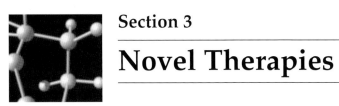

Section 3

Novel Therapies

9

Targeting nuclear receptors: PPARs as targets for drug design

Colin NA Palmer, Martin R Wilkins

SUMMARY

'Drugable' proteins are generally proteins whose normal function is to interact with small organic molecules. Enzymes involved in small molecule metabolism are obvious cases in point. Nuclear receptors may also be considered an ideal target for drugs as they are dedicated to the sensing of organic molecules of the size, range and structure that are ideal for the design of novel chemical entities. This chapter describes the development and pharmacology of peroxisome proliferator-activated receptor (PPAR) ligands as an example of targeting nuclear receptors. Moreover, the story of these ligands provides what has been described as a 'reverse endocrinology' in which potent chemical tools have been used to uncover the role of PPARs in human physiology and disease processes.

1. INTRODUCTION

1.1 Nuclear receptors as drug targets

Nuclear receptors form a large superfamily of zinc finger domain DNA-binding transcription factors (Fig. 9.1). This family includes the receptors for steroidal sex hormones such as oestrogen, progesterone and testosterone and it is these sex hormone receptors that have previously been targeted heavily for drug development. The two most notable drugs of this category are steroid antagonists, i.e. tamoxifen and RU486. Tamoxifen is an oestrogen receptor antagonist used in the secondary prevention of breast cancer[1] and RU486 is a progesterone receptor antagonist utilized in induction of parturition.[2]

The observation that tamoxifen reduces overall mortality in breast cancer has prompted interest in the development of cleaner oestrogen receptor antagonists. The development of the next generation of these drugs has been helped by the elucidation of the structure of the ligand-binding domain of the oestrogen receptor bound to agonists and antagonists.[3–5] These

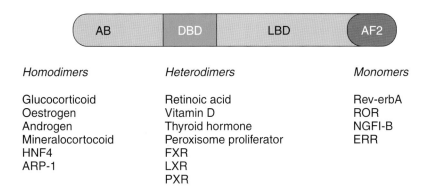

Homodimers	Heterodimers	Monomers
Glucocorticoid	Retinoic acid	Rev-erbA
Oestrogen	Vitamin D	ROR
Androgen	Thyroid hormone	NGFI-B
Mineralocortocoid	Peroxisome proliferator	ERR
HNF4	FXR	
ARP-1	LXR	
	PXR	

Fig. 9.1 Nuclear receptors: a large superfamily of ligand-activated transcription factors. Nuclear receptors share a common domain structure with a highly conserved zinc finger DNA-binding domain (DBD), a ligand-binding domain (LBD) and an activation domain (AF2).

structures have revealed the chemical interactions that are required to bind oestrogen receptors with a high affinity, providing insight into the way in which receptor activity can be selectively modified and permitting the in silico optimization of novel drugs.

1.2 Orphan receptors

As more and more lipophilic signalling molecules were found to have nuclear receptor targets, (such as vitamin A, vitamin D and thyroid hormone), the complexity of this family of proteins became apparent. Many groups began screening cDNA libraries with DNA probes encompassing the highly conserved zinc finger/DNA-binding domain. Screening with such a conserved motif resulted in the isolation of many new sequences that encoded proteins with no known hormone ligand – so-called orphan receptors.[6] With the complete sequence of the human genome now available it would appear that there are a total of 50 nuclear receptors encoded on the human chromosomes – although the efficiency of the previous screening programme meant that the human genome project did not find any additional genes.[7]

The discovery of so many orphan receptors has raised the possibility that a large body of unrecognized signalling compounds may exist that are ligands for such receptors; however, it is also possible that some members of this family are genuine hormone sensors and others may simply be constitutive transcription factors with no relevance to small molecule ligands.

Some members of the orphan receptor family have been characterized as important transcription factors, determining tissue- and cell-specific gene transcription. A key example of this is hepatic nuclear factor 4 (HNF4). This appears to be a constitutive transcription factor that directs liver-selective transcription of a number of genes, including several CYP genes, apolipoproteins, glucose transporters and bile acid transporters.[8]

It has been proposed that several orphan receptors are constitutively activated by endogenous ligands and their ligand-dependence can only be seen by using antagonists. This has been observed directly with CAR (constitutively-active androgen receptor), where CAR activity has been shown to be repressed in cell reporter systems by androgens.[9] CAR has recently been implicated in the regulation of hepatic CYP genes by a wide range of xenobiotics, including phenobarbital,[10,11] although it is still not clear if these effects are mediated by the binding of xenobiotics to CAR.[12] In a similar fashion, it has been suggested that HNF4 is regulated by a range of fatty acyl coA esters, suggesting that an endogenous ligand related to these esters may be responsible for in vivo constitutive activation of HNF-4.[13] Again this mechanism has been the subject of debate.[14] Other orphan receptors, such as rev-erbA, do not contain conserved transactivation domains and appear to function solely as repressor proteins for the feedback inhibition of the action of other nuclear receptors.[6,15,16]

1.3 The discovery of peroxisome proliferator-activated receptors (PPARs)

In order to identify ligands for orphan receptors, the ligand-binding domains of these receptors were fused to the DNA-binding domain of the glucocorticoid receptor. Using a chloramphenicol acetyl transferase gene controlled by a glucocorticoid-responsive enhancer it was possible to monitor transcriptional activity from the chimeric receptor (Fig. 9.2). Among the compounds screened by this strategy were drugs, herbicides and plasticizers that caused a distinct form of liver cancer in rodents. This group of compounds was known to promote liver cancer after a prolonged hyperplastic response, characterized by hepatocytes filled with large numbers of peroxisomes. Therefore, these compounds were known as peroxisome proliferators.[17] Upon screening the orphan receptor library, one receptor was consistently activated by peroxisome proliferators. This receptor was named the peroxisome proliferator-activated receptor (PPAR).[18] Studies in *Xenopus laevis* identified three forms of a receptor similar to the mouse PPAR.[19] The one that most closely related to the mouse form was named PPARα, and the other two were named PPARβ (now known as PPARδ) and PPARγ.

2. TISSUE DISTRIBUTION AND REGULATION OF PPARS

The three PPAR subtypes are the products of separate genes (see review in *Cell* 1999; Further reading), which show the highest similarity in their zinc finger DNA-binding domains (Fig. 9.3). Analysis of PPARα distribution in humans and rodents has shown high levels in metabolically active tissues, such as liver, heart, kidney and muscle.[20] PPARγ mRNA has been detected

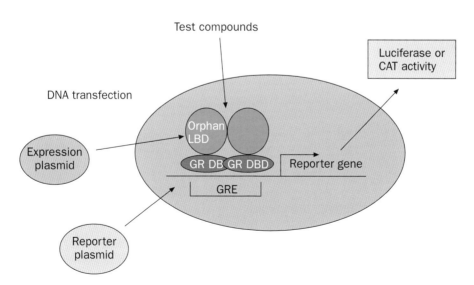

Fig. 9.2   Diagram of a chimeric transactivation assay. A common screen for compounds that activate orphan nuclear receptors utilized chimeric receptors, with the DNA-binding domain (DB) of the glucocorticoid receptor (GR) fused to the ligand-binding domain (LBD) of the orphan receptor. This allows for an output signal from a glucocorticoid-responsive reporter gene.

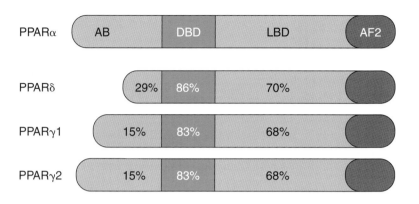

Fig. 9.3 PPAR subfamily. The PPAR subfamily is encoded by three genes. Percentages define degree of homology with PPARα. Abbreviations as for Fig. 9.1.

in three isoforms (PPARγ1, -2 and -3), which are the products of different promoters.[21–23] PPARγ1 and -3 encode identical proteins, and PPARγ2 encodes a protein that has an amino-terminal extension of 22 amino acids. PPARγ1 has the broadest tissue distribution, being found in adipose tissue, heart, large and small intestines, kidney, pancreas, spleen, skeletal muscle and macrophages. PPARγ2 is found mainly in adipose tissue and PPARγ3 in adipose tissue, colonic epithelium and macrophages. PPARδ is expressed widely, including liver, intestine, kidney, adipose tissue and skeletal muscle.[20]

PPARs are ligand-activated transcription factors; the binding of agonist ligands to the receptor results in changes in the level of mRNAs encoded by PPAR target genes. PPARs are activated by fatty acids.[24–26] PPARα binds a wide range of saturated fatty acids; indeed the absence of a single natural high-affinity ligand has given rise to the suggestion that PPARα senses the total flux of fatty acids in metabolically active tissues. PPARγ has a clear preference for polyunsaturated fatty acids, such as docosahexaenoic acid, eicosapentanoic acid, linolenic and arachidonic acids.[26,27] The J series of prostaglandins derived from PGD$_2$ have also been identified as PPARγ ligands.[28] PPARδ binds saturated and unsaturated fatty acids with a profile intermediate between PPARα and PPARγ and several eicosanoids, including perhaps PGI$_2$.[26]

PPARs play a central role in regulating the

storage and catabolism of dietary fats.[24] PPARs activate the transcription of genes involved in lipid homeostasis, such as peroxisomal acylCoA oxidase,[19] microsomal fatty acid φ-hydroxylases (CYP4A)[29] and fatty acid-binding proteins.[30] The PPAR responsiveness of target genes has been mapped to recognizable enhancer sequences known as peroxisome proliferator response elements (PPREs), which contain an imperfect repeat of the consensus nuclear receptor-binding sequence (AGGTCA) with a spacing of one nucleotide (Fig. 9.4). Sequences 5′ of this repeat are utilized to generate specificity in signalling.[31] PPARs do not bind to this element alone, as the N-terminal domain of PPARs inhibits the binding of monomeric PPARs to DNA; the DNA-binding activity is only seen in the presence of the promiscuous heterodimeric partner, retinoid X receptor (RXR).[32] PPARs bind to the 5′ repeat unit of the PPRE as a heterodimer with the RXR bound to the 3′ repeat. This arrangement has been shown to be required for co-operative signalling by PPAR ligands and RXR ligands. Other binding configurations, such as those seen with the thyroid hormone receptor and the vitamin D receptor, appear to silence the RXR partner. The binding of PPAR to RXR and thus to DNA has been shown to be facilitated by the binding of ligand,[33] and it has been shown that ligand binding is required to allow the binding of co-activator proteins,[34–36] which in turn interact with the RNA polymerase complex to transcribe the target gene (Fig. 9.4); therefore, the

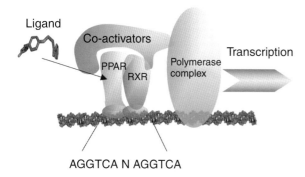

Ligand
Co-activators
Transcription
PPAR
RXR
Polymerase
complex

AGGTCA N AGGTCA

Fig. 9.4 PPARs act as molecular switches in control of gene transcription.

binding of ligand to PPAR is required for the assembly of the entire replication-competent enhancer/promoter complex. The co-activators may also represent drug targets, as they appear to have roles in the integration of metabolic processes. A good example of this is the control of gluconeogenesis by the PPARγ binding co-activator 1 (PGC-1).[37] Energy balance is also coordinated by AMP-activated kinase, partly through the phosphorylation of another PPAR co-activator known as CBP/p300.[38] Phosphorylation of CBP by AMP-K results in a reduced ability of PPARγ to activate transcription in response to ligand.

3. PPARS AS TARGETS FOR LIPID-LOWERING DRUGS

Consistent with a role in regulating lipid metabolism, it has emerged that one important class of synthetic ligands for PPARs are the hypolipidaemic fibrates, which include clofibrate, ciprofibrate, fenofibrate, bezafibrate and gemfibrozil,[36] (see also Willson et al, 2000). Clofibric acid and fenofibric acid, the active metabolites of clofibrate and fenofibrate, are dual PPARα and -γ ligands (with 10-fold selectivity for PPARα) while bezafibrate activates all three subtypes. Nonetheless, all these compounds require high micromolar concentrations to activate PPARα. More potent PPARα agonists have been identified and are under investigation.

Fibrates appear to mediate lipid-lowering by modulating apolipoprotein expression.[39] The ApoA1 gene is transcriptionally activated in the liver, allowing greater amounts of HDL assembly and a greater flow of reverse cholesterol transport. ApoCIII (a known inhibitor of VLL clearance) output is suppressed, limiting the formation of atherogenic, triglyceride-rich lipoproteins in the periphery.

It has also been suggested that fibrates may have direct beneficial effects on the vascular endothelium and smooth muscle cells in the control of inflammation, vasodilation and thrombolysis (see Bishop-Bailey, 2000; Further reading), but the concentrations required to produce these effects do not correlate very well with those required to activate PPARα. This discordance suggests that much has still to be learned regarding the mechanism of action of these drugs.

PPARγ agonists decrease plasma levels of triglycerides, cholesterol and non-esterified fatty acids in various animal models of dyslipidaemia. The changes in humans are less consistent. To quote one authority, 'PPARγ agonists have some utility in lowering triglycerides and free fatty acids ... [but] the pharmacological profile of these agents in a strictly dyslipidaemic setting is unknown' (Willson et al, 2000; Further reading).

Until recently, the role of PPARδ in lipid metabolism has been difficult to define because of the lack of specific agonists for this receptor. A novel PPARδ ligand developed by Glaxo Wellcome, GW1516, has a binding affinity for PPARδ of 1 nM, and binds PPARα and γ only at micromolar concentration.[40] Treatment of obese rhesus monkeys with GW1516 profoundly lowered triglyceride and LDL levels, and a corresponding increase in HDL cholesterol was observed. However, an increase in total serum cholesterol and an increase in apoCIII expression has also been noted in animals treated with GW1516. This increase in apoCIII expression is in contrast to the repression normally observed with fibrates, and apoCIII is associated with the formation of atherogenic forms of LDL. Interestingly, induction of apoCIII gene expression has been observed with ligands for the retinoid X receptor[41] and is potentially associated with the hypertriglyceridaemia that occurs as a common complication of retinoid therapy.[42,43] These observations suggest a novel mode of lipid-lowering by GW1516.

Indeed, it has been reported recently that a highly selective PPARδ agonist, compound F, promotes lipid-loading in human macrophages by oxidized LDL. It was also shown that over-expression of PPARδ in the human monocytic cell line, THP-1, provokes a profound increase in lipid accumulation in response to differentiation by phorbol esters. It is possible that PPARδ agonists may increase reverse cholesterol transport by HDL (by upregulation of ABCA1), but may massively increase macrophage activation and removal of lipids (LDL and triglycerides) from the serum (by increasing the scavenger receptors Class A and B (SRA and SRB) and decreasing apoE). In another recent study a novel lipid-lowering drug provoked massive foam cell accumulation in the spleen.[44] This suggests the possibility that the lipid-lowering mechanism of PPARδ ligands could be caused by increasing lipid accumulation in the periphery, which may result in a net increase in HDL-C formation. It is therefore of vital importance to determine the mechanism by which PPARδ ligands may have hypolipidaemic effects, to determine the suitability of PPARδ agonists for the management of dyslipidaemia in metabolic disease.

4. PPARS AS THE TARGET FOR INSULIN-SENSITIZING DRUGS

The thiazolidinedione family of insulin-sensitizing agents, such as troglitazone (Rezulin), pioglitazone (Actos) and rosiglitazone (Avandia), like the fibrates, were developed with no known target or receptor. Radioligand-binding studies with rosiglitazone had demonstrated that there was no membrane-associated receptor, but high affinity binding to nuclei isolated from adipocytes could be demonstrated. It was subsequently demonstrated that rosiglitazone binds and activates PPARγ.[45]

PPARγ was known to be a transcription factor responsible for controlling adipocyte-specific gene transcription.[30] The possibility that PPARγ was a mediator of the insulin-sensitizing actions of thiazolidinediones was surprising, as it was understood that skeletal muscle was the tissue principally responsible for determining insulin sensitivity. This has been partially clarified by the demonstration that, although less abundant in skeletal muscle, PPARγ is functional in this tissue.[46,47] Furthermore, novel neuroendocrine hormones have now been identified in adipocytes that contribute to the regulation of insulin sensitivity.[48,49] It is also evident that several steps in the signal transduction pathway of insulin are regulated by PPARγ. For example, PPARγ induces the expression of c-Cbl-associated protein in adipocytes, a potential signalling protein in insulin action. However, the actual mechanism of control of insulin sensitivity is still unknown.

The importance of PPARγ in regulating insulin sensitivity has been confirmed by human genetics. Several severely insulin-resistant individuals with mutations in the ligand-binding domain of PPARγ have been described.[50] These mutations appear to act as dominant negatives (i.e. to dominantly inhibit the wild-type receptor), although the mutant receptor does retain some function at higher concentrations of ligand (and so the disruption does not act as a true null mutation). This probably allows mutant individuals to survive, in contrast to the lethal phenotype observed with the homozygous murine knockout.[51,52] Interestingly, heterozygous null mice are more insulin-sensitive when compare with their wild-type littermates. This appears to be due to the size and number of adipocytes in those animals that contain 50% of the wild-type levels of PPARγ.[52]

Troglitazone was the first PPARγ ligand to be marketed for the management of type II diabetes. However, it was responsible for several deaths due to liver failure, and has subsequently been withdrawn (see review, Gale 2001; Further reading). Pioglitazone and rosiglitazone are now marketed in the USA and Europe as monotherapy or in combination therapy with the insulin secretagogue, metformin. The evidence to date suggests that these drugs are less liable to cause hepatotoxicity but there are a number of other concerns regarding their use, including weight gain and ankle oedema. The mechanism of these side-effects is not clear, but they confer a narrow therapeutic index on these drugs.

These concerns currently limit the use of PPARγ ligands in clinical practice and ensure that they are kept under close review by post-marketing surveillance groups. Nonetheless there is interest in their potential benefits in the management of the broader spectrum of insulin resistance syndrome – a term that acknowledges an association between reduced insulin sensitivity and other cardiovascular risk factors, (i.e. central obesity, hypertension and dyslipidaemia) – that predisposes to cardiovascular disease (i.e. myocardial infarction, stroke and systemic atherosclerosis).

5. PPAR LIGANDS, HYPERTENSION AND ATHEROSCLEROSIS

An interesting observation is that PPARγ ligands demonstrate hypotensive effects in some animal models. These include genetic models of hypertension – such as the Dahl S strain and spontaneously hypertensive rats – as well as one-kidney, one-clip Sprague-Dawley animals (see Bishop-Bailey, 2000; Further reading). The effect appears to be independent of their effect on insulin sensitivity but the mechanism is unknown. It is worth noting that PPARγ mutations were found in patients with profound early-onset hypertension as well as diabetes.[50]

Among the possible mechanisms are inhibition of vascular smooth muscle cell proliferation and structural remodelling of the blood vessel wall, as well as by reduction of vascular tone. PPARγ ligands influence the production of the vasodilator factor C-natriuretic peptide and the vasoconstrictor endothelin.[53,54] A direct effect mediated through inhibition of voltage-gated (L-type) calcium channels has also been proposed.[55] This property of PPARγ agonists adds to their potential therapeutic value in the management of insulin resistance.

The objective in the treatment of cardiovas-cular disease is to inhibit atherosclerosis. Both PPARα and PPARγ ligands appear to have protective effects on angiographically defined atherosclerosis.[56,57] While this may be due in part to the favourable effects of these drugs on lipids, insulin activity and hypertension, there is emerging evidence for a direct effect on the arterial wall. PPARα agonists downregulate adhesion molecule expression in human vascular endothelial cells. PPARγ ligands have been shown to block vascular smooth muscle cell proliferation and migration, and agonists for both subtypes promote apoptosis in macrophages (Bishop-Bailey, 2000; Further reading). These findings have prompted the speculation that combined PPARα/γ agonists may be useful in the prevention of atherosclerosis and this is likely to be the focus of future studies. Interestingly, the PPARδ isoform has been shown to mediate potentially atherogenic processes such as macrophage lipid accumulation and vascular smooth muscle proliferation, suggesting the possible utility of PPARδ antagonists in the management of atherosclerosis.[58,59]

6. PPARS AND THE CONTROL OF INFLAMMATION

PPARα null mice exhibit a prolonged inflammatory response in the archidonic acid ear-swelling test compared with wild-type mice. It was hypothesized that PPARα may regulate genes involved in eicosanoid catabolism but it is also clear that PPARα agonists directly modulate genes encoding inflammatory mediators in macrophages and vascular endothelium and smooth muscle.[60,61] This appears to be by the inhibition of activation of both the AP1 and NFκB pathways. Therefore PPARα ligands may both limit the production of inflammatory mediators and stimulate their clearance. Significantly, PPARα is a receptor for leukotriene B4 and pharmacological analogues while many potent leukotriene receptor antagonists are strong peroxisome proliferators.

Several inhibitors of ecosanoid synthesis, such as indomethacin, ibuprofen and fenoprofen, have been shown to be weak agonists at PPARγ receptors.[62] It is important to note that these compounds interact with PPARγ at concentrations significantly higher than those required for inhibition of cyclooxygenase. Interestingly, diclofenac, a NSAID commonly used in rheumatology, has recently been shown to be an antagonist of PPARγ at clinically relevant doses.[63] PPAR antagonism at low concentrations has also observed with for the COX-2 selective NSAIDs, nimesulide and NS398.[64]

The anti-inflammatory properties of PPAR ligands add weight to the arguments for using them in the management of atherosclerosis. There are, however, other clinical indications that merit investigation and PPARγ agonists have been utilized recently in the treatment of inflammatory bowel disease and psoriasis.[65,66]

7. PPARS AND ONCOLOGY

Paradoxically, given the role of PPARs in liver tumour formation in rodents, PPARs are under scrutiny as gene targets for preventing and/or treating cancer. The carcinogenic effect of PPAR ligands in rodents appears to be species-specific. Significantly, hepatic tumours have not been observed in a number of other laboratory animals, such as marmosets and guinea pigs, even with extreme doses of these compounds.[67] The possibility that PPARs may produce hepatic tumours in humans has been extensively studied and debated, but it appears that the rodent liver is hypersensitive to such compounds.[68–70]

On the contrary, activation of PPARα and PPARγ has anti-proliferative effects in a wide range of human epithelial cancer cell lines. PPARγ ligands in particular have received much attention. Troglitazone and rosiglitazone have been reported to have anti-proliferative effects in cancer cell lines from breast, lung, prostate, colon, bladder, pancreas and oesophagus.[71–75] The pharmacology of the anti-proliferative effects of thiazolidinediones does not correlate with their anti-diabetic activity or their ability to activate PPARγ. In most studies, rosiglitazone has no effects on cellular proliferation in cancer cell lines at concentrations under 1 μM. This is in contrast with an EC_{50} for adipogenesis of 50 nM in NIH3T3L1 cells and for

transactivation of PPARγ in transactivation assays. The potency of rosiglitazone in such assays is similar to troglitazone, a much weaker PPARγ ligand. It has been suggested that rosiglitazone has a blunted anti-proliferative effect in cancer cells owing to inhibition of PPAR signalling by the Ras/MAPK pathway,[75,76] but this should also inhibit the action of troglitazone to a similar extent.

In certain cancer types the action of thiazolidinediones provides a differentiation signal. This is most evident in the case of liposarcoma, where the adipocyte differentiation programme is reactivated by PPARγ.[77] This has also been observed in breast cancer cell lines, with marked lipid inclusions occurring in treated cells.[72] However, this is not the case in colon or pancreatic cells, where the role of PPARγ in the differentiation of these tissues is unclear.[71,75,78–80]

PPARδ has been implicated in the biology of colon cancer in transcriptional profiling analysis. Using serial analysis of gene expression (SAGE), PPARδ has been identified as a target of the APC/TCF/β-catenin pathway, and mutations in APC lead to a dramatic upregulation of PPARδ.[81] This places PPARδ at the centre of colon cancer growth regulation. In addition, ablation of the PPARδ gene in human colorectal cancer cells virtually abolishes the tumorigenic potential of these cells.[82] Sulindac, an NSAID with known anti-neoplastic properties in the human colon, has also been shown to be an antagonist of PPARδ activity.[81] Confusingly, activation of PPARδ with prostacyclin does not promote the growth of colon cancer cells and experiments have not been performed with selective PPARδ agonists to analyse their effects on growth.[83] It is therefore a matter of some importance to determine the action of selective activation of PPARδ in colon cancer cells, and compounds are now available that would be suitable for such experiments.[40,58,84]

8. DEVELOPMENT OF NEW PPAR LIGANDS

All PPAR ligands currently in use clinically were discovered before the discovery of PPARs. This will change soon. Many companies have screened large libraries of compounds and many patents and papers are now published that document the results of these screens. Some have described higher affinity ligands for PPARα and PPARγ with a view to generating more potent fibrates or insulin-sensitizers.[85] Some have described compounds that have mixed functions,[86,87] and some have reported ligands selective for PPARδ.[40,58,84]

PPARδ has been largely ignored in PPAR research until now. The availability of PPARδ-specific ligands is starting to reveal a role for PPARδ, particularly in physiological and patho-physiological functions.[40,58,88] Most of these screens have employed transactivation assays for the discovery of PPAR agonists that are similar to those described in Fig. 9.2. However, a new approach has been adopted for the rational design and optimization of PPAR ligands.

8.1 Rational design of PPAR ligands

The crystal structures of all three PPAR sub-types, including a structure of the PPARγ/RXR heterodimer, have been solved by researchers at Glaxo Wellcome and Astra Zeneca. Crystals have been described with various ligands, including antagonists bound.[26,89,90] This has taken the PPAR family from one of the least understood nuclear receptors to the most highly characterized subfamily, with documentation rivalling that of the oestrogen receptor.

A striking finding is that the PPAR ligand-binding pocket is much larger than that observed for other nuclear receptors, with fatty acids 'flip-flopping' around inside the cavity. However, it is clear that the three isoforms are different enough to rationalize observed pharmacological specificity and to predict the behaviour of novel chemical entities. This has been performed to optimize a third generation of specific PPAR agonists, with the isolation of very selective ligands for each form. Nonetheless it is still unclear as to how desirable clinically it would be to have such selective ligands.

One of the major strategies employed to increase the affinity of compounds has been to increase their size, thus making use of possible interactions within the large ligand-binding pocket. The common polar head group of PPAR ligands appears to fit within a restricted area between helix 3, 10 and the activation helix 12. This is the area that modulates the conformation of the 'charge clamp' required for interaction with co-activator proteins and therefore acts as the molecular switch for turning target genes 'on'.[26,89] This group is generally linked via a flexible region to a ring-based hydrophobic group, which is wrapped around helix 3 and occupies a larger cavity between helices 2', 3, 6 and 7. This is the large portion that allows the acyl chains of fatty acid ligands to 'flip-flop' as mentioned above. The helix 2' is not observed in other nuclear receptors and is responsible for the unusually large volume of the PPAR ligand-binding cavity.

Novel drugs such as GI262570[90] have larger groups that make many interactions in this large pocket and thus have much higher affinity for the receptor, providing binding at concentrations at between 50- and 1000-fold lower than that observed for first generation drugs (activation and binding can now be observed as low as picomolar concentrations). In the case of GI262570 the kd is 1 nM for PPARγ (cf 50 nM for rosiglitazone). This molecule is radically different from other ligands, as it has the functional carboxylic acid group in the middle of the molecule, interacting with the 'charge clamp' and large hydrophobic tails wrapping in both directions round helix 3 and projecting deep into the hydrophobic pockets in both directions. Incredibly this molecule still only fills 40% of the ligand-binding cavity, whereas rosiglitazone fills just 25% of the cavity. Selectivity has been generated by examining the internal space of the smaller cavity between helix 3 and helix 12, which has revealed residues that may hinder the binding of compounds to certain isoforms. Drugs could be designed with groups intended to 'bump' into these residues in specific isoforms and therefore discourage binding. This dual approach has yielded compounds with massively increased affinity and selectivity for individual PPAR isoforms.

As mentioned previously, the crystallization

of the oestrogen receptor with antagonists such as tamoxifen, raloxifene and ICI 164,384 has allowed a better understanding of how antagonists may work in nuclear receptors.[3–5] The situation is similar with PPARs. PPARγ was crystallized with a compound GW0072 buried in the ligand cavity (see review, Willson et al, 2000; Further reading). This compound makes no interactions with the activating helix 12 and therefore the 'charge clamp' is essentially in the conformation found in the apo-receptor. This appears to provide the molecular basis for partial agonism (Fig. 9.5). In contrast, binding of ICI 164,384 to the oestrogen receptor does alter the charge clamp configuration to a position that appears to be particularly non-permissive for the formation of the 'charge clamp' and binding of co-activators.[4] In this case a pure antagonist activity is observed. These different possibilities provide insight for the design of novel compounds that may have very sophisticated alterations in function that may be required for certain biological endpoints.

8.2 PPAR 'modulators'

Activation of PPARs has been the prevalent mind-set for the design of new ligands but the idea is emerging that drugs with a more complex interaction with the PPAR family may actually provide more clinical benefit. The major precedent for this approach comes from work involving the oestrogen receptor, where complex interactions between agonism and antagonism of ERα and ERβ may provide the key to a better anti-cancer drug.

Several groups have shown that insulin sensitization by PPARγ ligands is not directly related to their efficacy of activation of PPARγ in transactivation assays. It has been postulated that insulin sensitization may be a result of partial agonism or antagonism of PPARγ. Mice heterozygous for a PPARγ null allele, and expressing PPARγ at 50% of the level seen in wild-type mice, are in fact more sensitive to insulin than wild-type mice.[52,91] It would be interesting to investigate the utility of a combined PPARα agonist/PPARγ antagonist.

Taking another example from oestrogen receptor pharmacology, it may be possible to achieve tissue-specific modulation of PPAR activity. This would certainly be very desirable for the limitation of adverse side-effects and may be achieved by taking advantage of cell-specific expression of the co-activators. Drugs could be designed that allow binding of certain co-activators but not others and provide an additional layer of specificity to the pharmacological response.

One drug that appears to display some of these qualities is NC-2100.[87] This drug has been shown to activate PPARα and γ in transactivation assays. However, in vivo studies in obese mice have shown selective modulation of mitochondrial uncoupling protein UCP-1 in white adipose tissue, without apparent regulation of genes that are markers of PPARα and γ activation. This treatment effectively lowered plasma insulin and triglyceride levels without the increases in body weight that are a feature of treatment with other PPARγ agonists such as troglitazone and pioglitazone.

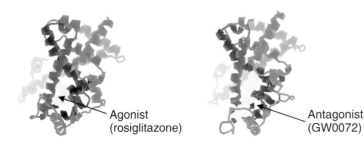

Fig. 9.5 Crystal structures of agonist and antagonist bound to PPARγ. The crystal structures corresponding to the coordinates deposited as 2PRG (agonist-bound) and 4PRG (antagonist-bound) are visualized using RasMAC version 2.6. The bound ligands are shown as blue space-filled models and are indicated by arrows.

Agonist (rosiglitazone)

Antagonist (GW0072)

9. CONCLUSIONS AND FUTURE DIRECTIONS IN THE CLINICAL USE OF PPAR LIGANDS

A greater understanding of the specific roles that PPARs play in individual organs/tissues/cells allows us to see future directions for clinical research. One such site of action is the heart. Recent studies have suggested that PPARα has an important role in the regulation of cardiomyocyte growth.[92,93] While PPARα null mice are outwardly healthy, their hearts are susceptible to mechanical overload and show a more marked trophic response. The data support previous work that had implicated PPARα in regulating fat metabolism as the main energy source in cardiac muscle. In hypertrophied cardiac muscle it had been observed that PPARα was downregulated and that the energy source was switched to glucose. These observations support the notion that PPARα agonists may be of use in the secondary prevention of myocardial infarction, independent of its effects on atherosclerosis/serum lipids. The fibrates may therefore be of use in patients diagnosed as suffering from heart enlargement and left ventricular hypertrophy in particular. This concept has been reinforced by the finding that common polymorphisms in the gene encoding PPARα are associated with left ventricular hypertrophy and excessive cardiac growth after exercise.[93]

PPARα and PPARβ/δ appear to modulate wound healing in skin. Both of these receptors are expressed in embryonic skin but are silent in normal adult skin.[94] Expression of PPARα and β/δ is reactivated upon wounding and genetic alterations in the PPARα or β genes in mice are associated with delayed wound healing. Clinical applications of this knowledge have yet to be proposed, but it is anticipated that PPAR agonists/antagonists may be used to accelerate healing or retard scarring in specific surgical scenarios. The discovery of anti-psoriasis activity of thiazolidenediones may prompt the investigation of topical/systemic administration of various PPAR ligands in the treatment of inflammatory skin disorders.[66]

The role of PPARs in the colon is unclear, but they may be involved in the correct programming of nutrient uptake, and the transfer of dietary lipid from the lumen to the bloodstream. Modulation of fat in rodent chow appears to modulate the expression of PPAR target genes such as those encoding fatty acid-binding proteins.[95] The use of PPAR ligands in inflammatory bowel disease may be rationalized in two ways in a similar manner to oncology. The first is a differentiation effect promoting the normal behaviour of the enterocyte and the second is an anti-inflammatory effect, opposing the unknown inflammatory stimulus that lies behind the origin of the disease. These two processes are inextricably linked; however, the details have yet to be elucidated.

Finally, an exciting finding is that PPARs are expressed in the brain and appear to modulate processes associated with response to injury and neurodegenerative disorders.[88,96,97] PPAR ligands have been found to protect neurons from ischaemia.[98] This may lead to investigation of the use of PPAR ligands in the prevention and treatment of stroke and dementia. The finding that PPARδ is involved in oligodendrocyte differentiation and demyelination would also suggest investigation into the use of PPAR ligands in the management of neuropathies such as multiple sclerosis.[88,99]

REFERENCES

Further reading

Anon. A unified nomenclature system for the nuclear receptor superfamily. *Cell* 1999; **97**: 161–3.

Bishop-Bailey D. Peroxisome proliferator-activated receptors in the cardiovascular system. *Br J Pharmacol* 2000; **129**: 823–34.

Gale EAM. Lessons from the glitazones: a story of drug development. *Lancet* 2001; **357**: 1870–5.

Willson TM, Brown PJ, Sternbach DD, Henke BR. The PPARs: from orphan receptors to drug discovery. *J Med Chem* 2000; **43**: 527–50.

Web-sites

■ http://www.cas.psu.edu/docs/CASDEPT/VET/jackvh/ppar/pparrfront.htm
The Peroxisome Proliferator-Activated Receptor Resource (PPARR) is a component of the Nuclear Hormone Receptor Resource (NRR)

project. The PPARR is designed to disseminate information about PPAR, including cDNA sequences, protein alignments, PPREs and sources of cDNAs and antibodies.

Scientific papers

1. Muss HB. Role of adjuvant endocrine therapy in early-stage breast cancer. *Semin Oncol* 2001; **28:** 313–21.

2. Spitz IM, Chwalisz K. Progesterone receptor modulators and progesterone antagonists in women's health. *Steroids* 2000; **65:** 807–15.

3. Brzozowski AM, Pike AC, Dauter Z et al. Molecular basis of agonism and antagonism in the oestrogen receptor. *Nature* 1997; **389:** 753–8.

4. Pike AC, Brzozowski AM, Walton J et al. Structural insights into the mode of action of a pure antiestrogen. *Structure (Camb)* 2001; **9:** 145–53.

5. Hubbard RE, Pike AC, Brzozowski AM et al. Structural insights into the mechanisms of agonism and antagonism in oestrogen receptor isoforms. *Eur J Cancer* 2000; **36 Suppl 4:** S17–S18.

6. Laudet V. Evolution of the nuclear receptor superfamily: early diversification from an ancestral orphan receptor. *J Mol Endocrinol* 1997; **19:** 207–26.

7. Maglich JM, Sluder A, Guan X et al. Comparison of complete nuclear receptor sets from the human, *Caenorhabditis elegans* and *Drosophila* genomes. *Genome Biol* 2001; **2**(8): RESEARCH0029.

8. Hayhurst GP, Lee YH, Lambert G, Ward JM, Gonzalez FJ. Hepatocyte nuclear factor 4alpha (nuclear receptor 2A1) is essential for maintenance of hepatic gene expression and lipid homeostasis. *Mol Cell Biol* 2001; **21:** 1393–403.

9. Forman BM, Tzameli I, Choi HS et al. Androstane metabolites bind to and deactivate the nuclear receptor CAR-beta. *Nature* 1998; **395:** 612–15.

10. Honkakoski P, Zelko L, Sueyoshi T, Negishi M. The nuclear orphan receptor CAR-retinoid X receptor heterodimer activates the phenobarbital-responsive enhancer module of the CYP2B gene. *Mol Cell Biol* 1998; **18:** 5652–8.

11. Waxman DJ. P450 gene induction by structurally diverse xenochemicals: central role of nuclear receptors CAR, PXR, and PPAR. *Arch Biochem Biophys* 1999; **369:** 11–23.

12. Zelko I, Sueyoshi T, Kawamoto T, Moore R, Negishi M. The peptide near the C terminus reg-

ulates receptor CAR nuclear translocation induced by xenochemicals in mouse liver. *Mol Cell Biol* 2001; **21:** 2838–46.

13. Hertz R, Magenheim J, Berman L et al. Fatty acyl-CoA thioesters are ligands of hepatic nuclear factor-4alpha. *Nature* 1998; **392:** 512–16.

14. Bogan AA, Dallas-Yang Q, Ruse MD, Jr et al. Analysis of protein dimerization and ligand binding of orphan receptor HNF4alpha. *J Mol Biol* 2000; **302:** 831–51.

15. Vu-Dac N, Chopin-Delannoy S, Gervois P et al. The nuclear receptors peroxisome proliferator-activated receptor alpha and Rev-erbalpha mediate the species-specific regulation of apolipoprotein A-I expression by fibrates. *J Biol Chem* 1998; **273:** 25713–20.

16. Gervois P, Chopin-Delannoy S, Fadel A et al. Fibrates increase human REV-ERBalpha expression in liver via a novel peroxisome proliferator-activated receptor response element. *Mol Endocrinol* 1999; **13:** 400–9.

17. Bentley P, Calder I, Elcombe C, Grasso P, Stringer D, Wiegand JH. Hepatic peroxisome proliferation in rodents and its significance for humans. *Food Chem Toxicol* 1993; **31:** 857–907.

18. Issemann I, Green S. Activation of a member of the steroid hormone receptor superfamily by peroxisome proliferators. *Nature* 1990; **347:** 645–50.

19. Dreyer C, Krey G, Keller H, Givel F, Helftenbein G, Wahli W. Control of the peroxisomal beta-oxidation pathway by a novel family of nuclear hormone receptors. *Cell* 1992; **68:** 879–87.

20. Braissant O, Foufelle F, Scotto C, Dauca M, Wahli W. Differential expression of peroxisome proliferator-activated receptors (PPARs): tissue distribution of PPAR-alpha, -beta, and -gamma in the adult rat. *Endocrinology* 1996; **137:** 354–66.

21. Fajas L, Auboeuf D, Raspe E et al. The organization, promoter analysis, and expression of the human PPARgamma gene. *J Biol Chem* 1997; **272:** 18779–89.

22. Mukherjee R, Jow L, Croston GE, Paterniti JR, Jr. Identification, characterization and tissue distribution of human peroxisome proliferator-activated receptor (PPAR) isoforms PPARγ2 versus PPARγ1 and activation with retinoid X receptor agonists and antagonists. *J Biol Chem* 1997; **272:** 8071–6.

23. Fajas L, Fruchart J-C, Auwerx J. PPARγ3 mRNA: a distinct PPARγ mRNA subtype transcribed from an independent promoter. *FEBS Lett* 1998; **438:** 55–60.

24. Gottlicher M, Widmark E, Li Q, Gustafsson JA. Fatty acids activate a chimera of the clofibric acid-activated receptor and the glucocorticoid receptor. *Proc Natl Acad Sci USA* 1992; **89:** 4653–4657.

25. Banner CD, Gottlicher M, Widmark E, Sjovall J, Rafter JJ, Gustafsson JA. A systematic analytical chemistry/cell assay approach to isolate activators of orphan nuclear receptors from biological extracts: characterization of peroxisome proliferator-activated receptor activators in plasma. *J Lipid Res* 1993; **34:** 1583–91.

26. Xu HE, Lambert MH, Montana VG et al. Molecular recognition of fatty acids by peroxisome proliferator-activated receptors. *Mol Cell* 1999; **3:** 397–403.

27. Palmer CNA, Wolf CR. *cis*-parinaric acid is a ligand for the human peroxisome proliferator activated receptor gamma: development of a novel spectrophotometric assay for the discovery of PPARgamma ligands. *FEBS Lett* 1998; **431:** 476–80.

28. Yu K, Bayona W, Kallne CB et al. Differential activation of peroxisome proliferator-activated receptors by ecosanoids. *J Biol Chem* 1995; **270:** 23975–83.

29. Palmer CNA, Hsu MH, Muerhoff AS, Griffin KJ, Johnson EF. Interaction of the peroxisome proliferator-activated receptor alpha with the retinoid X receptor alpha unmasks a cryptic peroxisome proliferator response element that overlaps an ARP-1-binding site in the CYP4A6 promoter. *J Biol Chem* 1994; **269:** 18083–9.

30. Tontonoz P, Hu E, Graves RA, Budavari AI, Spiegelman BM. mPPAR gamma 2: tissue-specific regulator of an adipocyte enhancer. *Genes Dev* 1994; **8:** 1224–34.

31. Palmer CNA, Hsu MH, Griffin HJ, Johnson EF. Novel sequence determinants in peroxisome proliferator signaling. *J Biol Chem* 1995; **270:** 16114–21.

32. Kliewer SA, Umesono K, Noonan DJ, Heyman RA, Evans RM. Convergence of 9-cis retinoic acid and peroxisome proliferator signalling pathways through heterodimer formation of their receptors. *Nature* 1992; **358:** 771–4.

33. Forman BM, Chen J, Evans RM. Hypolipidemic drugs, polyunsaturated fatty acids, and eicosanoids are ligands for peroxisome proliferator-activated receptors alpha and delta. *Proc Natl Acad Sci USA* 1997; **94:** 4312–17.

34. Zhu Y, Qi C, Calandra C, Rao MS, Reddy JK. Cloning and identification of mouse steroid receptor coactivator-1 (mSRC-1), as a coactivator of peroxisome proliferator-activated receptor gamma. *Gene Expr* 1996; **6:** 185–95.

35. Zhu Y, Qi C, Jain S, Rao MS, Reddy JK. Isolation and characterization of PBP, a protein that interacts with peroxisome proliferator-activated receptor. *J Biol Chem* 1997; **272:** 25500–6.

36. Krey G, Braissant O, L'Horset F et al. Fatty acids, eicosanoids, and hypolipidemic agents identified as ligands of peroxisome proliferator-activated receptors by coactivator-dependent receptor ligand assay. *Mol Endocrinol* 1997; **11:** 779–91.

37. Spiegelman BM, Puigserver P, Wu Z. Regulation of adipogenesis and energy balance by PPARgamma and PGC-1. *Int J Obes Relat Metab Disord* 2000; **24**(Suppl. 4): S8–S10.

38. Yang W, Hong YH, Shen XQ, Frankowski C, Camp HS, Leff T. Regulation of transcription by AMP-activated protein kinase: phosphorylation of p300 blocks its interaction with nuclear receptors. *J Biol Chem* 2001; **276:** 38341–4.

39. Gervois P, Torra IP, Fruchart JC, Staels B. Regulation of lipid and lipoprotein metabolism by PPAR activators. *Clin Chem Lab Med* 2000; **38:** 3–11.

40. Oliver WR, Jr, Shenk JL, Snaith MR et al. A selective peroxisome proliferator-activated receptor delta agonist promotes reverse cholesterol transport. *Proc Natl Acad Sci USA* 2001; **98:** 5306–11.

41. Vu-Dac N, Gervois P, Torra IP et al. Retinoids increase human apo C-III expression at the transcriptional level via the retinoid X receptor. Contribution to the hypertriglyceridemic action of retinoids. *J Clin Invest* 1998; **102:** 625–32.

42. Lee JS, Newman RA, Lippman SM et al. Phase I evaluation of all-trans-retinoic acid in adults with solid tumors. *J Clin Oncol* 1993; **11:** 959–66.

43. Redlich CA, Chung JS, Cullen MR, Blaner WS, Van Bennekum AM, Berglund L. Effect of long-term beta-carotene and vitamin A on serum cholesterol and triglyceride levels among participants in the Carotene and Retinol Efficacy Trial (CARET). *Atherosclerosis* 1999; **145:** 425–32.

44. Feldman DL, Sawyer WK, Jeune MR, Mogelesky TC, Von Linden-Reed J, Forney Prescott M. CGP 43371 paradoxically inhibits development of rabbit atherosclerotic lesions while inducing extra-arterial foam cell formation. *Atherosclerosis* 2001; **154:** 317–28.

45. Lehmann JM, Moore LB, Smith OT, Wilkison WO, Willson TM, Kliewer SA. An antidiabetic thiazolidinedione is a high affinity ligand for peroxisome proliferator-activated receptor gamma (PPAR gamma). *J Biol Chem* 1995; **270:** 12953–6.

46. Kruszynska YT, Mukherjee R, Jow L, Dana S, Paterniti JR, Olefsky JM. Skeletal muscle peroxisome proliferator-activated receptor-gamma expression in obesity and non-insulin-dependent diabetes mellitus. *J Clin Invest* 1998; **101**: 543–8.

47. Furnsinn C, Brunmair B, Meyer M et al. Chronic and acute effects of thiazolidinediones BM13.1258 and BM15.2054 on rat skeletal muscle glucose metabolism. *Br J Pharmacol* 1999; **128**: 1141–8.

48. Steppan CM, Bailey ST, Bhat S et al. The hormone resistin links obesity to diabetes. *Nature* 2001; **409**: 307–12.

49. Way JM, Gorgun CZ, Tong Q et al. Adipose tissue resistin expression is severely suppressed in obesity and stimulated by peroxisome proliferator-activated receptor gamma agonists. *J Biol Chem* 2001; **276**: 25651–3.

50. Barroso I, Gurnell M, Crowley VE et al. Dominant negative mutations in human PPARgamma associated with severe insulin resistance, diabetes mellitus and hypertension [see comments]. *Nature* 1999; **402**: 880–3.

51. Barak Y, Nelson MC, Ong ES et al. PPAR gamma is required for placental, cardiac, and adipose tissue development. *Mol Cell* 1999; **4**: 585–95.

52. Kubota N, Terauchi Y, Miki H et al. PPAR gamma mediates high-fat diet-induced adipocyte hypertrophy and insulin resistance. *Mol Cell* 1999; **4**: 597–609.

53. Itoh H, Doi K, Tanaka T et al. Hypertension and insulin resistance: role of peroxisome proliferator-activated receptor γ. *Clin Exp Pharmacol Physiol* 1999; **26**: 558–60.

54. Satoh H, Tsukamoto K, Hashimoto Y et al. Thiazolidinediones suppress endothelin-1 secretion from bovine vascular endothelial cells: a new possible role for PPARγ on vascular endothelial function. *Biochem Biophys Res Commun* 1999; **254**: 757–63.

55. Zhang F, Sowers JR, Ram JL, Standley PR, Peuler JD. Effects of pioglitazone on calcium channels in vascular smooth muscle. *Hypertension* 1994; **24**: 170–5.

56. Ericsson CG. Results of the Bezafibrate Coronary Atherosclerosis Intervention Trial (BECAIT) and an update on trials now in progress. *Eur Heart J* 1998; **19**(Suppl. H): H37–H41.

57. Koshiyama H, Shimono D, Kuwamura N, Minamikawa J, Nakamura Y. Rapid communication: inhibitory effect of pioglitazone on carotid arterial wall thickness in type 2 diabetes. *J Clin Endocrinol Metab* 2001; **86**: 3452–6.

58. Vosper H, Patel L, Graham TL et al. The peroxisome proliferator-activated receptor delta promotes lipid accumulation in human macrophages. *J Biol Chem* 2001; **276**: 44258–65.

59. Zhang J, Fu M, Zhu X et al. Peroxisome proliferator-activated receptor delta is upregulated during vascular lesion formation and promotes post-confluent cell proliferation in vascular smooth muscle cells. *J Biol Chem* 2002; **277**: 11505–12.

60. Staels B, Koenig W, Habib A et al. Activation of human aortic smooth-muscle cells is inhibited by PPARalpha but not by PPARgamma activators. *Nature* 1998; **393**: 790–3.

61. Chinetti G, Lestavel S, Bocher V et al. PPAR-alpha and PPAR-gamma activators induce cholesterol removal from human macrophage foam cells through stimulation of the ABCA1 pathway. *Nat Med* 2001; **7**: 53–8.

62. Lehmann JM, Lenhard JM, Oliver BB, Ringold GM, Kliewer SA. Peroxisome proliferator-activated receptors alpha and gamma are activated by indomethacin and other non-steroidal anti-inflammatory drugs. *J Biol Chem* 1992; **272**: 3406–10.

63. Adamson DJ, Frew D, Tatoud R, Wolf CR, Palmer CNA. Diclofenac antagonizes peroxisome proliferator-activated receptor-gamma signaling. *Mol Pharmacol* 2002; **61**: 7–12.

64. Kalajdzic T, Faour WH, He QW et al. Nimesulide, a preferential cyclooxygenase 2 inhibitor, suppresses peroxisome proliferator-activated receptor induction of cyclooxygenase 2 gene expression in human synovial fibroblasts: evidence for receptor antagonism. *Arthritis Rheum* 2002; **46**: 494–506.

65. Su CG, Wen X, Bailey ST et al. A novel therapy for colitis utilizing PPAR-gamma ligands to inhibit the epithelial inflammatory response. *J Clin Invest* 1999; **104**: 383–9.

66. Ellis CN, Varani J, Fisher GJ et al. Troglitazone improves psoriasis and normalizes models of proliferative skin disease: ligands for peroxisome proliferator-activated receptor-gamma inhibit keratinocyte proliferation. *Arch Dermatol* 2000; **136**: 609–16.

67. Cattley RC, DeLuca J, Elcombe C et al. Do peroxisome proliferating compounds pose a hepatocarcinogenic hazard to humans? *Regul Toxicol Pharmacol* 1998; **27**: 47–60.

68. Chevalier S, Roberts RA. Perturbation of rodent hepatocyte growth control by nongenotoxic hepatocarcinogens: mechanisms and lack of

relevance for human health (review). *Oncol Rep* 1998; **5**: 1319–27.

69. Palmer CNA, Hsu MH, Griffin KJ, Raucy JL, Johnson EF. Peroxisome proliferator activated receptor-alpha expression in human liver. *Mol Pharmacol* 1998; **53**: 14–22.

70. Holden PR, Tugwood JD. Peroxisome proliferator-activated receptor alpha: role in rodent liver cancer and species differences. *J Mol Endocrinol* 1999; **22**: 1–8.

71. Kubota T, Koshizuka K, Williamson EA et al. Ligand for peroxisome proliferator-activated receptor gamma (troglitazone) has potent antitumor effect against human prostate cancer both in vitro and in vivo. *Cancer Res* 1998; **58**: 3344–52.

72. Mueller E, Sarraf P, Tontonoz P et al. Terminal differentiation of human breast cancer through PPAR gamma. *Mol Cell* 1998; **1**: 465–70.

73. Guan YF, Zhang YH, Breyer RM, Davis L, Breyer MD. Expression of peroxisome proliferator-activated receptor gamma (PPARgamma) in human transitional bladder cancer and its role in inducing cell death. *Neoplasia* 1999; **1**: 330–9.

74. Tsubouchi Y, Sano H, Kawahito Y et al. Inhibition of human lung cancer cell growth by the peroxisome proliferator-activated receptor-gamma agonists through induction of apoptosis. *Biochem Biophys Res Commun* 2000; **270**: 400–5.

75. Mueller E, Smith M, Sarraf P et al. Effects of ligand activation of peroxisome proliferator-activated receptor gamma in human prostate cancer. *Proc Natl Acad Sci USA* 2000; **97**: 10990–5.

76. Shao D, Rangwala SM, Bailey ST, Krakow SL, Reginato MJ, Lazar MA. Interdomain communication regulating ligand binding by PPAR-gamma. *Nature* 1998; **396**: 377–80.

77. Tontonoz P, Singer S, Forman BM et al. Terminal differentiation of human liposarcoma cells induced by ligands for peroxisome proliferator-activated receptor gamma and the retinoid X receptor. *Proc Natl Acad Sci USA* 1997; **94**: 237–41.

78. DuBois RN, Gupta R, Brockman J, Reddy BS, Krakow SL, Lazar MA. The nuclear eicosanoid receptor, PPARgamma, is aberrantly expressed in colonic cancers. *Carcinogenesis* 1998; **19**: 49–53.

79. Lefebvre AM, Chen I, Desreumaux P et al. Activation of the peroxisome proliferator-activated receptor gamma promotes the development of colon tumors in C57BL/6J-APCMin/+ mice. *Nat Med* 1998; **4**: 1053–7.

80. Sarraf P, Mueller E, Jones D et al. Differentiation and reversal of malignant changes in colon

cancer through PPARgamma. *Nat Med* 1998; **4**: 1046–52.

81. He TC, Chan TA, Vogelstein B, Kinzler, KW. PPARdelta is an APC-regulated target of non-steroidal anti-inflammatory drugs. *Cell* 1999; **99**: 335–45.

82. Park BH, Vogelstein B, Kinzler KW. Genetic disruption of PPARdelta decreases the tumorigenicity of human colon cancer cells. *Proc Natl Acad Sci USA* 2001; **98**: 2598–603.

83. Gupta RA, Tan J, Krause WF et al. Prostacyclin-mediated activation of peroxisome proliferator-activated receptor delta in colorectal cancer. *Proc Natl Acad Sci USA* 2000; **97**: 13275–80.

84. Brown PJ, Smith-Oliver TA et al. Identification of peroxisome proliferator-activated receptor ligands from a biased chemical library. *Chem Biol* 1997; **4**: 909–18.

85. Guerre-Millo M, Gervois P, Raspe E et al. Peroxisome proliferator-activated receptor alpha activators improve insulin sensitivity and reduce adiposity. *J Biol Chem* 2000; **275**: 16638–42.

86. Shibata T, Takeuchi S, Yokota S, Kakimoto K, Yonemori F, Wakitani K. Effects of peroxisome proliferator-activated receptor-alpha and -gamma agonist, JTT-501, on diabetic complications in Zucker diabetic fatty rats. *Br J Pharmacol* 2000; **130**: 495–504.

87. Fukui Y, Masui S, Osada S, Umesono K, Motojima K. A new thiazolidinedione, NC-2100, which is a weak PPAR-gamma activator, exhibits potent antidiabetic effects and induces uncoupling protein 1 in white adipose tissue of KKAy obese mice. *Diabetes* 2000; **49**: 759–67.

88. Saluja I, Granneman JG, Skoff RP. PPAR delta agonists stimulate oligodendrocyte differentiation in tissue culture. *Glia* 2001; **33**: 191–204.

89. Nolte RT, Wisely GB, Westin S et al. Ligand binding and co-activator assembly of the peroxisome proliferator-activated receptor-gamma. *Nature* 1998; **395**: 137–43.

90. Gampe RT, Jr, Montana VG, Lambert MH et al. Asymmetry in the PPARgamma/RXRalpha crystal structure reveals the molecular basis of heterodimerization among nuclear receptors. *Mol Cell* 2000; **5**: 545–55.

91. Miles PD, Barak Y, He W, Evans RM, Olefsky JM. Improved insulin-sensitivity in mice heterozygous for PPAR-gamma deficiency. *J Clin Invest* 2000; **105**: 287–92.

92. Barger PM, Brandt JM, Leone TC, Weinheimer CJ, Kelly DP. Deactivation of peroxisome proliferator-activated receptor-alpha during cardiac

hypertrophic growth. *J Clin Invest* 2000; **105:** 1723–30.

93. Jamshidi Y, Montgomery HE, Hense HW et al. Peroxisome proliferator-activated receptor alpha gene regulates left ventricular growth in response to exercise and hypertension. *Circulation* 2002; **105:** 950–5.

94. Michalik L, Desvergne B, Tan NS et al. Impaired skin wound healing in peroxisome proliferator-activated receptor (PPAR)α and PPARβ mutant mice. *J Cell Biol* 2001; **154:** 799–814.

95. Poirier H, Niot I, Monnot MC et al. Differential involvement of peroxisome-proliferator-activated receptors alpha and delta in fibrate and fatty-acid-mediated inductions of the gene encoding liver fatty-acid-binding protein in the liver and the small intestine. *Biochem J* 2001; **355:** 481–8.

96. Basu-Modak S, Braissant O, Escher P, Desvergne B, Honegger P, Wahli W. Peroxisome proliferator-activated receptor beta regulates acyl-CoA synthetase 2 in reaggregated rat brain cell cultures. *J Biol Chem* 1999; **274:** 35881–8.

97. Kitamura Y, Shimohama S, Koike H et al. Increased expression of cyclooxygenases and peroxisome proliferator-activated receptor-gamma in Alzheimer's disease brains. *Biochem Biophys Res Commun* 1999; **254:** 582–6.

98. Uryu S, Harada J, Hisamoto M, Oda T. Troglitazone inhibits both post-glutamate neurotoxicity and low-potassium-induced apoptosis in cerebellar granule neurons. *Brain Res* 2002; **924:** 229–36.

99. Granneman J, Skoff R, Yang X. Member of the peroxisome proliferator-activated receptor family of transcription factors is differentially expressed by oligodendrocytes. *J Neurosci Res* 1998; **51:** 563–73.

10

The use of antisense oligonucleotides as therapeutic agents

Punit Ramrakha

SUMMARY

For over a decade, antisense oligonucleotides have been used to downregulate gene expression. Although some impressive successes have been reported, it can still be difficult to rationally design a specific antisense inhibitor and demonstrate effective suppression of target protein expression. This review discusses some of the issues involved in the rational design of an antisense oligonucleotide. A variety of chemical modifications of the basic phosphodiester backbone of the DNA oligonucleotides have been tested in vitro and in vivo, and advances in medicinal chemistry have allowed the production of potent antisense molecules with good bioavailability and little systemic toxicity. There is much optimism surrounding the field of antisense therapeutics at the present time, as the first of many antisense oligonucleotides has finally received the licence for routine clinical use.

1. INTRODUCTION

Antisense nucleic acids are single-stranded RNAs or DNAs that are complementary to the sequence of their target genes. Antisense agents can be thought of as inhibitors of the intermediary metabolism of RNA. This process begins with transcription of pre-messenger RNA and ends when the mature mRNA is used to produce a protein and the RNA is degraded. The antisense agents have the potential to block any of these steps – transcription, RNA processing, mRNA transport, translation or mRNA stability (Fig. 10.1).

The seductiveness of the antisense concept derives from three basic attributes of the technology. Watson-Crick base-pairing provides affinity and specificity that are many orders of magnitude higher than can be achieved in traditional 'drug–receptor' pharmacology. Furthermore, since the factors that determine the interactions between nucleic acids are well characterized, the rational design of the antisense agent should be relatively straightforward. Finally, the technology can potentially be used to design antisense inhibitors for any RNA molecule whose

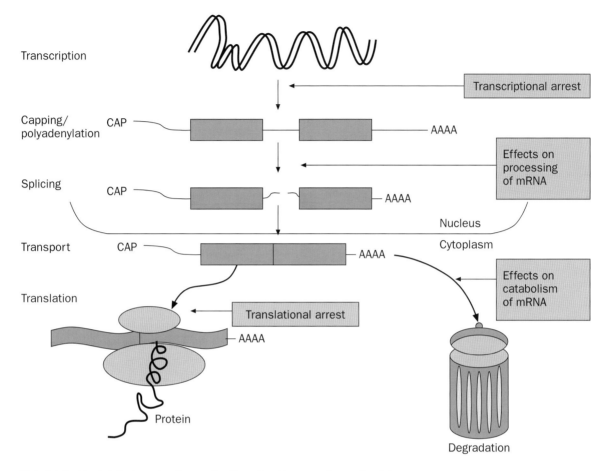

Fig. 10.1 Postulated mechanisms of action of antisense oligonucleotides.

sequence is known. Two basic approaches are outlined in Table 10.1.

It has been recognized for many years that natural antisense transcripts are used to regulate gene expression in both prokaryotes and eukaryotes.[1,2] The vast majority of antisense regulation is at the level of translation. In most cases, the regulatory RNA hybridizes to the mRNA across the Shine-Delgarno sequence and/or translation start codon, thus preventing ribosome binding and translation (class I in the Inouye classification[3]). In some cases, translation is blocked by the binding of antisense RNA to the 5′ end of the mRNA upstream of the ribosome binding site, and locking the mRNA into a secondary structure unfavourable for

translation (class II). Messenger RNA processing can also be affected by binding of the antisense RNA to sequences that interfere with the splice donor or acceptor sites, or blocking mRNA transport from the nucleus to the cytoplasm.[4]

Antisense oligonucleotides have a number of advantages. Based on the estimated size of the genome, oligonucleotides of >13 bases complementary to nucleotide sequences of mRNA should be able to inhibit the expression of the cellular protein in a sequence-specific manner. The first clear elaboration of the antisense concept was the elegant work by Zamecnik and Stephenson.[5] A synthetic deoxyoligonucleotide that was complementary to a sequence in the

Table 10.1   Comparison of the advantages and disadvantages of antisense reagents

Approach	Advantages	Disadvantages
DNA oligonucleotides	• No transformation required • RNAase H target destruction • Good heteroduplex formation • Stability and delivery may be improved with modifications of bases/backbone • Reactive groups for cleavage, intercalation or modification • Target RNA or DNA	• Unstable and inefficient • Transient inhibition • Non-specific toxicity
Antisense RNA	• Constitutive and regulated expression • Permanent or inducible	• Potentially short lifetime • Inefficient • Depends on DNA-mediated transformation to introduce plasmid into cells

Rous sarcoma virus genome produced selective inhibition of gene expression in cells in culture. They postulated that this oligomer inhibited replication by binding to viral RNA – a mechanism that has since been used to define the antisense approach.

The best characterized mechanism of action of antisense nucleotides, however, involves the enzyme RNAase H. This enzyme is present during DNA replication and is responsible for digesting the RNA primers needed for synthesis of Okazaki fragments. Hybridization of a DNA oligomer to the message RNA activates this enzyme and results in cleavage of the target RNA. The 5′ cleavage fragment lacks a poly-A tail, and so is usually degraded by cellular nucleases. The 3′ cleavage fragment lacks a guanosine cap, and so is also degraded.[6–8] As long as the oligonucleotide remains intact, a single antisense sequence can mediate multiple rounds of destruction of the target.

As the antisense field has developed, the rationale and experimental approaches needed for defining the antisense approach are being defined. Certain regions of the RNA, especially the translation initiation domain of mRNAs, have been shown to be more susceptible to inhibition by antisense oligonucleotides than other sites in the molecule, and the advantages of using DNA analogues, specifically phosphate-modified derivatives, to solve problems such as nuclease susceptibility inherent in natural DNA are now established.[9,10]

However, their large molecular weights, relative instability in the biological milieu (short half-lives) and the charged nature of DNA oligonucleotides pose major challenges to the successful delivery of antisense molecules to their intracellular sites of action. Upon administration (by any route), these molecules need to remain stable, and not degrade within the extracellular environment, for a period of time long enough to allow sufficient of the antisense oligonucleotide to enter the cells and exert the desired biological activity. Furthermore, once inside the cells, these molecules also need to avoid degradation until or after they have exerted the desired biological effect. Intracellular stability of the oligonucleotides becomes especially important when chosen targets have a slow turnover. In this case, biological activity of the oligonucleotides against the target needs to be maintained for long periods of time until the pre-existing levels of protein product are allowed to decay.

The list of proteins whose expression has been significantly, reproducibly and convincingly downregulated has grown to include *c-myc* and *c-myb*,[11] protein kinase C-α (PKC-α),[12] c-raf kinase,[13] Ha-ras,[14] bcl-2,[15,16] bcl-xL,[17,18] IL-2, IL-4[19] and IL-5[20], and human and murine endothelial cell adhesion molecules[21,22] – to name a few (for reviews see refs 23–25).

A number of theoretical considerations apply when planning to inhibit the expression of a specific gene with antisense agents (Box 10.1). Even once the antisense sequences have been designed, there are factors as yet undetermined that influence whether the antisense agent will produce the desired effect. Thus the correlation between the theoretical suitability of an antisense agent and its potency is not perfect. This review will discuss some of these issues, highlighting some of the successes and pitfalls in the application of antisense oligonucleotides as therapeutic agents.

2. RATIONAL DESIGN OF AN ANTISENSE AGENT

2.1 Choice of target sequence for the antisense oligonucleotide

The minimal length for specificity depends on the number of transcribed sequences within the

---

> **Box 10.1 Theoretical considerations for the design of an antisense agent: rational design of an 'antisense' oligonucleotide or RNA**
>
> - Biological stability
> - Intracellular availability
> - Gene suppression potency
> - Specificity
> - Lack of toxicity and non-specific effects

---

cell. On a statistical basis, an AT sequence 19 nucleotides long is unique in the human genome at DNA level. For a GC sequence the figure is 15 nucleotides.[26] The difference between the two numbers originates in the over-representation of AT pairs (60%) in the human genome. If we assume that only 0.5% of DNA is transcribed, uniqueness at the RNA level is reached with 15-mer and 11-mer for AT and GC targets, respectively. Initial experiments demonstrated that certain regions of RNA, especially the translation initiation domain of mRNAs, are more susceptible to inhibition by antisense oligonucleotides than other sites in the molecule.[9,10]

However, as yet there are no established rules to identify the optimal target site on mRNA to which an antisense reagent (DNA oligonucleotide or RNA) should hybridize. Most successful reports target the AUG transcription initiation codon, but greater potency may be achieved by targeting other sites such as the 5'-untranslated region, exon–intron boundaries and 3'-untranslated region.[22] For example, Manson et al[27] reported that an antisense oligonucleotide to the 5'-untranslated region of the IL-1β gene inhibited IL-1β expression. Daaka and Wickstrom[28] determined that out of three target sites on the *c-Ha-ras* mRNA, an oligonucleotide that hybridized to the 5'-cap site was more effective than an oligonucleotide designed to hybridize to the AUG codon or 5'-untranslated region.

RNA is not a linear molecule. The cellular RNAs have tertiary structures where most of the sequence elements are not accessible as targets for an antisense oligonucleotide. Systematic screening of target mRNAs with large numbers of antisense oligomers reveals that most of the molecule is not accessible towards antisense-mediated cleavage, and a naïve approach based on sequence alone is unlikely to yield an effective antisense agent. Most successful reports of antisense reagent discovery have involved the analysis of a large number of oligonucleotides directed to various regions of the target mRNA to identify the ones that are most effective.[22]

The use of computer programs to determine

the most likely base-paired folding pattern of mRNA sequences based on thermodynamic parameters can reveal possible accessible single-stranded regions.[29] Chiang and co-workers[21] identified two regions of ICAM-1 mRNA predicted by computer modelling to form stable stem-loop structures. Although it is not known whether these structures actually exist in the mRNA or if they play a regulatory role in ICAM-1 expression, targeting these two regions with antisense oligonucleotides resulted in marked inhibition of ICAM-1 expression. Furthermore, targeting sequences upstream or downstream from these putative stem-loop structures resulted in significant loss of activity.[21] Mir and Southern[30] have suggested that optimum target sites contain a small single-stranded region at which nucleation takes place, plus a double-stranded, helically ordered stem that is invaded by the antisense molecule with displacement of one of the strands. This largely eliminates the unfavourable energetics consequent to reforming a double helix from what essentially would be two single strands.

Another promising technique is that of oligonucleotide arrays.[31] Using arrays of oligonucleotides that are complementary to extensive regions of the target mRNA, it is possible to determine which antisense oligonucleotides bind to the RNA optimally. Furthermore, there appears to be good correspondence between the ability of an oligonucleotide to bind to the target mRNA and its activity as an antisense agent, both in vitro and in vivo.[31] More recently Patzel et al[32,33] have developed a very promising 'in silico' approach to the selection of active sequence.

When coupled with the large number of genome sequences that are now available, one can imagine that with the help of these empirical approaches, it will soon be possible to identify potential targets for antisense oligonucleotides to study the function of undefined genes via an antisense approach.

2.2 Factors affecting the efficacy of antisense oligonucleotide therapy

2.2.1 Physicochemical properties determining stability of the molecule

The initial successful demonstration of the antisense strategy in cell culture employed unmodified DNA oligodeoxynucleotides.[5,34] However, it was rapidly recognized that unmodified phosphodiester oligonucleotides were easily degraded in cell culture medium containing serum, and that biological effects could be obtained only if large concentrations of oligonucleotide were used (up to 100 μM).[35] Nucleases are virtually ubiquitous, being found both in plasma and intracellularly. Digestion of a phosphodiester oligonucleotide appears to occur primarily by 3'-5'-exonucleolytic activity,[36] but there is also some evidence for endonucleolytic digestion. Equally unfortuitously, the nucleoside monophosphate digestion products can also be toxic.[37] Batch-to-batch variations in commercially available serum, and the fact that nuclease activity is not completely destroyed by heat inactivation procedures, may account for much of the variability in biological effect observed by many investigators using unmodified oligonucleotides.

A number of chemical modifications have been made to the conventional deoxyribonucleic acid structure to improve the stability of these analogues toward nucleases.[38] The most commonly used are the first-generation analogues that possess modifications within the phosphodiester inter-nucleoside linkages (see Fig. 10.2). The most widely used modifications are the phosphorothioate (substitution of a sulphur atom for a non-bridging oxygen at each phosphorus) and the methylphosphonate oligonucleotides (substitution of a non-bridging oxygen at each phosphorus in the oligodeoxynucleotide chain by a methyl group; MP-oligo). Phosphorothioate oligonucleotides retain a repeating negative charge in the phosphodiester backbone, and are polyanionic, whereas MP-oligonucleotides are neutral. These modifications determine not only the intrinsic physicochemical properties of the analogues, but also may influence cellular uptake and degradation.

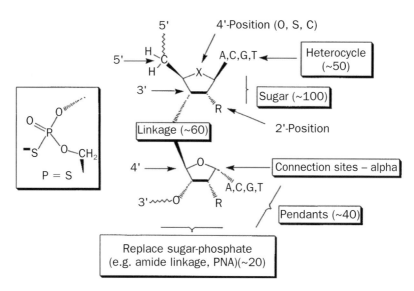

Fig. 10.2 Modifications of the phosphodiester backbone of oligonucleotides that have been employed to improve the biological stability of the molecules, showing the sites and numbers of modifications that have been synthesized and tested. The initial modifications concentrated on the phosphate linkage, substituting a non-bridging oxygen by a sulphur atom (phosphorothioate, shown as P = S above) or a methyl group (methylphosphonate). Many other modifications have been tried, and as shown above, nearly every portion of the molecule has been tried.[39] PNA, peptide nucleic acid.

The methylphosphonate oligonucleotides, in contrast to the isosequential phosphodiesters, are uncharged, and this dramatically reduces their aqueous solubility, resulting in formulation difficulties. In fact, none of the substitutions that result in uncharged oligomers have much activity in experiments in tissue culture in the absence of heroic methods of delivery. Uncharged molecules depend on steric blockade of translation for their effect. This is usually inefficient because the 80S elongating ribosomes have an intrinsic unwinding ability, and can read through the steric block.

The phosphorothioate modification has become the standard choice for most antisense attempts[40] as it offers stability against nucleases, ability to recruit RNAase H (an enzyme thought to play a key role in mediating the 'antisense effect', see above), and ease of synthesis. However, this modification appears to reduce the affinity for RNA (perhaps due to the presence of stereoisomers) and increase protein binding (and thus non-specific side-effects).

The most recent target for modification is the ribose portion of the oligonucleotides.[41] The ribose ring has been appended and substituted, conformationally restricted and even replaced by hexose. However, modification of the 2′ position appear to be the most promising, and the introduction of the 2′-methoxyethoxy group both confers nuclease stability to phosphodiester oligonucleotides and retains excellent binding affinity.[42]

Complete modification of the molecule may not be necessary. Tidd and colleagues showed that incorporation of as few as two terminal MP linkages at the 3′ end (3′ end-capping) of a conventional phosphodiester oligonucleotide resulted in significant protection against degradation by 3′ phosphodiesterase, the predominant nuclease of fetal calf serum.[35,43] Similar protection can be afforded by 3′ end-capping with other modifications such as phosphorothioate or phosphoramidate linkages, and by having an inverted nucleotide conjugated to the oligomers via a 3′–3′ linkage at the 3′-terminal.[44]

Combination of the modifications to produce mixed-backbone oligonucleotides (MBOs) have been demonstrated to produce molecules with affinities greater than the unmodified phosphodiester analogue, and long half-lives, both in vitro and in vivo, and – coupled with advances in large-scale production of these modified oligomers – this should lead to rapid advances in the antisense field.

2.2.2 Intracellular availability

For an oligonucleotide to be an effective therapeutic agent, it must be bioavailable in vivo. Their large molecular weights, relative instability in the biological milieu (short half-lives) and the charged nature of oligonucleotides pose major challenges to the successful delivery of antisense molecules to their intracellular sites of action. Upon administration (by any route), these molecules need to remain stable, and not degrade within the extracellular environment, for a period of time long enough to allow sufficient antisense oligonucleotide to enter cells and exert the desired biological activity. Furthermore, once inside the cells, these molecules also need to avoid degradation until or after they have exerted the desired biological effect. Intracellular stability of the oligonucleotides becomes especially important when chosen targets have a slow turnover. In this case, biological activity of the oligonucleotides against the target needs to be maintained for long periods of time until the pre-existing levels of protein product are allowed to decay.

Phosphorothioate oligonucleotides degrade from both the 3' end and the 5' end in a time- and tissue-dependent manner. The pharmacokinetic profile is similar after subcutaneous, intradermal or intraperitoneal administration, but with lower maximum plasma concentrations.[45] They are well absorbed from all parental sites, are distributed rapidly and reside for long periods in the tissues. They have a broad peripheral tissue distribution, but are not distributed to the brain, and are cleared by metabolism over a prolonged period ($>50\%$ over 10 days). There are minimal differences between sequences.

End-modified mixed-backbone oligonucleotides (MBOs) containing nuclease-resistant 2'-0-alkylribonucleotides or methylphosphonate internucleoside linkages at both the 3' and 5' ends have better stability in vivo, and these MBOs demonstrate up to 20–30% oral bioavailability. Oral administration of end-modified MBO targeted to the RIα subunit of protein kinase A in tumour-bearing mice (xenografts of human breast and colon cancer) produced an anti-tumour effect, demonstrating that clinically significant levels of antisense oligonucleotide could be achieved.

These observations are important. Until Zamecnik and Stephenson's demonstration of an antisense effect of oligonucleotides,[5] it was believed that charged molecules did not cross cell membranes. However, since then numerous studies have demonstrated that antisense oligonucleotides, containing either unmodified phosphodiester inter-nucleoside linkages or modifications of the backbone designed to improve stability of the molecules in the biological milieu, inhibit expression of viral and host gene products. It is inferred from these studies that oligonucleotides are capable of entering cells and achieving sufficient concentrations, within the same cellular compartment as the target mRNA or pre-mRNA, to inhibit expression of target protein.

However, most investigators agree that cellular permeation of oligonucleotides is usually extremely inefficient. Early work, almost without exception, showed that DNA was delivered transiently to cytoplasmic vesicles followed by release to the surrounding media without delivery in detectable amounts to the cytoplasm or nucleus. Simple chemical modifications of the phosphodiester backbone did not improve delivery: neutral backbone oligonucleotides (e.g. methylphosphonates) are not taken up more readily than their charged counterparts.

Charged or uncharged, oligonucleotides enter cells essentially by two processes – adsorptive endocytosis and fluid-phase endocytosis (pinocytosis).[46] Initial studies investigating the mechanism of cellular uptake of the oligonucleotides suggested that molecules with charged backbones (e.g. phosphodiester or phosphorothioate oligomers) enter the cell by an endocytic process, whereas molecules with a neutral backbone (e.g. methylphosphonates) entered cells by passive diffusion.[47–50] These conclusions were based on concentration, temperature and energy dependence of oligonucleotide uptake, binding of the phosphodiester oligonucleotides to a specific membrane protein, and localization of fluorescent probe-labelled oligonucleotides in a punctate pattern within the cytoplasm of the cells, presumably in lysosomes. However, it is now recognized not only that uncharged oligonucleotides are too large, but also that the presence of the nucleobases renders these molecules too polar for passive diffusion.[51]

Polycationic polymers (e.g. L-lysine) have shown some potential in improving the cytoplasmic delivery of the oligonucleotides. Phosphodiester oligonucleotides (15–17-mers) chemically conjugated to poly (L-lysine) were 50–100-fold more efficient than unconjugated material in several biological models.[52] The increased efficiency essentially arose from increased membrane association and subsequent internalization, and to some extent from increased nuclease resistance. Cytotoxicity in some cell lines in vitro, and more importantly, complement activation in vivo, will unfortunately limit the use of poly (L-lysine)-based delivery vehicles for systemic delivery of antisense oligonucleotides.

Liposomes provide an alternative solution.[53] These are microscopic closed vesicles composed of bilayered phospholipid membranes surrounding aqueous spaces in which various drugs (including oligonucleotides) can be entrapped for delivery to cells. Cationic liposomes, rather than entrapping the nucleotides, complex the molecules by ionic interactions between the negative charges of the phosphate groups of the oligonucleotide and the positive charges on the surface of the liposome. The cationic liposomes have interesting cell fusogenic properties,[54] but create the disadvantage of complexing the nucleotides at the liposomal surface, which may potentially be susceptible to degradation by nucleases. However, with some modification of the in vitro conditions, oligonucleotides can be delivered to the cell with high efficiency.[53] Lipid toxicity, stability of pH-sensitive liposomes in the presence of serum, efficiency of encapsidation and the preferential uptake of particulate material by macrophages are the main limitations.

A necessary prerequisite for an intracellular biological effect is the efflux of the oligonucleotides from the endosomes and/or lysosomes (see Fig. 10.3). Poor escape from the endocytic compartments can severely limit the activity in intact cells. This may occur by a combination of destabilization of the vesicles (e.g. with pH-sensitive liposomal preparations) and slow diffusion into the cytoplasm. The subsequent localization of the oligonucleotides is variable. Microinjection of labelled oligonu-

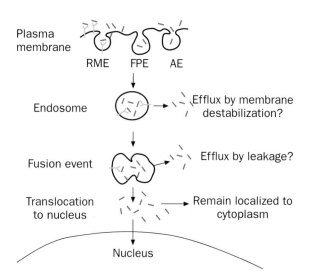

Fig. 10.3 Cellular uptake of oligonucleotides. Unmodified phosphodiester and phosphorothioate analogues are thought to enter cells by receptor-mediated endocytosis (RME), whereas uncharged analogues (e.g. methylphosphonates) are thought to enter cells by either adsorptive (AE) or fluid-phase (FPE) endocytosis. On entry, oligonucleotides become enclosed within membrane vesicles (endosomes). In order to exert a biological effect, the oligonucleotides need to escape this acidic compartment, by simple diffusion, transient membrane destabilization or simple leakage during fusion with lysosomes. Free cytosolic oligonucleotides may then either remain in the cytoplasm or translocate to the nucleus.

cleotides has shown that the molecules rapidly diffuse into and localize within the nucleus,[55,56] although there are some that localize predominantly to the cytoplasm.[57] Exploiting the cellular membrane-crossing ability of some cellular or viral proteins (e.g. 16 amino acids of the *Drosophila* protein Antennapedia, and 35 amino acids of the HIV protein TAT) might represent an interesting alternative.[58,59]

Substantial inhibition of protein expression by a single addition or a few applications of antisense molecules can be achieved only if the turnover rate of the target protein is sufficiently high. The amount of protein needs to decrease rapidly enough so that the lack of protein synthesis can produce functional effects. The turnover of nuclear receptors such as the members of the *jun*, *fos* and *myc* families have very rapid turnover and are thus good targets for antisense mediated suppression. The turnover of membrane receptor proteins is generally much lower. Thus, theoretically, inhibition of their expression with externally applied antisense molecules might not lead to physiological effects as quickly and/or as effectively.

2.3 Non-specific effects

In addition to their sequence-specific effects, many 'antisense' oligonucleotides have been found to show non-sequence-specific effects; this may in part be due to their polyanionic backbones.[60] Substitution of sulphur for oxygen in the phosphorothioate oligonucleotides not only improves nuclease resistance, but also creates a molecule with very different properties as compared with the phosphodiester equivalent.

Phosphorothioate oligonucleotides bind in a length- and somewhat sequence-independent manner to heparin-binding proteins (Table 10.2).[61–63] These include platelet-derived growth factor (PDGF), acidic and basic fibroblast growth factors (aFGF and bFGF), vascular endothelial growth factor (VEGF) and its receptors, the epidermal growth factor receptor (EGFR), fibronectin, laminin, Mac-1 (CD11–CD18), CD4, HIV gp120, HIV reverse transcriptase, certain forms of protein kinase C (PKC), to

name but a few. For EGFR, phosphorothioate oligonucleotides have been shown to induce autophosphorylation in the absence of EGF, and under certain circumstances, phosphorothioates have been shown to activate transcription factors such as Sp1. Phosphorothioate oligonucleotides with four contiguous guanosine nucleotides can form quadruple-stranded tetraplexes and other higher order structures that can be extremely biologically active, but their activity may have little if anything to do with an antisense effect.

As described earlier, the antisense effect of antisense oligonucleotides is probably mediated by RNAase H. This enzyme cleaves the mRNA strand at the site of hybridization with a complementary strand of DNA. Another source of non-specific activity can be the low stringency of RNAase H. Very short heteroduplexes (four base pairs for the *Escherichia coli* enzyme I) are substrates for RNAase H. The human RNAase HI is even able to cleave at the level of a single ribo-residue in a DNA context for both strands of the duplex.[64] Moreover, mismatches are tolerated by RNAase H.[65] Ideally the antisense oligonucleotide should hybridize only with the target mRNA, but the chance of a mismatch increases with the length of oligonucleotide used, leading to the counter-intuitive proposal that oligonucleotide specificity is actually inversely related to its length.

The minimal length for specificity depends on the number of transcribed sequences within the cell. On a statistical basis, an AT sequence 19 nucleotides long is unique in the human genome at DNA level. For a GC sequence the figure is 15 nucleotides.[26] The difference between the two numbers originates in the over-representation of AT pairs (60%) in the human genome. If we assume that only 0.5% of DNA is transcribed, uniqueness at RNA level is reached with 15-mer and 11-mer for AT and GC targets, respectively. Longer sequences might be expected to increase the non-specific effects of the molecules, as longer sequences would theoretically produce a larger number of partially complementary sequences. Such long duplexes would tolerate mismatches and mismatched complexes might be a substrate for

Table 10.2   Non-sequence-specific effects of phosphorothioate oligonucleotides

Oligonucleotide	Target/effect
S-dC$_n$	Blockade of binding of gp120 to CD4; prevention of HIV-1-induced syncitia formation
	Binding to v3 loop of HIV-1 gp120
	Inhibition of HIV-1 reverse transcriptase activity
	Inhibition of DNA polymerases activity
	Competitive inhibition of PKC α1 and other isoforms of protein kinase C
	Inhibition of binding of bFGF to all surface receptors
	Inhibition of titriated thymidine uptake in NIH3T3 cells
	Inhibition of PDGF stimulation of u-PA activity
	Binding to aFGF, FGF-4 and VEGF
	Binding to extracellular matrix derived from NIH3T3 cells
	Inhibition of fibronectin binding to cell surface receptors
	Inhibition of laminin binding to sulphatide
	Non-specific induction of Sp1 activity
	Inhibition of proton pumping activity of vacuolar H'-ATPase
	Inhibition of some tyrosine kinases
S-dT$_{28}$	Inhibition of Taq polymerase activity
S-dT$_n$; G-quartet	Inhibition of binding of bFGF to all surface receptors
	Inhibition of titriated thymidine uptake in NIH3T3 cells
	Binding to extracellular matrix derived from NIH3T3 cells
CpG motif	Lymphocyte activation

Adapted from Stein and Krieg.[63] S-dCn refers to polynucleotide of dCTP with phosphorothioate modification of each base.

RNAase H. This was clearly demonstrated for an antisense sequence targeted to the point mutated region of the *Ha-ras* gene: a 17-mer allowed discrimination between the mutated and wild-type sequences whereas a 19-mer did not.[66]

'Irrelevant cleavage' by RNAase-H is easily eliminated if RNAase-H activity is eliminated, for example, by reducing the charge of the backbone. However, this poses difficulties in the solubility and formulation of the antisense molecule, as well as its delivery to the site of activity. Chimeric or 'winged' oligonucleotides have been designed to preserve the ability to mediate the cleavage of the target site on the

one hand and to reduce the activity of RNAase H at non-complimentary sequences on the other. Oligonucleotides in which a central 'window' of unmodified phosphodiester nucleotides is placed between two stretches of methylphosphonates residues have been shown to display a higher specificity than the homologous unmodified patent sequence.[67,68]

Given the possibility of non-specific effects, it is important that experiments are conducted with the appropriate controls. This begs the question, what are the most appropriate controls? The short answer is several, based on the length and base sequence of the oligonucleotide of interest.

1. Sense sequence. The base composition is not conserved. In addition, this sequence might be a binding site for some factor playing a role in the regulation of the target gene. Thus, additional controls are necessary.
2. Scrambled sequences. The same base composition is arranged in a different order. In this case, internal structural features are lost.
3. Mismatched sequences. The introduction of one or several mismatches in the antisense sequence should weaken the binding, and consequently the amplitude, of the antisense effect. The base composition is lost.
4. Mixed sequences. A mixture of all possible sequences is achieved by the introduction of the four bases at each position. Some sequences are expected to display a strong effect but this will be averaged by the number of different molecules (a mixed 20-mer corresponds to $4^{20} = 10^{12}$ sequences).
5. The inverted sequence (5′–3′). It is the only one that keeps constant the base composition and most of the structural peculiarities. However, this cannot be used for palindromic or quasi-palindromic sequences.

3. CLINICAL APPLICATION OF ANTISENSE TECHNOLOGY

The goal of antisense therapeutics is of course to produce a safe, specific and effective treatment. Most experience has been reported with phosphorothioate oligonucleotides. The pharmacokinetic and toxicological effects of these oligomers have been characterized in many species and in humans. Vitravene™, an antisense phosphorothioate oligonucleotide against cytomegalovirus (CMV), is the first antisense drug to be licensed in the USA, and demonstrates that this class of molecules can yield clinically useful drugs.

The unravelling of the molecular events that lead to malignancy and the identification of key genes involved in that process have provided investigators with a number of targets for antisense therapy of cancer. The preclinical development of several antisense compounds targeting cancer-related genes has proceeded relatively rapidly. Many have shown convincing in vitro reduction in target gene expression and promising activity against a wide variety of tumours. The clinical testing of the most promising oligonucleotides has taken place over the last several years, although, until recently, few studies have reached completion. Current studies involve antisense oligonucleotides targeted to p53, bcl-2, c-raf, H-ras, protein kinase C-alpha and protein kinase A. Most studies have tested first-generation oligonucleotide compounds that contain a phosphorothioate backbone, which accounts for the great similarity in toxicity profiles.

Clinical toxicological studies have demonstrated that phosphorothioate oligonucleotides have no significant subacute toxicity in rodents and monkeys after intravenous doses of up to 100 mg/kg. Single and multiple doses have been demonstrated to be safe in humans. High doses (>80 mg/kg per day) result in cytokine release, inhibit coagulation, activate complement and can result in thrombocytopenia. Given that doses as low as 0.06 mg/kg per day have been shown to be effective in some models, the therapeutic index would appear to be satisfactory. Inhibition of target genes by the antisense compounds has not been verified by assay in all clinical studies. When these assays have been performed, reductions in target gene expression in peripheral blood cells have been modest, at most, and variable from patient to patient.

Combinations of antisense and chemotherapy thus far have not shown unexpected pharmacokinetic interactions, and suggest that antisense-chemotherapy combinations might be administered safely. GEM®231 is an antisense inhibitor of the RIα subunit of protein kinase A that is known to be increased in the cells of many human cancers. In preclinical cancer models, GEM®231 has been studied alone and in combination with Taxol®, Taxotere®, Camptosar®, Adriamycin® and IMC-225. In each model, results demonstrated enhanced antitumour activity of each drug when used in combination with GEM®231. It was the first advanced chemistry antisense drug candidate to be investigated in oncology patients. Initial studies are investigating the effect of GEM®231 in patients with malignant solid tumours who have failed other therapies. As an advanced chemistry antisense agent, GEM®231 has also demonstrated activity in human cancer models when administered by the oral route.

Antisense drugs have also been developed for viral targets such as CMV (CMV retinitis – Vitravene™), human papilloma virus (HPV) and hepatitis C virus (HCV). Endothelial cell adhesion molecules (ICAM) play a key role in inflammatory disorders such as inflammatory bowel disease and ischaemia-reperfusion injury. ISIS 2302 inhibits the expression of ICAM-1 and is undergoing Phase III clinical trials in patients with Crohn's disease.

Some of the limitations of the first-generation compounds will be overcome with additional modifications. These newer generation compounds offer hope that current dose-limiting side-effects might be avoided and that greater inhibition of target genes could be achieved. ISIS 104838 is the first antisense oligonucleotide based on second-generation chemistry. The compound is an antisense inhibitor of tumour necrosis factor-alpha (TNF-α), a molecule known to play a role in a variety of inflammatory diseases such as rheumatoid arthritis (RA) and psoriasis. Phase II trials of ISIS 104838, administered intravenously and subcutaneously in patients with RA are currently underway and are due to report in 2002. In addition, a Phase II clinical trial of topically administered ISIS 104838 in patients with psoriasis is ongoing, and oral formulations are being studied in humans to identify a suitable delivery system.

GEM®92 is another second-generation antisense drug candidate that is targeted to the *gag* gene of the human immunodeficiency virus (HIV-1). Based on the insights gained with a previous molecule (GEM®91), modifications were made in GEM®92 to overcome undesirable properties. It is the first antisense agent to be administered orally in a clinical study. The initial single-dose Phase I study of GEM®92 orally at three dose levels and by injection shows excellent safety results and successfully con-

firms oral delivery of advanced chemistry antisense agents.

4. CONCLUSIONS AND FUTURE DIRECTIONS

Among researchers in the antisense field, the enthusiasm for antisense oligonucleotides as therapeutic agents has passed through several phases ranging from extreme optimism, primarily because of the simplistic nature of the concept, to considerable scepticism, when difficulties arose on many fronts, such as poor uptake of the oligomers, lack of biological activity by most oligonucleotides tested and difficulties encountered in interpreting the results.

These problems exist primarily because oligomers cause many cellular effects, not through antisense mechanisms, but because these molecules are polyanionic or have sequence elements that stimulate non-antisense-mediated biochemical events. Oligonucleotides have been shown to stimulate cytokine release, bind to and inhibit enzymes, and inhibit transcription of chromosomal DNA by direct interaction with the double-helix. In principle, any oligonucleotide may have any of these activities, depending on the relative values of K_d for the different oligonucleotide binding sites, and on the intracellular localization of the oligonucleotide. Rather than focusing on the oligonucleotide as an 'antisense' agent, it is perhaps more important to accurately investigate the biological effect of the oligonucleotide as compared to the toxic effects of the molecule, at both the cellular level and the systemic level.

Appreciating the problems has led to solutions and novel approaches to the discovery and analysis of antisense agents, and the list of antisense oligonucleotides undergoing clinical evaluation grows steadily (Table 10.3) – a reflection of the intense research activity that has been devoted to this field over the past 10 years. Advances in medicinal chemistry, the evolution of backbone modifications described earlier, and novel techniques for screening for suitable targets on the RNA molecule should produce new chemical classes with improved potency, pharmacokinetic and toxicological properties for the clinic. Clearly, as more is

Table 10.3   Antisense drugs in development and clinical trials

Product (delivery route)	Target	Indication	Company	Status
Vitravene (I)	Antiviral	CMV retinitis	ISIS/Novartis	On market
ISIS 3521 (P)	PKC-α	Cancer: non-SCLC, others	ISIS/Lilly	Phase III
GEM®92 (O)	HIV (*gag*)	HIV disease	Hybridon	Phase II
GEM®231 (P)	PKA	Cancer	Hybridon	Phase II
ISIS 2302 (P)	ICAM-1	Crohn's disease	ISIS	Phase II
ISIS 2302 (T)	ICAM-1	Topical psoriasis	ISIS	Phase II
ISIS 2303 (E)	ICAM-1	Ulcerative colitis	ISIS	Phase II
ISIS 14803 (P)	Antiviral	Hepatitis C	ISIS/Elan	Phase II
ISIS 2503 (P)	Ha-*ras*	Cancer: pancreatic, others	ISIS	Phase II
ISIS 5132 (P)	*c-raf*	Cancer: ovarian, others	ISIS	Phase II
ISIS 104838 (P, O)	TNF-α	RA, Crohn's disease	ISIS/Elan	Phase II
ISIS 104838 (T)	TNF-α	Topical psoriasis	ISIS	Phase II
GTI 2040 (P)	Ribonucleotide reductase	Cancer: renal	Lorus	Phase II
MG98 (P)	DNA methyl transferase	Cancer	MethylGene Inc.	Phase II
EPI-2010	Adenosine A1 receptor	Asthma	Epigenesis	Phase II
G3139 (P)	bcl-2	NHL, prostate, melanoma	Genta	Phase I/II
ISIS 113715 (P, O)	PTP-1B	Diabetes	ISIS/Merck	Phase I
ISIS 13650 (I)	*c-raf*	Diabetic retinopathy, AMD	ISIS	Phase I
ISIS 107248 (P, O)	VLA-4	MS	ISIS	Phase I
OGX-011 (P, O)	Clusterin	Cancer: prostate, others	OncoGenex/ISIS	Phase I
GTI 2501 (P)	Ribonucleotide reductase	Cancer: renal	Lorus	Phase I
ORI-1001 (T)	HPV	Papilloma	Origenix	Phase I
OL(1)p53 (P)	p53	AML, MDS	ISIS	Phase I
LR-3001 (P)	c-myb	CML, AML	Lynx	Phase I

Data as available Jan 2002. (*Routes of delivery*: I, intravitreal; P, parenteral; E, enema; T, topical; O, oral).
Abbreviations: AMD = ageing macular degeneration; AML = acute myeloid leukaemia; CML = chronic myeloid leukaemia; CMV = cytomegalovirus; MDS = myelodysplasia; MS = multiple sclerosis; NHL = non-Hodgkin's lymphoma; RA = rheumatoid arthritis; SCLC = small cell carcinoma.

learned we will be in a position to perform more sophisticated studies and to understand more of the factors that determine whether an oligonucleotide actually works via an antisense mechanism.

Since this article was written, there has been an explosion of interest in a novel mechanism of RNA-mediated gene suppression termed 'RNA interference' (RNAi). Double-stranded RNA (dsRNA), expressed in or introduced into a cell of interest, is converted into short RNAs that direct ribonucleases to homologous mRNA targets. This process appears to be related to the normal defense against viruses and may provide an efficient alternative to antisense for tissue- and stage-specific gene targeting.[69–71]

REFERENCES

Further reading

Cohen JS. *Oligonucleotides: Antisense Inhibitors of Gene Expression.* London: Macmillan Press, 1989.

Erickson RP, Izant JG. *Gene Regulation: Biology of Antisense RNA and DNA.* New York: Raven Press, 1992.

Crooke ST, Lebleu B. *Antisense Research & Applications.* Boca Raton, FL: CRC Press, 1993.

Chadwick DJ, Cardew G. *Oligonucleotides as Therapeutic Agents.* Chichester: Wiley, 1997.

Web-sites

■ http://www.liv.ac.uk/~giles/index.htm
The Antisense Research Group at Liverpool University, UK – an overview of theory and practice.

■ http://www.cem.msu.edu/~cem181h/
projects/97/antisense/home.htm
Michigan State University site on Antisense Technology in AIDS Research.

■ http://www.isip.com/index.html
ISIS Pharmaceuticals – antisense technology and drugs in development.

■ http://www.hybridon.com/
Hybridon, Inc. – clinical programme of drug development.

■ http://www.epigenesispharmaceuticals.com
Epigenesis Pharmaceuticals – antisense drugs in respiratory disease.

Scientific papers

1. Kimelman D. Regulation of eukaryotic gene expression by natural antisense transcripts: the case of the modifying reaction. In: Erickson RP, Izant JG, eds. *Gene Regulation: Biology of Antisense RNA and DNA.* New York: Raven Press, 1992: 1–10.

2. Krystal GW. Regulation of eukaryotic gene expression by naturally occurring antisense RNA. In: Erickson RP, Izant JG, eds. *Gene Regulation: Biology of Antisense RNA and DNA.* New York: Raven Press, 1992: 11–20.

3. Inouye M. Antisense RNA: its function and applications in gene regulation – a review. *Gene* 1988; **72:** 25–34.

4. Liu Z, Batt DB, Carmichael GD. Targeted nuclear antisense RNA mimics natural antisense-induced degradation of polyoma virus early RNA. *Proc Natl Acad Sci USA* 1994; **91:** 4258–62.

5. Zamecnik P, Stephenson M. Inhibition of Rous sarcoma virus replication and cell transformation by a specific oligodeoxynucleotide. *Proc Natl Acad Sci USA* 1978; **75:** 280–4.

6. Dash P, Lotan M, Knapp M, Kandel ER, Goelet P. Selective elimination of mRNAs *in vivo*: complementary oligonucleotides promote RNA degradation by an RNase H-like activity. *Proc Natl Acad Sci USA* 1987; **84:** 7896–900.

7. Shuttleworth J, Colman A. Antisense oligonucleotide-directed cleavage of mRNA in *Xenopus* oocytes and eggs. *EMBO J* 1988; **7:** 427–34.

8. Smith RC, Dworkin MB, Dworkin-Rastl E. Destruction of a translationally controlled mRNA in *Xenopus* oocytes delays progesterone-induced maturation. *Genes Dev* 1988; **2:** 1296–306.

9. Barrett JC, Miller PS, Ts'o POP. Inhibitory effect of complex formation with oligodeoxyribonucleotide ethyl phosphotriesters on transfer ribonucleic acid aminoacylation. *Biochemistry* 1974; **13:** 4897–910.

10. Ts'o POP, Miller PS, Greene JJ. Nucleic acid analogues with targeted delivery as chemotherapeutic agents. In: Cheng YC, Goz B, Minkoff M, eds. *Development of Target-Orientated Anticancer Drugs.* New York: Raven Press, 1983: 189–206.

11. Venturelli D, Travali S, Calabretta B. Inhibition of T-cell proliferation by a MYB antisense oligomer is accompanied by selective down-regulation of DNA polymerase alpha expression. *Proc Natl Acad Sci USA* 1990; **87:** 5963–7.

12. Geiger T, Muller M, Dean NM, Fabbro D. Antitumor activity of a PKC-alpha antisense oligonucleotide in combination with standard chemotherapeutic agents against various human tumors transplanted into nude mice. *Anticancer Drug Des* 1998; **13:** 35–45.

13. Monia BP. First- and second-generation antisense inhibitors targeted to human c-raf kinase: in vitro and in vivo studies. *Anticancer Drug Des* 1997; **12:** 327–39.

14. Cowsert LM. In vitro and in vivo activity of antisense inhibitors of ras: potential for clinical development. *Anticancer Drug Des* 1997; **12:** 359–71.

15. Ziegler A, Luedke GH, Fabbro D, Altmann KH, Stahel RA, Zangemeister-Wittke U. Induction of apoptosis in small-cell lung cancer cells by an antisense oligodeoxynucleotide targeting the Bcl-2 coding sequence. *J Natl Cancer Inst* 1997; **89:** 1027–36.

16. Cotter FE. Antisense therapy of hematologic malignancies. *Semin Hematol* 1999; **36:** 9–14.

17. Leech SH, Olie RA, Gautschi O et al. Induction of apoptosis in lung-cancer cells following bcl-xL anti-sense treatment. *Int J Cancer* 2000; **86:** 570–6.

18. Taylor JK, Zhang QQ, Monia BP, Marcusson EG, Dean NM. Inhibition of Bcl-xL expression sensitizes normal human keratinocytes and epithelial cells to apoptotic stimuli. *Oncogene* 1999; **18:** 4495–504.

19. Harel BA, Durum S, Muegge K, Abbas AK, Farrar WL. Specific inhibition of lymphokine biosynthesis and autocrine growth using antisense oligonucleotides in Th1 and Th2 helper T cell clones. *J Exp Med* 1988; **168:** 2309–18.

20. Karras JG, McGraw K, McKay RA et al. Inhibition of antigen-induced eosinophilia and late phase airway hyperresponsiveness by an IL-5 antisense oligonucleotide in mouse models of asthma. *J Immunol* 2000; **164:** 5409–15.

21. Chiang MY, Chan H, Zounes MA, Freier SM, Lima WF, Bennett CF. Antisense oligonucleotides inhibit intercellular adhesion molecule 1 expression by two distinct mechanisms. *J Biol Chem* 1991; **266:** 18162–71.

22. Bennett CF, Condon TP, Grimm S, Chan H, Chiang MY. Inhibition of endothelial cell adhesion molecule expression with antisense oligonucleotides. *J Immunol* 1994; **152:** 3530–40.

23. Helene C, Toulme JJ. Specific regulation of gene expression by antisense, sense and antigene nucleic acids. *Biochim Biophys Acta* 1990; **1049:** 99–125.

24. Carter G, Lemoine NR. Antisense technology for cancer therapy: does it make sense? *Br J Cancer* 1993; **67:** 869–76.

25. Lebedeva I, Stein CA. Antisense oligonucleotides: promise and reality. *Annu Rev Pharmacol Toxicol* 2001; **41:** 403–19.

26. Helene C, Toulme JJ. Antigene oligonucleotides. In: Cohen JS, ed. *Oligonucleotides: Antisense Inhibitors of Gene Expression*. London: Macmillan Press, 1989: 137–72.

27. Manson J, Brown T, Duff G. Modulation of interleukin 1 beta gene expression using antisense phosphorothioate oligonucleotides. *Lymphokine Res* 1990; **9:** 35–42.

28. Daaka Y, Wickstrom E. Target dependence of antisense oligodeoxynucleotide inhibition of c-Ha-ras p21 expression and focus formation in T24-transformed NIH3T3 cells. *Oncogene Res* 1990; **5:** 267–75.

29. Zuker M. On finding all suboptimal foldings of an RNA molecule. *Science* 1989; **244:** 48.

30. Mir KU, Southern EM. Determining the influence of structure on hybridisation using oligonucleotide arrays. *Nat Biotechnol* 1999; **17:** 788–92.

31. Southern EM, Milner N, Mir KU. Discovering antisense reagents by hybridization of RNA to oligonucleotide arrays. *Ciba Found Symp* 1997; **209:** 38–44.

32. Patzel V, Steidl U, Kronenwett R, Haas R, Sczakiel G. A theoretical approach to select effective antisense oligodeoxyribonucleotides at high statistical probability. *Nucleic Acids Res* 1999; **27:** 4328–34.

33. Scherr M, Rossi JJ, Sczakiel G, Patzel V. RNA accessibility prediction: a theoretical approach is consistent with experimental studies in cell extracts. *Nucleic Acids Res* 2000; **28:** 2455–61.

34. Blake KR, Murakami A, Miller PS. Inhibition of rabbit globin mRNA translation by sequence specific oligodeoxynucleotides. *Biochemistry* 1985; **24:** 6139–45.

35. Tidd DM. A potential role for antisense oligonucleotide analogues in the development of oncogene targeted cancer chemotherapy. *Anticancer Res* 1990; **10:** 1169–82.

36. Eder P.S, DeVine RJ, Dagle JM, Walder JA. Substrate specificity and kinetics of degradation of antisense oligonucleotides by a 3′ exonuclease in plasma. *Antisense Res Dev* 1991; **1:** 141–51.

37. Vaerman JL, Moureau P, Deldime F et al. Antisense oligodeoxyribonucleotides suppress hematologic cell growth through stepwise release of deoxyribonucleotides. *Blood* 1997; **90:** 331–9.

38. Matteucci, M. Oligonucleotide analogues: an overview. In: Chadwick DJ, Cardew G, eds. *Oligonucleotides as Therapeutic Agents*. Chichester: Wiley, 1997: 5–18.

39. Verma S, Eckstein F. Modified oligonucleotides: synthesis and strategy for users. *Annu Rev Biochem* 1998; **67:** 99–134.

40. Cohen JS. Phosphorothioate oligodeoxynucleotides. In: Crooke ST, Lebleu B, eds. *Antisense Research, Applications*. Boca Raton, FL: CRC Press, 1993: 205–21.

41. De Mesmaeker AD, Haner R, Martin P, Moser HE. Antisense oligonucleotides. *Acc Chem Res* 1995; **28:** 366–74.

42. Altmann KH, Dean NM, Fabbro D. Second generation of antisense oligonucleotides: from nuclease resistance to biological efficacy in animals. *Chimia* 1996; **50:** 168–76.

43. Tidd D, Warenius HM. Partial protection on oncogene, antisense oligodeoxynucleotides against serum nuclease degradation using terminal methylphosphonate groups. *Br J Cancer* 1989; **60:** 343–50.

44. Shaw JP, Kent K, Bird J, Fishback J, Froehler B. Modified deoxyoligonucleotides stable to exonuclease digestion in serum. *Nucleic Acids Res* 1991; **19:** 747–50.

45. Agrawal S, Zhang RL. Pharmacokinetics of oligonucleotides. In: Chadwick DJ, Cardew G. *Oligonucleotides as Therapeutic Agents*. Chichester: Wiley, 1997: 60–78.

46. Tonkinson JL, Stein CA. Patterns of intracellular compartmentalization, trafficking and acidification of 5′-fluorescein labeled phosphodiester and phosphorothioate oligodeoxynucleotides in HL60 cells. *Nucleic Acids Res* 1994; **22**: 4268–75.

47. Miller PS. Oligonucleoside methylphosphonates as antisense reagents. *Biotechnology* 1991; **9**: 358–62.

48. Loke SL, Stein CA, Zhang XH et al. Characterisation of oligonucleotide transport into living cells. *Proc Natl Acad Sci USA* 1989; **86**: 3474–8.

49. Crooke RM. *In vitro* toxicology and pharmacokinetics of antisense oligonucleotides. *Anticancer Drug Des* 2000; **6**: 609–46.

50. Yakubov LA, Deeva EA, Zarytova VF et al. Mechanism of oligonucleotide uptake by living cells: involvement of receptors? *Proc Natl Acad Sci USA* 1989; **86**: 6454–8.

51. Akhtar S, Kole R, Juliano RL. Stability of antisense DNA oligodeoxynucleotide analogs in cellular extracts and sera. *Life Sci* 1991; **49**: 1793–801.

52. Lebleu B, Bastide L, Bisbal C. Poly (L-lysine)-mediated delivery of nucleic acids. In: Gregoriadis G, McCormack B, eds. *Targeting of Drugs: Strategies for oligonucleotide and gene delivery in therapy.* New York: Plenum Press, 1997: 115–22.

53. Bennett CF, Chiang MY, Chan H, Shoemaker JE, Mirabelli CK. Cationic lipids enhance cellular uptake and activity of phosphorothioate antisense oligonucleotides. *Mol Pharmacol* 1992; **41**: 1023–33.

54. Malone RW, Felgner PL, Verma IM. Cationic liposome-mediated RNA transfection. *Proc Natl Acad Sci USA* 1989; **86**: 6077–81.

55. Chin DJ, Green GA, Zon G, Szoka FC, Straubinger RM. Rapid nuclear accumulation of injected oligodeoxynucleotides. *New Biol* 1990; **9**: 1091–100.

56. Leonetti JP, Mechti N, Degols G, Gagnor C, Lebleu B. Intracellular distribution of microinjected oligodeoxynucleotides. *Proc Natl Acad Sci USA* 1991; **88**: 2702–6.

57. Cerruzzi M, Draper K, Schwartz J. Natural and phosphorothioate-modified oligodeoxynucleotides exhibit a non-random cellular distribution. *Nucleosides and Nucleotides* 1990; **9**: 679–95.

58. Vives E, Brodin P, Lebleu B. A truncated HIV-1 Tat protein basic domain rapidly translocates through the plasma membrane and accumulates in the cell nucleus. *J Biol Chem* 1997; **272**: 16010–17.

59. Derossi D, Calvert S, Trembleau A, Brunissen A, Chassaing G, Prochiantz A. Cell internalization of the third helix of the *Antennapedia* homeodomain is receptor-independent. *J Biol Chem* 1996; **271**: 18188–93.

60. Stein CA, Cheng YC. Antisense oligonucleotides as therapeutic agents – is the bullet really magical? *Science* 1993; **261**: 1004–12.

61. Guvakova MA, Yakubov LA, Vlodavsky I, Tonkinson JL, Stein CA. Phosphorothioate oligodeoxynucleotides bind to basic fibroblast growth factor, inhibit its binding to cell surface receptors, and remove it from low affinity binding sites on extracellular matrix. *J Biol Chem* 1995; **270**: 2620–7.

62. Fennewald SM, Rando RF. Inhibition of high affinity basic fibroblast growth factor binding by oligonucleotides. *J Biol Chem* 1995; **270**: 21718–21.

63. Stein CA, Krieg AM. Non-antisense effects of oligodeoxynucleotides. In: Lichtenstein C, Nellen W, eds. *Antisense Technology: A Practical Approach.* Oxford: Oxford University Press, 1997: 241–64.

64. Eder PS, Walder JA. Ribonuclease H from K562 human erythroleukemia cells. Purification, characterization, and substrate specificity. *J Biol Chem* 1991; **266**: 6472–9.

65. Cazenave C, Stein CA, Loreau N et al. Comparative inhibition of rabbit globin mRNA translation by modified antisense oligodeoxynucleotides. *Nucleic Acids Res* 1989; **17**: 4255–73.

66. Freier, SM. Antisense oligonucleotides. In: Lebleu B, Crooke ST, eds. *Antisense Research and Applications.* Boca Raton: CRC Press, 1993: 67–82.

67. Giles RV, Tidd DM. Increased specificity for antisense oligodeoxynucleotide targeting of RNA cleavage by RNase H using chimeric methylphosphonodiester/phosphodiester structures. *Nucleic Acids Res* 1992; **20**: 763–70.

68. Larrouy B, Blonski C, Boiziau C et al. Toulme RNase H-mediated inhibition of translation by antisense oligodeoxyribonucleotides: use of backbone modification to improve specificity. *Gene* 1992; **121**: 189–94.

69. Hannon GJ. RNA interference. *Nature* 2002; **418**:244–51.

70. Carthew RW. Gene silencing by double-stranded RNA. *Curr Opin Cell Biol* 2001; **13**:244–8.

71. Fjose A, Ellingsen S, Wargelius A, Seo HC. RNA interference: mechanisms and applications. *Biotechnol Annu Rev* 2001; **7**:31–57.

11

Gene therapy: theoretical and practical aspects

Rebecca Kristeleit, Martin R Wilkins

Summary • Introduction • Gene transfer systems • Viral vectors • Non-viral systems • Gene therapy in practice • Conclusions • References

SUMMARY

Gene therapy has just passed its tenth anniversary. It was introduced with great excitement and promise but at the present time there are questions about whether it can deliver and concerns over its safety. This chapter reviews the current status of gene transfer systems and discusses the practical aspects of conducting gene-based therapeutics.

1. INTRODUCTION

Gene therapy can be defined as the deliberate transfer of genetic material into human somatic cells for therapeutic, prophylactic or diagnostic purposes.[1] The technology to conduct germline engineering is imminent but the ethical aspects of such manipulation remain the subject of considerable debate at present.[2-5]

The gene-based approach to the treatment of disease represents one of the most important developments in medicine, with far-reaching possibilities for a wide range of conditions, both inherited and acquired. Such a system offers superior cell-, tissue- or organ-specific targeting (thus improving therapeutic index) and a prolonged duration of action. It is also aimed at treating or eliminating the underlying cause of a disease process and not just the symptoms.

Revolutionary advances in molecular biology and genetics have enabled translation of gene transfer technology into clinical research over the last decade. Candidate diseases have included monogenic disorders such as cystic fibrosis, severe combined immunodeficiencies and haemophilia B as well as cancers, coronary disease and rheumatoid arthritis. Although the first patient trial was opened in 1990,[6] it is only within the past 2 years that clinical benefit has been demonstrated clearly for the first time.[7-9] There are now over 600 gene therapy clinical trials that have been approved worldwide, the majority of which (63%) are cancer studies.

2. GENE TRANSFER SYSTEMS

The main obstacle in the development of gene therapy as an effective clinical tool has been the difficulty in identifying a suitable vector system that can deliver genetic material efficiently to the target tissue. While much progress has been

---

Box 11.1 Desirable properties of an ideal vector

The ideal vector should:

- Be able to accommodate large transgenes
- Be able to transduce active and quiescent cells in vivo
- Be able to target specific tissues with minimal local tissue damage
- Be immunologically inert
- Integrate into the host genome or reside as an episome within the nucleus
- Produce sustained expression
- Be subject to post-transduction regulation
- Permit large-scale reliable commercial production

---

made and several systems have been developed, this still remains the limiting step as regards the broad application of gene therapy to a wide range of diseases. The desirable properties of an ideal vector are summarized in Box 11.1.

An ideal vector is capable of targeting specific cells types without stimulating an inflammatory response in the host. It should also be amenable to any size of genetic insert (the coding sequence lengths of therapeutic genes vary enormously and there should also be flexibility to add regulatory sequences for transduction and expression) and be integrated into the host chromosome at a specific site or reside as an episome within the nucleus (random integration into the host chromosome is undesirable as control of expression is then compromised). It should also be capable of production on a commercial scale. Simply stated, such a vector has not yet been developed.

Current vector systems can be broadly categorized as either viral (e.g. adenovirus, retrovirus) or non-viral (e.g. naked DNA, liposomes) (Box 11.2). The advantages of using the latter group are: decreased immunogenicity, ease of large-scale production, simplicity of use and unlimited insert size; but the drawbacks are inefficient gene transfer and transient expression.[10] Viral vectors currently give the most effective levels of transfection and can result in long-term expression but they are markedly immunogenic, have insert size limitations (inability to package the genetic material into the viral capsid) and are difficult to produce reliably on a large scale.[11,12] To date, non-cardiovascular applications of gene therapy have relied predominantly on viral vectors, whereas cardiovascular studies have used non-viral vectors, mainly naked plasma DNA or liposome carriers.

3. VIRAL VECTORS

Viruses are obligate intracellular parasites that often have specificity for a particular cell type. The viral life cycle has two distinct phases of infection and replication. During infection the viral genome is introduced into the cell, fol-

---

Box 11.2 Current vectors

Properties	Viral	Non-viral
Transfection efficiency	Potentially high	Low
Length of expression	Potentially long	Transient
Insert size	Limited	Large
Ease of use	Difficult	Straightforward
Immunogenicity	High	Low
Ease of production	Difficult	Straightforward

lowed rapidly by the production of viral regulatory products and later, structural genes are expressed, resulting in the assembly of new viral particles. Gene therapy vectors have a modified genome that contains a therapeutic gene cassette in place of expendable (non-essential, i.e. needed for the replication phase of the life cycle) viral sequences. To produce such a recombinant viral vector, the non-essential genes are provided in trans either integrated into the 'producer' cell genome or within a plasmid. The viral *cis*-acting regulatory sequences attached to the therapeutic gene are then introduced into the same producer cell, leading to the generation of replication-defective particles that have the capacity to transduce the desired genetic information into the target cell.

Each viral vector system is characterized by an individual set of properties that determines its suitability for the treatment of specific diseases. For example, therapies designed to inhibit the growth of cancer cells by the reintroduction of inactivated tumour suppressor genes will require gene transfer into a large proportion of the abnormal cells to have a useful effect. In contrast, strategies based on genes encoding proteins that are excreted or the conversion of anti-tumour pro-drugs to toxic chemicals can be successful when more limited numbers of cells are transfected by making use of the bystander effect (a process where even cells that are not transduced are killed or their biology is modified because of the local effects of the secreted toxin or cytokine around the transduced cell) (Fig. 11.1).[13,14] Another strategy employs a genetically engineered virus to replicate selectively within tumour cells, owing to specific properties of the abnormal cells, which then results in cell lysis. These agents (which do not contain transgenes) are known as oncolytic viruses.[15]

The viral vectors can be divided into two groups according to the integration or non-integration of the introduced gene into the host cell. Retroviral (including lentiviral) and adeno-associated viral vectors integrate into recipient cells, while the adenoviral vector genome is maintained as an episome within the cell

nucleus. The most frequently used vector to date has been the retrovirus (38% of clinical studies), closely followed by adenoviral vector trials (25%), but newer agents such as adeno-associated virus (AAV), herpes simplex and pox viruses are being brought more to the fore (www.wiley.co.uk/genetherapy).

3.1 Non-replicating

3.1.1 Retrovirus (including lentivirus)

Retroviruses are a class of enveloped viruses containing a single-stranded RNA molecule as the genome. Reverse transcriptase transcribes this molecule into double-stranded DNA, which can integrate into the host genome and express proteins. Vectors are usually based on the Moloney murine leukaemia virus (Mo-MLV), an amphotropic virus capable of both mouse and human infection, thus enabling vector development in mouse models to be translated directly into treatment for humans.

Vectors based on retroviruses were among the first to be researched and have, therefore, been important in the developmental process of engineering viral transfer agents.[12,16] Their ability to integrate into the target cell chromosome gives the possibility of prolonged transgene

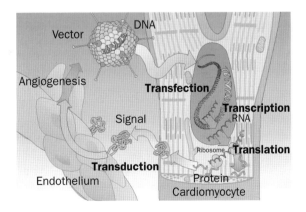

Fig. 11.1 Transfection of cardiomyocyte with viral vector leading to the production of a secreted protein that stimulates angiogenesis in surrounding tissue (used with permission of Collateral Therapeutics Inc.).

Table 11.1 Non-replicating viral vectors		
Virus	**Advantages**	**Disadvantages**
Retrovirus	Broad cell tropism Stable integration Low immunogenicity High ex vivo transfection efficiency	Transfects dividing cells only Poor in vivo transfection rates Limited insert size (8 kb) Large-scale production difficult Doubts about long-term safety
Lentivirus	Broad cell tropism Transfects active and quiescent cells Stable integration	Limited insert size (10 kb) Doubts about long-term safety
Adenovirus	Transfects active and quiescent cells High transfection efficiency Reasonable tissue targeting Commercial production possible	Limited insert size Transient expression Immunogenic
Adeno-associated virus	Transfects active and quiescent cells Long-term expression Tissue specificity Non-pathogenic, non-toxic	Small insert size High titres difficult to produce

expression (days to weeks shorter in vivo) but at a reduced level. The process that turns expression off is not well understood but may be due to methylation around the promoter site, resulting in inaccessibility of the transgene to transcriptional machinery.[17] The main advantages of using this type of vector are stable integration leading to potential long-term expression in comparison with other systems, relatively high transfection efficiency ex vivo and decreased immunogenicity (although there is still a cytotoxic T-lymphocyte (CTL) response to heterologous transgenes that extinguishes transduced cells but less than that for adenovirus), as most retroviruses do not express residual viral genes.

However, there are a number of important disadvantages.[11,18] First, the virus can only penetrate the nucleus of a target cell at mitosis, so transfection is limited to dividing cells. Normal tissues (tumour cells in these tissues do remain

vulnerable as they are dividing) within, for example, the eye, brain, lung and pancreas, are not amenable to direct in vivo gene delivery. Second, the insert size capacity is limited to 8 kb, which is relatively small and restricts potential modifications. Third, serum complement rapidly inactivates the retroviral vector in vivo, resulting in poor transfection rates. Fourth, while tissue-specific promoters work well in retroviruses,[19,20] retargeting is proving more challenging and the host range for some retroviruses is still limited. The technology is available to retarget transfection to cell surface proteins other than the natural receptor (pseudotyping) but efficient transmission in humans has not yet been reported. Fifth, the possibility of integrative inactivation of tumour suppressor genes, the transformation of a cell by integration close to a cellular proto-oncogene or recombination with a cryptic retrovirus resident in the human genome have raised doubts about the long-term safety of these vectors, particularly in non-cancer indications. Finally, large-scale production remains difficult and retaining infectivity in storage has also been challenging.

Given these drawbacks it is not difficult to see why the most extensive use of retroviral vectors has been in ex vivo work. This approach requires only small amounts of virus, cells can be cultured to allow efficient transfection, it avoids inactivation by serum complement and the genetic information is already within the host cell when it enters the body.

Despite these problems, recent advances in the manufacture of retrovirus vectors, including the use of envelope proteins from other viruses (vesicular stomatitis virus) to package the recombinant genomes, promises higher viral titres, greater complement resistance, transfection of a wider range of cell types and more efficient transfection in vivo.[21] In the meantime, retroviruses continue to be used extensively for introducing genes into dividing cells such as tumours and haematopoietic cells.

Lentiviruses (HIV, SIV) are a subset of the retroviral family but have a significant advantage in that they are capable of transducing non-dividing cells.[22,23] These viruses have a considerably more complex genome with an additional six coding sequences (tat, rev, nef, vif, vpu, vpr) above the three (gag, pol, env) found in more simple retroviruses. First-generation lentiviral vectors had vesicular stomatitis virus G protein (VSVG) in place of the viral env protein,[24] which enabled targeting of cells other than those positive for CD4 such as neurones, hepatocytes, muscle fibres and retinal cells. Owing to the possibility of these first-generation vectors undergoing recombination and generating infectious HIV particles, research groups have attempted deletion of as many accessory viral genes as possible, while safeguarding the ability of the virus to infect non-dividing cells.[25,26] While lentiviral vectors have some advantages over their retroviral relations, they have not yet been used within clinical trials. They will still have the disadvantage of non-site-specific integration (i.e. possible insertional mutagenesis) into the host genome and

the durability of any resulting transformation remains to be seen.

3.1.2 Adenovirus

The use of recombinant adenovirus as a genetic delivery vehicle received much attention in the early development of gene therapy as a system to transfer a therapeutic gene sequence to the respiratory epithelium of cystic fibrosis sufferers. It soon became apparent that these viruses were also capable of infecting other tissue types efficiently[27–29] regardless of the mitotic status of the cell.

Adenoviruses cause a benign respiratory tract infection in humans and are non-enveloped viruses that contain a linear double-stranded DNA genome. There are over 50 serotype strains of human adenovirus but current vectors are derived predominantly from subgroup C, types 2 and 5, the serotypes to which most adults (55%) will have already have been exposed.[30] Because of this prior exposure many adults have a pre-existing immunity to these strains and there are now efforts to engineer other serotypes or even non-human adenoviruses to avoid the potentially reduced efficacy resulting from a pre-programmed immune response.[31] Another technique being developed in animal models to bypass host immunity during re-administration of the virus is to use a different serotype for each repeat treatment.[32]

Following cell entry the viral genome enters the nucleus but remains as an episome (i.e. the DNA does not integrate into chromosomal DNA) thus reducing the risk of insertional mutagenesis. The early region genes (E1) regulate the transcription process and, in combination with E2 and E4 regions, are required for genome replication. The structural proteins are made late in the life cycle and provide the capsid shell for the newly replicated genomes, which are then released by viral-induced cell lysis. The E3 region is involved in monitoring host immunity and it is likely that it has a role in protection against immune-mediated response against the vector or vector-transduced cells but this remains controversial owing to variations in animal species and vectors used for the studies.[33,34] It is important to establish the precise role of E3, as removal of this region increases the space available for insertion of new genetic material.

First-generation adenovirus vectors were disabled through removal of the E1 region in an attempt to prevent transcription of the downstream genes involved in viral replication. Despite E1 deletion there was still low-level expression of the remaining genes used for replication and these attracted early cytokine responses from the host as well as later antigen-dependent destruction of transduced cells.[35] This adversely affected gene expression and other ways of rendering the virus replication incompetent were investigated. Next-generation viruses had deletions of E1 with either E2 or E4, which conferred a reduced toxicity profile in animals.[36,37] However, an intrahepatic E1/E4 deleted virus was responsible for the first gene therapy death in an 18-year-old boy (Jesse Gelsinger) with partial ornithine transcarbamylase deficiency.

To circumvent the host immune responses more efficiently, attempts are under way to produce a 'gutless' (helper-dependent) adenovirus vector. This involves removal of virtually all residual adenoviral genes and increases insert capacity to 30 kb.[38,39] These newer vectors do show a greatly reduced immunogenicity in comparison with the earlier-generation constructs and a significantly more prolonged expression of transgenes in mice,[38] producing therapeutic quantities of protein, but there are additional problems in terms of manufacture and the amounts of recombinant virus particles generated.

The advantages of adenovirus as a vector are several. They can transfect both quiescent and dividing cells, which immediately opens up a wide range of target diseases. The transfection efficiency is very high in both ex vivo and in vivo models compared with other systems. The cytomegalovirus (CMV) promoter used most commonly with adenovirus (and all other vectors) gives very good expression in many tissues and other promoter systems give preferential transcription to certain cell types with retention of specificity in the context of adenovirus.[38] This virus can also be re-targeted to a range of tissues through several cell surface proteins while maintaining efficacy.[40] Commercial manufacture is relatively straightforward, yielding high viral titres. Finally, there is also a wealth of clinical experience with this vector, which is critical when designing constructs that will ultimately be used to treat humans.

The disadvantages are dominated by the strong immunogenicity of this virus and the fact that at high doses it can spark an inflammatory response. The host generates neutralizing antibodies that target the viral particles and prevent binding to the cell and reduce the efficiency of gene transfer on repeat dosing. Several strategies to evade the neutralizing antibodies are being tried. Methods such as oral tolerization,[41] disguising key epitopes with hydrophilic polymers[42,43] or blockade of the co-stimulatory molecule CD40 ligand[44] are still at an early stage. The CTL responses also inhibit transgene expression, contributing to silencing of the therapeutic insert and manoeuvres such as macrophage depletion,[44] blockade of co-stimulatory molecules[35] or of inflammatory cytokines[45] are being investigated as possible counteractive mechanisms. Repeat dosing in the presence of a neutralizing immune response is also problematic but the option of treating with different serotypes on repeat administration is a feasible approach to protect transgene expression.[32] Other than immunogenicity issues, transgene expression – although initially very high – is transient in comparison with other systems, becoming low or undetectable in most tissues after 2 weeks, predominantly as a result of the episomal nature of the viral genome. The insert size is limited to 7.5 kb (8 kb without E3), which restricts manipulation of the genome.

Therefore, given the properties above, adenovirus vectors are most useful for direct cell killing, immunotherapy strategies and some acute diseases and have been used in preclinical animal studies to transduce liver, skeletal muscle, heart, brain, lung, pancreas and tumours.[46] Currently, adenovirus vectors are being used widely in cancer trials,[15,47] not only because of their high transduction rates, but also as a result of their cellular toxicity and immune response stimulation, which enhance the antitumour effects. There have also been recent trials for peripheral vascular and coronary artery disease with these vectors. Many of the clinical studies that are showing encouraging signs of efficacy are utilizing adenovirus vectors.

3.1.3 Adeno-associated virus

Adeno-associated virus (AAV) is a small, non-pathogenic, single-stranded DNA parvovirus that has shown encouraging signs of being an effective gene delivery vehicle.[48] It normally requires a helper virus, such as adenovirus, to provide extra genes to mediate a productive infection.[49] Most constructs are developed from AAV-2, one of the six identified human serotypes. AAV is not associated with any human disease, which adds to its suitability as a gene therapy vector. The virus has two genes (*rep* and *cap*) flanked by viral inverted terminal repeat (ITR) sequences. The packaging capacity is only 4.5 kb, which is a major disadvantage of this system. The wild-type virus integrates easily into the human chromosome at a specific site on chromosome 19, but this stability is unfortunately lost in recombinants owing to the absence of the *rep* gene and integration is a much more random process whereby some recombinant genomes persist in unintegrated forms.[50] Recombinants are produced by replacing *rep* and *cap* with the therapeutic gene. *Rep* and *cap* are provided in trans in the packaging cell along with the adenoviral proteins needed for replication. Large-scale production is currently difficult, inefficient and labour-intensive, yielding only low viral titres.

AAV appears to be capable of long-term transgene expression in vivo with evidence of expression being detected several months after injection in humans.[51] This suggests that these vectors may be ideal vehicles for the treatment of chronic disease. Another distinct advantage is the absence of viral coding sequences, which minimizes the stimulation of host immunity. This accounts for the weak or absent CTL response and thus, lack of inflammatory response or detectable toxicity. However, some data estimate that 32% of adults have pre-existing neutralizing antibodies and that injection of doses sufficient to generate transgene expression do increase the levels of neutralizing antibody that may decrease subsequent efficacy.[30,52] Transfer of the therapeutic gene can occur in quiescent or dividing cells and tissue-targeted promoters retain their specificity in AAV. Preliminary data also show that efficient retargeting of this vector is likely.[53]

The main disadvantages of AAV vectors are their complex manufacturing process and very small insert size (4.5 kb). Despite this, several clinical trials are under way with this vector and are demonstrating some very encouraging results, particularly in haemophilia, muscular dystrophy and cystic fibrosis.[9,51,54,55]

3.1.4 Herpes simplex virus

The attractive features of herpesvirus as a vector are the harnessing of their ability to persist after primary infection in a latent state and that re-activation even in an immunocompromised host is unlikely once the virus has been modified. Herpes simplex virus (HSV) is an enveloped double-stranded DNA virus of approximately 152 kb and the serotype most used for engineering is HSV-1.[56] It contains a number of genes with identified essential and non-essential functions (in vitro) whose expression is regulated in a complex manner. HSV has a natural tropism for neuronal and mucosal cells. Techniques have been developed for genetic engineering and it is possible to replace some genes to create up to 30 kb of space for multiple inserts (coordinately or simultaneously expressed) or a single large gene.[57] It has a built-in safety mechanism through its *tk* gene; antiviral agents such as acyclovir and gancyclovir can be administered to halt the spread of the virus.

The role of pre-existing immunity to HSV-1 has been assessed in rodent tumour models[58] and it was shown not to ablate gene expression from the virus or its efficacy, although gene expression was reduced by 80%. HSV-1 gene deletion vectors can be grown efficiently in complementing cell lines without generating replication-competent virus, are non-cytotoxic, efficiently infect a large number of cell types and are capable of latency in both neurones and non-neuronal tissues.[59] They are also highly efficient gene transducers, a property that does not seem to be affected by immune response on repeat dosing.

The disadvantages of using this category of gene delivery vehicle are lack of clinical experience (unlike adenoviruses and retroviruses), poor long-term transgene expression in some tissues (including brain) and complex attachment and entry processes that make retargeting very challenging.

Treatment of animal models for cancer, peripheral neuropathy, brain disease and pain involving this vector have all demonstrated efficacy.[60–62] Given the natural tropism towards sensory neurones, these may well be the most appropriate target for HSV in the future. In humans there have been two Phase I clinical trials using selectively replicating HSV mutants in patients with either glioblastoma multiforme or anaplastic astrocytomas.[63,64] No significant toxicity was reported but further trials are needed before efficacy can be assessed.

3.1.5 Pox virus, vaccinia virus and baculovirus

Avipox viral vectors are used predominantly for vaccination against disease, given their ability to infect and express recombinant proteins in human cells without replication.[65] They have become the third most frequently used viral vector in the context of clinical trials (6.4%).

Vaccinia vectors are generated by homologous recombination and are able to accommodate large inserts. Their application has been mainly in the delivery of interleukins (IL) such as IL-1β and the co-stimulatory molecules B7-1 and B7-2 in both in vitro and ex vivo models.[66,67]

Baculovirus is an insect virus that has been used in vitro primarily for protein expression and is now being investigated for its utility in gene therapy because of this property.[68]

3.1.6 Other

New vectors are continually being investigated, driven by the need for different properties for the treatment of a range of diseases. Those currently in the early stages of development are based on SV-40,[69] α-viruses,[70] hepatitis viruses,[71] negative strand RNA viruses (e.g. influenza and Ebola)[72] and Epstein–Barr virus.[73]

3.2 Replicating

Replication-selective viruses for the treatment of tumours are an emerging therapeutic platform within the field of gene therapy and within oncology. The need for agents that select more effectively for cancer cells, have greater potency and, critically, have novel mechanisms of action (to avoid cross-resistance with currently available approaches) led to the development of this new category of vector with the potential for targeted oncolysis. The advantages conferred by the retention of selective replication are amplification of the input dose at the site of disease, decreased toxicity and efficient clearance (as normal cells are not infected) and a variety of mechanisms to induce cell death (induction of T-cell immunity, inflammatory cytokines, toxic proteins and increased cell sensitivity to these effects) other than apoptosis, which avoids cross-resistance with chemotherapeutics or radiation.[15,74]

The viral species used over the last decade for tumour selectivity have been adenovirus, herpesvirus and vaccinia. Those that have inherent tumour selectivity have also been identified and added to this list, i.e. reovirus, autonomous parvoviruses, Newcastle disease virus, measles virus strains and vesicular stomatitis virus.[75] Tumour selectivity has been demonstrated both in vitro and in vivo with many of these agents after intratumoral, intraperitoneal and intravenous routes of administration.

In designing such an agent and rational engineering of the inherent properties, an understanding of the genes modulating infection, replication or pathogenesis is necessary. In addition, the virus should be capable of infecting both cycling and non-cycling cells, as most solid tumours have a low growth fraction and the receptors for viral entry must be expressed on the target tumours in patients. The safety aspects require the viral vector to be amenable to high-titre production and purification, cause only mild, well-characterized human disease and have a non-integrating genome for greater genetic stability.

Five main approaches are currently being employed to develop tumour-selective replicating viral vectors:

1. The use of virus that already has inherent tumour selectivity (e.g. reovirus, Newcastle disease virus).[76,77]
2. Engineering tissue/tumour-specific promoters (e.g. prostate-specific antigen (PSA) for prostate cancer) into viruses (e.g. HSV or adenovirus) to limit expression of the genes necessary for replication to specific cells and tissues.[78,79]
3. Deletion of entire genes that are necessary for efficient replication and/or toxicity in normal cells but are expendable in tumour cells (e.g. deletion of the E1B adenoviral region, thereby removing the ability of the virus to inactivate p53 in normal cells while maintaining their ability to infect tumour cells that are negative for p53).[80]
4. Deletion of functional gene regions that are necessary for efficient replication and/or toxicity in normal cells but are expendable in tumour cells. For example, mutation of the E1A adenoviral region such that it can no longer induce cell cycling in normal cells (and therefore cannot replicate) but can target tumour cells that are already cycling using their machinery for replication.[81]
5. The viral coat can be modified to target uptake selectively to tumour cells (e.g. poliovirus and adenoviruses).[82]

Each system of modification has its own advantages and disadvantages. Exploiting the inherent selectivity in some viruses is an attractive option because of its ease but optimization of these agents will be difficult if the molecular mechanisms of selectivity are unknown. Complete gene deletion definitely augments safety but it is usually at the cost of reduced potency, as many viral genes are multifunctional. Viral mutants with partial gene deletions

are showing promising signs of retaining potency as well as demonstrating selectivity and have a similar safety profile to mutants with complete gene deletions.[81] The success of the tumour/tissue-specific promoter system will depend on factors such as promoter activity in target versus normal tissues exposed to the virus and modification of viral coat proteins as a technique is still in the early stages.

Clinical experience with these agents is now plentiful and is most extensive with adenoviral mutants, particularly dl1520 (originally Onyx 015) in both Phase I and Phase II clinical trials.[83] Selectively replicating herpesviruses (e.g. G207) have been used particularly for the treatment of brain tumours[63,64] and vaccinia viruses encoding various proteins (GM-CSF, IL-2, CEA) have been used in the treatment of malignant melanoma, bladder cancer, metastatic adenocarcinoma, prostate cancer and mesothelioma.[84–88] All results have been encouraging as regards safety and toxicity. In addition, tumour regression has been seen but these responses have not been maintained for a durable period.

Second-generation agents are now being developed with a focus on increasing potency while maintaining safety and selectivity. This is likely to involve the inclusion of therapeutic genes into the virus,[47] modifying viral coats and suppressing the host humoral immune response. In addition, identification of the mechanism determining observed positive interaction between chemotherapy and replicating vectors could lead to an understanding of how to augment this process. These agents do hold true therapeutic promise for patients with cancer.

4. NON-VIRAL SYSTEMS

Non-viral systems have been developed to avoid some of the safety concerns applicable to the use of viral vectors. They offer simplicity of use and ease of production and do not generate specific immune responses (Box 11.3).

4.1 Naked DNA (plasmids)

This is the simplest concept in non-viral delivery systems. In 1990, Wolff and colleagues

---

Box 11.3   Non-viral vectors

Naked DNA

Efficient gene transfer in vivo with long-term expression in some tissues but poor for targeting tissues

Cationic lipids

Good transfection rates ex vivo but formulations and unstable and heterogeneous, poor tissue targeting and short duration of expression

Condensed DNA particles

Transfection efficiency similar to naked DNA and manufacture is reliable but at the developmental stage

Gene gun

Small quantities of DNA can be targeted directly to the tissue but experience is limited

Cell-based systems

---

made the discovery that exogenous genes could be expressed following direct injection into muscle.[89] This led to the development of naked DNA vaccines (injecting a plasmid encoding a protein antigen to activate an immune response), which have been used in a recent Phase I study to encode a gene of *Plasmodium falciparum* with evidence of stimulation of a cytotoxic T-lymphocyte response.[90,91] There have also been some very encouraging results with the use of naked DNA encoding angiogenic factors in muscle tissue of people suffering from ischaemic vascular disease.[7] The molecular events leading to antigen presentation are not yet fully understood.

Naked DNA is an efficient gene transfer vehicle in vivo (particularly in muscle and skin) but gives no transfection ex vivo. There are reports of gene expression lasting for months in skeletal muscle (in mice) but only days in skin.[92] The disadvantages of this system are low gene delivery efficiency compared with adenovirus

or AAV, lack of experience with these agents, brief expression in most tissues and unsuitability for targeting. However, the successes with DNA vaccination make this a promising concept for future applications.

4.2 Cationic lipids

Cationic lipids are a synthetic gene delivery system comprising DNA/lipid complexes held together by electrostatic interaction. This technique was first used successfully in 1987 and subsequent generations of vector have now been developed.[93,94] They give particularly good transfection ex vivo and have also been used extensively for delivery of the *CFTR* (cystic fibrosis transmembrane receptor) gene when administered to the nose and lungs of cystic fibrosis patients, although the expression was neither prolonged enough nor sufficient for clinical benefit.[95]

The main disadvantages with this gene delivery system are instability and heterogeneity of formulation, inactivation in blood, relatively low transfection efficacy, poor targeting, relatively short duration of gene expression and, at present, a limited understanding of the mechanisms of transfection and cellular interaction.[93] Transfection activity seems to be affected by poor uptake and inefficient trafficking of DNA to the nuclear site of gene expression, although a promising development utilizing cationic polymers to compact the DNA before mixing it with the lipid component may improve the efficacy of this group of synthetic vectors.[96]

Although progress in some areas has been slow, two strategies using 'lipoplexes' have now successfully entered Phase II clinical trials for the treatment of cancer.

4.3 Molecular conjugates (condensed DNA particles)

These cationic polymer-based gene delivery systems are far more efficient at condensing DNA than cationic lipids, which may enhance their uptake and protect the DNA from degradation. The polymers showing the most potential for clinical application at present are the polyethylenimines (PEI), which have been shown to give significant transfection in vivo in lung and kidney tissue and via intracerebral or intravenous injection.[97] However, the transfection rate is not better than that of naked DNA.

These types of formulation tend to aggregate in physiological conditions into particles that are too large for efficient cellular uptake and some agents (not PEI) require endosomal disruption compounds (e.g. chloroquine) to enable transfection in vitro. However, the advantages are reliable manufacture and the potential for developing more specific and efficient vectors through targeting or administration in conjunction with intracellular trafficking enhancers. This approach has not yet progressed to clinical trials and remains in the early stages of development.

4.4 Gene gun

This is a procedure that enables delivery of DNA without the use of a needle. A high-pressure stream of helium delivers DNA-coated gold particles directly into cell cytoplasm.[98] This approach gives reasonable transfection in a variety of cells ex vivo and gives similar results for skin cells in vivo. Susceptible skin cells include Langerhans cells, antigen-presenting cells that signal to naive T cells to elicit primary immune responses. This property suggests that gene gun delivery of plasmids bearing protein antigens to the skin could be an effective alternative to naked DNA injection into muscle for genetic vaccination.[99] The advantage of the gene gun in this situation is that much smaller quantities of DNA are required.

4.5 Cell-based gene transfer

Gene delivery by administering cells that have been transfected ex vivo has the potential to reduce vector loss, by protecting the vector from immune inactivation and non-specific adhesion, and to improve tissue targeting.[100] The cells can be derived from the patient for autologous transplantation and be packaged with mechanisms to regulate expression of the gene. The best candidates for the stealthy delivery of tumour-targeted vectors would be immune cells, such as macrophages and T-cells, but there is also considerable interest in stem cells. A disadvantage of this approach is that the transplanted cells may secrete a variety of other proteins.

5. GENE THERAPY IN PRACTICE

5.1 Clinical experience

There have been over 600 approved gene therapy trials worldwide targeted at a range of diseases (Box 11.4) since the first opened in 1990.[6] These have involved around 3500 patients and have been predominantly small Phase I/II studies, although approval for some Phase III studies has already been granted. Initial clinical trials have been directed at medical disorders

---

Box 11.4 Examples of diseases in which gene therapy studies are being conducted

Monogenic diseases
- X-linked severe combined immunodeficiency (SCID)
- ADA deficiency (ADA-SCID)
- Mucopolysaccharidosis
- Familial hypercholesterolaemia
- Cystic fibrosis
- Haemophilia B (factor IX deficiency)
- Chronic granulomatous disease

Cancer
- Adenocarcinoma of the prostate, colon and breast
- Mesothelioma
- Metastatic liver disease

Infectious diseases
- AIDS
- Vaccines

Vascular diseases
- Peripheral vascular disease
- Myocardial ischaemia
- Heart failure

for which conventional therapeutic options have been exhausted. The standard approach for investigating any novel therapy is to enrol patients who are so severely ill that they have nothing to lose from participation. This philosophy is important to minimize the risk to otherwise healthy patients with a reasonable life expectancy while gaining experience with the treatment. However, it compromises both mortality data and the analysis of the treatment with respect to differentiating adverse effects caused by the transgene from the disease itself. In general, the safety profile of these treatments has been acceptable but the outcome – in terms of gene transfer, expression, biological consequences and clinical benefit – has been less effective than initially hoped.

The major challenges remain targeting the right gene to the right location in the right cell and obtaining sufficient expression while minimizing any adverse reactions. Much of the work in gene transfer concentrates on viral vectors but there is a view that the future of gene therapy lies with safer non-viral vectors.

The death of Jesse Gelsinger during clinical trials at the University of Pennsylvania in 1999 and the recent discovery of a leukaemia-like disorder in a child treated for SCID have focused public attention on the risks of gene therapy and emphasized the need for cautious progress. Gene therapy remains a highly sensitive issue, tightly regulated and closely scrutinized. The regulations governing gene therapy vary with each country but are concerned with the safe use of genetically modified organisms, the quality and safety of the manufactured product and the conduct of clinical trials.[101] There is clear recognition of the need for the long-term follow-up of recipients of gene therapy (and perhaps any subsequent offspring) for evidence of adverse effects, particularly the acceleration of proliferative lesions such as neoplasia, atherosclerosis and retinopathy (Box 11.5). It has been suggested that tissue is archived so that molecular events can be traced.

In the UK, trials of gene therapy are subject to the same regulations as any new drug, with the additional requirement for approval by the Gene Therapy Advisory Committee (GTAC).

5.2 Gene Therapy Advisory Committee (GTAC)

Gene therapy in the UK requires the prior approval of GTAC (www.doh.gov.uk/genetics/gtac.htm). This committee regards gene therapy as research and not innovative treatment. Approval should be sought where any part of gene therapy research takes place in the UK.

The committee considers studies involving the use of most of the established techniques for delivering genes into cells, including xenotransplantation of genetically modified animal cells (but not solid organs). The possibility of genetically modifying germ cells needs to be carefully assessed during preclinical studies – GTAC will not consider research aimed at interfering with the germline of subjects.

The GTAC submission requires information on the following:

(i) The objectives of and background to the study. This should include information about the disease and alternative options for treatment together with data on preclinical and prior clinical experience with the gene construct and delivery system.

(ii) The study protocol. The study population must be well defined and the therapy should not put patients at disproportionate risk. Particular attention is given to choice of dose and any plans for dose escalation. The arrangements for monitoring patients for toxicity need to be stated.

Box 11.5 Morbidity concerns regarding cardiovascular gene therapy

- Accelerated atherosclerosis
- Vascular malformations
- Neoplasms
- Retinopathy
- Oedema
- Hypotension
- Arrythmias

<table>
<tr><td>

Box 11.6   Recommended screening for adenovirus studies

Recommended minimum for all studies:
- Anti-adenovirus antibody titres before and after dosing
- Pre-treatment assessment of T-cell population

For intravascular administration:
Before treatment and daily for the first 3–4 days after treatment (longer if abnormalities persist)
- Full blood count 6–8-hourly for the first 24 hours
- C-reactive protein 6–8-hourly for the first 24 hours
- Complement C3
- Coagulation studies
- Fibrinogen
- Fibrin split products
- Liver enzymes (AST/AT/ALP/γGT)
- Bilirubin
- Creatinine, urea and electrolytes
- Urine microscopy
- Proteinuria
- Consider monitoring serum cytokines (e.g. IL-6/IL-10/TNF-α)

http://www.doh.gov.uk/pdfs/gtacwpreport.pdf

</td></tr>
</table>

(microbiology and infection control, etc.) and demonstrate procedures for the safe disposal of waste. The arrangements to safeguard research staff, relatives and visitors must be explained.

There is particular sensitivity with respect to the use of viral vectors. The recommendations for laboratory screening and surveillance with respect to the use of adenoviruses are outlined in Box 11.6.

Researchers are required by law to report all serious adverse reactions in gene therapy studies to the Medicines and Healthcare products Regulatory Agency (MHRA), formerly MCA. Summaries of adverse events must be reported to GTAC on an annual basis and to the Local Research Ethics Committee (LREC). GTAC does not replace the work of LRECs. At present, where the study is being conducted in five or more centres, GTAC does act as the Multi-Centre Ethics Committee (MREC) but this may change. Appropriate approval must also be gained from the MHRA (Clinical Trial Certificate, Clinical Trial Exemption or Doctors and Dentists Exemption) and details of their role are provided on a website (http://www.open.gov.uk/mca/mcahome.htm). If a novel medical device is employed to deliver the product, approval must be obtained from the Medical Devices Agency (http://www.medical-devices.gov.uk/).

6. CONCLUSIONS

The initial view of gene therapy was that of a treatment for monogenic diseases such as cystic fibrosis in which a normal gene could be introduced to replace the function of a mutated gene. The implicit requirement of such a strategy is the availability of vectors that can provide robust gene replacement in a large population of cells for an extended if not indefinite period of time. At present this is not achievable. The approach in cardiovascular gene therapy has been to recognize disorders in which transient gene expression may be sufficient to stimulate the appropriate response. For example, 2–3 weeks of gene expression may be all that is required to promote neovascularization

(iii) Details of the therapeutic gene construct and its manufacture and supporting technical information.

(iv) The information that will be given to patients. Considerable thought has been given to this and the design of the Patient Information Sheet and any recommended wording should be followed.

(v) The experience of the investigators. GTAC wishes to be satisfied that gene therapy is conducted only in centres of excellence, with the appropriate staff.

(vi) The suitability of the centre. The centre must have the necessary infrastructure or inhibit restenosis. Moreover, using genes that encode proteins that are naturally secreted exploits the paracrine effect of such molecules and overcomes the need to transfect large numbers of cells.

The past 2 years have seen a marked improvement in vector manufacturing and production and this is no longer a major constraint on choice of vector when considering clinical studies. The vectors described above are not an exhaustive list and it is likely that new agents will continue to emerge with a variety of complementary properties. Of particular interest is the possibility of regulating expression of the transgene after cell transduction. This would allow for activation of the transgene when it is needed, maintaining its expression within a defined therapeutic window and silencing it if necessary.

It is unlikely that any one vector will be suitable for all potential gene therapy applications, given the range of properties that would be required. At present, the concepts proving to be the most promising are the use of adenoviruses for the delivery of genes for the direct killing of tumour cells, the use of naked DNA for vaccination and the delivery of angiogenesis genes for the treatment of cardiovascular disease, and AAV gene delivery for chronic disorders such as haemophilia.

As with many novel therapeutic strategies, gene therapy promised much quickly and has delivered little. The major challenges remain targeting the right gene to the right location in the right cell and obtaining sufficient expression while minimizing any adverse reactions. Much of the work in gene transfer concentrates on viral vectors but there is a view that the future of gene therapy lies with safer non-viral vectors. There have been some scares. This has resulted in some loss in confidence and raised concerns among the general public. Nonetheless gene therapy is happening and the expectation is that it will find a place in our therapeutic armoury. It is important that it is evaluated with the same degree of scientific and ethical scrutiny that is applied to other therapeutic interventions.

REFERENCES

Further reading

Isner JM. Myocardial gene therapy. *Nature* 2002; **415:** 234–9.

Leiden JM. Human gene therapy: the good, the bad and the ugly. *Circ Res* 2000; **86:** 923–5.

Mountain A. Gene therapy: the first decade. *Trends Biotechnol* 2000; **18:** 119–28.

Rubanyi GM. The future of gene therapy. *Mol Aspects Med* 2001; **22:** 113–42.

Web-sites

■ www.wiley.co.uk/genetherapy
The Journal of Gene Medicine Clinical Trial site, the most comprehensive source of information on gene therapy clinical trials available on the internet.

■ http://www.doh.gov.uk/genetics/gtac/index.htm
The Gene Therapy Advisory Committee (GTAC) advises on the ethical acceptability of proposals for gene therapy research on humans taking account of the scientific merits and the potential benefits and risks, and provides advice to UK Health Ministers on developments in gene therapy research.

Scientific papers

1. Gene Therapy Advisory Committee (GTAC) Seventh Annual Report, January 2000–December 2000. (www.doh.gov.uk/genetics/gtac/gtac7th annualreport.pdf).
2. Wadman M. Germline gene therapy 'must be spared excessive regulation'. *Nature* 1998; **392:** 317.
3. Billings PR. *In utero* gene therapy – the case against. *Nat Med* 1999; **5:** 255–6.
4. Schneider H, Coutelle C. *In utero* gene therapy – the case for. *Nat Med* 1998; **5:** 256–7.
5. Walsh CE. Fetal gene therapy. *Gene Ther* 1999; **6:** 1200–1.
6. Blaese RM, Culver KW, Miller D et al. T lymphocyte-directed gene therapy for ADA-SCID: initial trial results after 4 years. *Science* 1995; **270:** 475–80.
7. Baumgartner I, Pieczek A, Manor O et al. Constitutive expression of phVEGF$_{165}$ following intramuscular gene transfer promotes collateral

vessel development in patients with critical limb ischaemia. *Circulation* 1998; **97:** 1114–23.

8. Cavazzana-Calvo M, Hacein-Bey S, de Saint Basile G et al. Gene therapy of human severe combined immunodeficiency (SCID)-XI disease. *Science* 2000; **288:** 669–72.

9. Kay MA, Manno CS, Ragni MV et al. Evidence for gene transfer and expression of blood coagulation factor IX in patients with severe haemophilia B treated with an AAV vector. *Nature Genet* 2000; **24:** 257–61.

10. Li S, Huang L. Nonviral gene therapy: promises and challenges. *Gene Ther* 2000; **7:** 31–4.

11. Kay MA, Glorioso JC, Naldini L. Viral vectors for gene therapy: the art of turning infectious agents into vehicles of therapeutics. *Nat Med* 2001; **7:** 33–40.

12. Somia N, Verma IM. Gene therapy: trials and tribulations. *Nat Genet Rev* 2000; **1:** 91–9.

13. Aghi M, Hochberg F, Breakefield XO. Prodrug activation enzymes in cancer gene therapy. *J Gene Med* 2000; **2:** 148–64.

14. Cao L, Kulmburg P, Veelken H et al. Cytokine gene transfer in cancer therapy. *Stem Cells* 1998; **16**(Suppl. 1): 1251–60.

15. Heise C, Kirn DH. Replication-selective adenoviruses as oncolytic agents. *J Clin Invest* 2000; **105:** 1169–1172.

16. Anderson WF. Human gene therapy. *Nature* 1998; **392**(6679 Suppl.) 25–30**.**

17. Kuriyama S, Sakamoto T, Kikukawa M et al. Expression of a retrovirally transduced gene under control of an internal housekeeping gene promoter does not persist due to methylation and is restored partially by 5-azacytidine treatment. *Gene Ther* 1998; **5:** 1299–305.

18. Hodgson CP. The vector void in gene therapy: can viral vectors and transfection be combined to permit safe, efficacious and targeted gene therapy? *Biotechnology* 1995; **13:** 222–5**.**

19. Diaz RM, Eisen T, Hart IR, Vile RG. Exchange of viral promoter/enhancer elements with regulatory sequences generated targeted hybrid long terminal repeat vectors for gene therapy of melanoma. *J Virol* 1998; **72:** 789–95.

20. Miller N, Whelan J. Progress in transcriptionally targeted and regulatable vectors for genetic therapy. *Hum Gene Ther* 1997; **8:** 803–15**.**

21. Ory DS, Neugeboren BA, Mulligan RC. A stable human derived packaging cell line for production of high titre retrovirus/vesicular stomatitis virus G pseudotypes. *Proc Natl Acad Sci USA* 1996; **93:** 11400–6.

22. Lewis P, Hensel M, Emerman M. Human immunodeficiency virus infection of cells arrested in the cell cycle. *EMBO J* 1992; **11:** 3053–8.

23. Bukrinsky MI, Haggerty S, Dempsey MP et al. A nuclear localisation signal within HIV-1 matrix protein that governs infection of non-dividing cells. *Nature* 1993; **365:** 666–9.

24. Naldini L, Blomer U, Gallay P et al. In vivo gene delivery and stable transduction of non-dividing cells by a lentiviral vector. *Science* 1996; **272:** 263–7.

25. Kafri T, Blomer U, Peterson DA, Gage FH, Verma IM. Sustained expression of genes delivered directly into liver and muscle by lentiviral vectors. *Nat Genet* 1997; **17:** 314–17.

26. Zufferey R, Nagy D, Mandel RJ, Naldini L, Trono D. Multiply attenuated lentiviral vector achieves efficient gene delivery in vivo. *Nat Biotechnol* 1997; **15:** 871–5.

27. Benihoud K, Yeh P, Perricaudet M. Adenovirus vectors for gene delivery. *Curr Opin Biotechnol* 1997; **10:** 440–7.

28. Kovesdi I, Brough DE, Bruder JT, Wickham TJ. Adenoviral vectors for gene transfer. *Curr Opin Biotechnol* 1997; **8:** 583–9.

29. Hitt MM, Addison CL, Graham FL. Human adenovirus vectors for gene transfer into mammalian cells. *Adv Pharmacol* 1997; **40:** 137–206.

30. Chirmule N, Propert K, Magosin S, Qian Y, Qian R, Wilson J. Immune responses to adenovirus and adeno-associated virus in humans. *Gene Ther* 1999; **6:** 1574–83.

31. Loser P, Hillgenberg M, Arnold W, Both GW, Hofmann C. Ovine adenovirus vectors mediate efficient gene transfer to skeletal muscle. *Gene Ther* 2000; **7:** 1491–8.

32. Parks R, Evelegh C, Graham F. Use of helper-dependent adenoviral vectors of alternative serotypes permits repeat vector administration. *Gene Ther* 1999; **6:** 1565–73.

33. Ilan Y, Droguett G, Chowdhury NR et al. Insertion of the adenoviral E3 region into a recombinant viral vector prevents antiviral humoral and cellular immune responses and permits long-term gene expression. *Proc Natl Acad Sci USA* 1997; **94:** 2587–92.

34. Schowalter DB, Himeda CL, Winther BL, Wilson CB, Kay MA. Implication of interfering antibody formation and apoptosis as two different mechanisms leading to variable duration of adenovirus-mediated transgene expression in immune-competent mice. *J Virol* 1999; **73:** 4755–66.

35. Yang Y, Li Q, Ertl HC, Wilson JM. Cellular and humoral immune responses to viral antigens create barriers to lung-directed gene therapy with recombinant adenoviruses. *J Virol* 1995; **69:** 2004–115.

36. Lusky M, Christ M, Rittner K et al. *In vitro* and *in vivo* biology of recombinant adenovirus vectors with E1, E1/E2a or E1/E4 deleted. *J Virol* 1998; **72:** 2022–32.

37. Christ M, Louis B, Stoeckel F et al. Modulation of the inflammatory properties and hepatotoxicity of recombinant adenovirus vectors by the viral E4 gene products. *Hum Gene Ther* 2000; **11:** 415–27.

38. Schiedner G, Morral N, Parks RJ et al. Genomic DNA transfer with a high capacity adenovirus vector results in improved in vivo gene expression and decreased toxicity. *Nat Genet* 1998; **18:** 180–3.

39. Morsy MA, Caskey CT. Expanded-capacity adenoviral vectors – the helper-dependent vectors. *Mol Med Today* 1999; **5:** 18–24.

40. Searle PF, Mautner V. Adenoviral vectors: not to be sneezed at. *Gene Ther* 1998; **5:** 725–7.

41. Ilan Y, Prakash R, Davidson A et al. Oral tolerization to adenoviral antigens permits long-term gene expression using recombinant adenoviral vectors. *J Clin Invest* 1997; **99:** 1098–106.

42. Beer SJ, Matthews CB, Stein CS, Ross BD, Hilfinger JM, Davidson BL. Poly (lactic-glycolic) acid copolymer encapsulation of recombinant adenovirus reduces immunogenicity *in vivo*. *Gene Ther* 1998; **5:** 740–6.

43. Chillon M, Lee JH, Fasbender A, Welsh MJ. Adenovirus complexed with polyethylene glycol and cationic lipid is shielded from neutralising antibodies *in vitro*. *Gene Ther* 1998; **5:** 995–1002.

44. Stein CS, Pemberton JL, van Rooijen N, Davidson BL. Effects of macrophage depletion and anti-CD40 ligand on transgene expression and redosing with recombinant adenovirus. *Gene Ther* 1998; **5:** 431–9.

45. Benihoud K, Saggio I, Opolon P et al. Efficient repeated adenovirus-mediated gene transfer in mice lacking both tumour necrosis factor alpha and lymphotoxin alpha. *J Virol* 1998; **72:** 9514–25.

46. Bramson JL, Graham FL, Gauldie J. The use of adenoviral vectors for gene therapy and gene transfer in vivo. *Curr Opin Biotechnol* 1995; **6:** 590–5.

47. Hermiston T. Gene delivery from replication-selective viruses: arming guided missiles in the war against cancer. *J Clin Invest* 2000; **105:** 1169–72.

48. Monahan PE, Samulski RJ. AAV vectors: is clinical success on the horizon? *Gene Ther* 2000; **7:** 24–30.

49. Muzyczka N. Use of adeno-associated virus as a general transduction vector for mammalian cells. *Curr Top Microbiol Immunol* 1992; **158:** 97–129.

50. Balague C, Kalla M, Zhang WW. Adeno-associated virus Rep78 protein and terminal repeats enhance integration of DNA sequences into the cellular genome. *J Virol* 1997; **71:** 3299–306.

51. Wagner JA. Efficient and persistent gene transfer of AAV-CFTR in maxillary sinus. *Lancet* 1998; **351:** 1702–3.

52. Xiao W, Chirmule N, Berta SC, McCullough B, Gao G, Wilson JM. Gene therapy vectors based on adeno-associated virus type 1. *J Virol* 1999; **73:** 3994–4003.

53. Bartlett JS, Kleinschmidt J, Boucher RC, Samulski RJ. Targeted adeno-associated virus vector transduction of non-permissive cells mediated by a bispecific F(ab'gamma)₂ antibody. *Nat Biotechnol* 1999; **17:** 181–6.

54. Stedman H, Wilson JM, Finke R, Kleckner AL, Mendell J. Phase I clinical trial utilising gene therapy for limb girdle muscular dystrophy: α-, β-, γ- or Δ-sarcoglycan gene delivered with intramuscular instillations of adeno-associated vectors. *Hum Gene Ther* 2000; **11:** 777–90.

55. Wagner JA, Messner AH, Moran ML et al. Safety and biological efficacy of an adeno-associated virus vector-cystic fibrosis transmembrane regulator (AAV-CFTR) in the cystic fibrosis maxillary sinus. *Laryngoscope* 1999; **109:** 266–74.

56. Martuza R. Conditionally replicating herpes vectors for cancer therapy. *J Clin Invest* 2000; **105:** 841–6.

57. Krisky DM, Marconi PC, Oligino TJ et al. Development of herpes simplex virus replication-defective multigene vectors for combination gene therapy applications. *Gene Ther* 1998; **5:** 1517–30.

58. Herrlinger U, Kramm CM, Aboody-Guterman KS et al. Pre-existing herpes simplex virus 1 (HSV-1) immunity decreases, but does not abolish, gene transfer to experimental brain tumors by a HSV-1 vector. *Gene Ther* 1998; **5:** 809–19.

59. Samaniego LA, Neiderhiser L, DeLuca NA. Persistence and expression of the herpes simplex virus genome in the absence of immediate-early proteins. *J Virol* 1998; **72:** 3307–20.

60. Burton EA, Glorioso JC. Herpes simplex virus vector-based gene therapy for malignant glioma. *Gene Ther Mol Biol* 2000; **5:** 1–17.

61. Yenari MA, Fink SL, Sun GH et al. Gene therapy with HSP72 is neuroprotective in rat models of stroke and epilepsy. *Ann Neurol* 1998; **44:** 584–91.

62. Goss JR, Mata M, Goins WF et al. Antinociceptive effect of a genomic herpes simplex virus-based vector expressing human proenkephalin in rat dorsal root ganglion. *Gene Ther* 2001; **8:** 551–6.

63. Rampling R, Cruickshank G, Papanastassiou V et al. Toxicity evaluation of replication-competent herpes simplex virus (ICP 34.5 null mutant 1716) in patients with recurrent malignant glioma. *Gene Ther* 2000; **7:** 859–66.

64. Markert JM, Medlock MD, Rabkin SD et al. Conditionally replicating herpes simplex virus mutant, G207 for the treatment of malignant glioma: results of a Phase I trial. *Gene Ther* 2000; **7:** 867–74.

65. Wilkinson GW, Borysiewicz LK. Gene therapy and viral vaccination: the interface. *Br Med Bull* 1995; **51:** 205–16.

66. Peplinski GR, Tsung K, Whitman ED, Meko JB, Norton JA. Construction and expression in tumour cells of a recombinant vaccinia virus encoding human interleukin-1 beta. *Ann Surg Oncol* 1995; **2:** 151–9.

67. Hodge JW, Abrams S, Schlom J, Kantor JA. Induction of antitumour immunity by recombinant vaccinia viruses expressing B7–1 or B7–2 costimulatory molecules. *Cancer Res* 1994; **54:** 5552–5.

68. Forstova J, Krauzewicz N, Sandig V et al. Polyoma virus pseudocapsids as efficient carriers of heterologous DNA into mammalian cells. *Hum Gene Ther* 1995; **6:** 297–306.

69. Strayer DS. Gene therapy using SV-40 derived vectors: what does the future hold. *J Cell Physiol* 1999; **181:** 375–84.

70. Hewson R. RNA viruses: emerging vectors for vaccination and gene therapy. *Mol Med Today* 2000; **6:** 28–35.

71. Chaisomonit S, Tyrrell DL, Chang LJ. Development of replicative and non-replicative hepatitis B virus vectors. *Gene Ther* 1997; **4:** 1330–40.

72. Palese P, Zheng H, Engelhardt OG, Pleschka S, Garcia-Sastre A. Negative-strand RNA viruses: genetic engineering and applications. *Proc Natl Acad Sci USA* 1996; **93:** 11354–8.

73. Sclimenti CR, Calos MP. Epstein–Barr virus vectors for gene expression and transfer. *Curr Opin Biotechnol* 1998; **9:** 476–9.

74. Kirn DH. Replication-selective oncolytic adenoviruses: virotherapy aimed at genetic targets in cancer. *Oncogene* 2000; **19:** 6660–9.

75. Kirn DH. Replication-selective microbiological agents: fighting cancer with targeted germ warfare. *J Clin Invest* 2000; **105:** 837–9.

76. Norman K, Lee P. Reovirus as a novel oncolytic agent. *J Clin Invest* 2000; **105:** 1035–8.

77. Coffey MC, Strong JE, Forsyth PA, Lee PW. Reovirus therapy of tumours with activated ras pathway. *Science* 1998; **282:** 1332–4.

78. Hallenbeck P. Oncolytic adenovirus driven by alfa-feto protein promoter. *Hum Gene Ther* 1999; **10:** 1721–33.

79. Rodriguez R, Schuur ER, Lim HY, Henderson GA, Simons JW, Henderson DR. Prostate attenuated replication competent adenovirus (ARCA) CN706: a selective cytotoxic for prostate-specific antigen-positive prostate cancer cells. *Cancer Res* 1997; **57:** 2559–63.

80. Heise C, Sampson-Johannes A, Williams A, McCormick F, Von Hoff DD, Kirn DH. ONYX-015, an E1B gene-attenuated adenovirus, causes tumor-specific cytolysis and antitumoral efficacy that can be augmented by standard chemotherapeutic agents. *Nat Med* 1997; **3:** 639–45.

81. Heise C. An adenovirus E1A mutant that demonstrates potent and selective antitumoral efficacy. *Nat Med* 2000; **6:** 1134–9.

82. Roelvink PW, Mi Lee G, Einfeld DA, Kovesdi I, Wickham TJ. Identification of a conserved receptor-binding site on the fiber proteins of CAR-recognizing adenoviridae. *Science* 1999; **286:** 1568–71.

83. Kirn DH. Clinical research results with dl1520 (Onyx-015), a replication-selective adenovirus for the treatment of cancer: what have we learned? *Gene Ther* 2001; **8:** 89–98.

84. Mastrangelo MJ, Eisenlohr LC, Gomella L, Lattime EC. Poxvirus vectors: orphaned and underappreciated. *J Clin Invest* 2000; **105:** 1031–4.

85. Mastrangelo MJ, Maguire HC, Jr, Eisenlohr LC et al. Intratumoral recombinant GM-CSF-encoding virus as gene therapy in patients with cutaneous melanoma *Cancer Gene Ther* 1999; **6:** 409–22.

86. Mukherjee S, Haenel T, Himbeck R et al. Replication-restricted vaccinia as a cytokine gene therapy vector in cancer: persistent transgene expression despite antibody generation. *Cancer Gene Ther* 2000; **7:** 663–70.

87. Conry RM, Khazaeli MB, Saleh MN et al. Phase I trial of a recombinant vaccinia virus encoding carcinoembryonic antigen in metastatic adenocarcinoma: comparison of intradermal versus

subcutaneous administration. *Clin Cancer Res* 1999; **5:** 2330–7.

88. Eder JP, Kantoff PW, Roper K et al. A phase I trial of a recombinant vaccinia virus expressing prostate-specific antigen in advanced prostate cancer. *Clin Cancer Res* 2000; **6:** 1632–8.

89. Wolff JA, Malone RW, Williams P et al. Direct gene transfer into mouse muscle *in vivo*. *Science* 1990; **247:** 1465–8.

90. Ulmer JB, Donnelly JJ, Parker SE et al. Heterologous protection against influenza by injection of DNA encoding a viral protein. *Science* 1993; **259:** 1745–9.

91. Wang R, Doolan DL, Le TP et al. Induction of antigen-specific cytotoxic T-lymphocytes in humans by a malaria DNA vaccine. *Science* 1998; **282:** 476–80.

92. Li S, Huang L. Nonviral gene therapy: promises and challenges. *Gene Ther* 2000; **7:** 31–4.

93. Felgner PL, Gadek TR, Holm M et al. Lipofection: a highly efficient, lipid-mediated DNA-transfection procedure. *Proc Natl Acad Sci USA* 1987; **84:** 7413–17.

94. Lee ER, Marshall J, Siegel CS et al. Detailed analysis of structures and formulations of cationic lipids for efficient gene transfer to the lung. *Hum Gene Ther* 1996; **7:** 1701–17.

95. Caplen NJ, Alton EW, Middleton PG et al. Liposome-mediated CFTR gene transfer to the nasal epithelium of patients with cystic fibrosis. *Nat Med* 1995; **1:** 39–46.

96. Li S, Huang L. In vivo gene transfer via intravenous administration of cationic lipid-protamine-DNA (LPD) complexes. *Gene Ther* 1997; **4:** 891–900.

97. Boussif O, Lezoualc'h F, Zanta MA et al. A versatile vector for gene and oligonucleotide transfer into cells in culture and in vivo: polyethylenimine. *Proc Natl Acad Sci USA* 1995; **92:** 7297–301.

98. Yang NS, Burkholder J, Roberts B, Martinell B, McCabe D. In vivo and in vitro gene transfer to mammalian somatic cells by particle bombardment. *Proc Natl Acad Sci USA* 1990; **87:** 9568–72.

99. Condon C, Watkins SC, Celluzzi CM, Thompson K, Falo LD, Jr. DNA-based immunisation by in vivo transfection of dendritic cells. *Nat Med* 1996; **2:** 1122–8.

100. Harrington K, Alvarez-Vallina L, Crittenden M et al. Cells as vehicles for cancer gene therapy: the missing link between targeted vectors and systemic delivery. *Hum Gene Ther* 2002; **13:** 1263–80.

101. Cohen-Haguenauer O, Rosenthal F, Gansbacher B et al. Opinion paper on the current status of the regulation of gene therapy in Europe. *Hum Gene Ther* 2002; **13:** 2085–110.

Index

Note: references in *italics* denote illustrations and tables